Neurovascular Imaging: Advanced Techniques

Neurovascular Imaging: Advanced Techniques

Edited by Holden Ray

hayle
medical

New York

Hayle Medical,
750 Third Avenue, 9th Floor,
New York, NY 10017, USA

Visit us on the World Wide Web at:
www.haylemedical.com

ISBN: 978-1-63241-582-0

Cataloging-in-Publication Data

Neurovascular imaging : advanced techniques / edited by Holden Ray.
    p. cm.
Includes bibliographical references and index.
ISBN 978-1-63241-582-0
1. Neurovascular diseases--Imaging. 2. Diagnostic imaging. 3. Medical radiology.
4. Radiography, Medical--Digital techniques. I. Ray, Holden.
RC349.D52 N48 2019
616.804 754--dc23

Table of Contents

Preface

The advances in optical and MRI based imaging technology have expanded the frontiers of neuroscience and neurovascular research. Some common neurovascular imaging techniques include computed tomography (CT) scan, magnetic resonance imaging (MRI), magnetoencephalography (MEG), positron emission tomography (PET), and cerebral angiography. In a computed tomography (CT) scan, there is a use of computer-processed combinations of X-ray measurements taken from different angles to produce cross-sectional images of a specific body organ or the scanned object. In a magnetic resonance imaging, there is a use of nuclear magnetic resonance to form pictures of the anatomy and the physiological processes of the body. A CT scan of the head is useful in the detection of tumors, calcifications, infarction bone trauma, and haemorrhage, whereas, an MRI of the head is useful in diagnosing nuerological cancers, cerebrovascular disease, epilepsy, Alzheimer's disease, demyelinating diseases, etc. This book studies, analyzes and upholds the pillars of neurovascular imaging and its utmost significance in modern times. It includes some of the vital pieces of work being conducted across the world, on various topics related to the advanced techniques of neurovascular imaging. This book will serve as a reference to a broad spectrum of readers.

This book is the end result of constructive efforts and intensive research done by experts in this field. The aim of this book is to enlighten the readers with recent information in this area of research. The information provided in this profound book would serve as a valuable reference to students and researchers in this field.

At the end, I would like to thank all the authors for devoting their precious time and providing their valuable contribution to this book. I would also like to express my gratitude to my fellow colleagues who encouraged me throughout the process.

Editor

Computational fluid dynamics of computed tomography angiography to detect the hemodynamic impact of intracranial atherosclerotic stenosis

Xinyi Leng[1], Fabien Scalzo[2], Albert K Fong[2], Mark Johnson[2], Hing Lung Ip[1], Yannie Soo[1], Thomas Leung[1], Liping Liu[3], Edward Feldmann[4], Ka Sing Wong[1] and David S Liebeskind[2,5*]

Abstract

Background: In symptomatic intracranial atherosclerotic stenosis (ICAS), its hemodynamic impact may affect the risk of stroke recurrence, in addition to the degree of luminal stenosis. We therefore conducted a pilot study to evaluate the feasibility to delineate the hemodynamic impact of symptomatic ICAS lesions using computational fluid dynamics (CFD) models reconstructed based on computed tomography angiography (CTA) source images.

Methods: Three-dimensional CFD models were reconstructed based on routine CTA source images of patients with a symptomatic ICAS lesion. The anatomic features and hemodynamic impact of target ICAS lesions were evaluated on the CFD models. The hemodynamic impact of a lesion was evaluated using distal to proximal pressure ratio (PR) and pressure gradient (PG) across the lesion. PG was defined as pressure drop across the lesion divided by length of the lesion.

Results: Among the 10 cases recruited, CTA source images of 9 cases were successfully processed to CFD models. The hemodynamic characteristics of the ICAS lesions could be quantitatively evaluated on the CFD models, such as the pressures, blood flow velocities, wall shear stress and shear strain rates. The median PR was 0.58 and the median PG was 93 mmHg/cm. PRs and PGs varied in cases with similar degrees of stenoses with different lesion lengths and proximal vessel diameters.

Conclusions: This pilot study demonstrated the feasibility to quantitatively assess the hemodynamic impact of ICAS using CFD models reconstructed based on routine CTA. Further studies are required to improve the models built in this pilot study, and to evaluate the ultimate value of this technique in clinical assessment and risk stratification of patients with symptomatic ICAS.

Keywords: Cerebral hemodynamics, Cerebrovascular disease, Stroke, Computational flow dynamics, Computed tomography angiography

Background

As the most common cause of ischemic stroke and transient ischemic attack in Asian populations and an important cause of stroke as well in other populations, intracranial atherosclerotic stenosis (ICAS) has attracted attention both in clinical practice and relevant research fields in recent decades [1-3]. The degree of anatomic stenosis was

* Correspondence: davidliebeskind@yahoo.com
[2]UCLA Stroke Center, University of California, CA 90095 Los Angeles, USA
[5]UCLA Department of Neurology, Neuroscience Research Building, Suite 225, Los Angeles, CA 90095-7334, USA
Full list of author information is available at the end of the article

noted as an independent predictor for recurrent ischemic stroke in the territory of the index artery (SIT), for instance, in the Warfarin-Aspirin Symptomatic Intracranial Disease (WASID) trial [4]. However, the fact also existed that nearly half of the SIT occurred in patients with 50-69% ICAS in the WASID trial [4]. According to the Chinese IntraCranial AtheroSclerosis Study, recurrent stroke also occurred in a considerable percentage of patients with <50% ICAS [5]. On the other hand, factors affecting hemodynamics of ICAS, for instance, collateralization, have been found to dramatically alter subsequent stroke risks in the WASID and the Stenting and Aggressive Medical Management for Preventing Recurrent stroke in Intracranial Stenosis (SAMMPRIS) trial [6,7]. Therefore, hemodynamics plays an important role in the case of ICAS, concerning subsequent risk of SIT. Evaluation of hemodynamic impact of ICAS will probably facilitate in the risk stratification of patients with symptomatic ICAS.

Computational fluid dynamic (CFD) techniques, when applied in simulation of blood flow, can quantitatively reveal hemodynamic characteristics of arterial stenosis. Noninvasive fractional flow reserve (FFR), which is the distal to proximal pressure ratio (PR) across a stenosis, measured through CFD reconstruction of coronary computed tomography angiography (CTA), has been identified of high diagnostic accuracy for the hemodynamic significance of stenosed coronary arteries as compared with FFR obtained invasively, and this is promising in guiding patient selection for percutaneous coronary intervention [8,9]. More recently, virtual FFR obtained from CFD models based on coronary angiograms by assigning averaged generic downstream boundary conditions without simulating hyperemic conditions, was also found to be substantially accurate to define hemodynamically significant coronary lesions (accuracy of 97%), as compared with invasively measured FFR under induced hyperemia [10]. In addition, CFD could also be used to reveal the hemodynamic effects of ICAS [11,12]. In the present pilot study, we evaluated the feasibility to discern hemodynamic impact of ICAS using CFD models reconstructed from routinely obtained CTA images with a small sample size, to pave the way for generalized application of this technique in larger clinical studies in the near future.

Methods
Subjects
This was a retrospective observational study. Ten patients, each with a symptomatic ICAS lesion (50-99% luminal stenosis, WASID criteria [13]) of a major intracranial artery [intracranial portion of internal carotid artery (ICA); M1 segment of middle cerebral artery (MCA-M1); or basilar artery (BA)] identified on CTA, were retrospectively selected from a prospective clinical study at Prince of Wales Hospital in Hong Kong. All patients had given written informed consent for the previously approved prospective clinical study, and the current retrospective study was also approved by the Joint Chinese University of Hong Kong-New Territories East Cluster Clinical Research Ethics Committee (the Joint CUHK-NTEC CREC). Patients' characteristics were collected from clinical records. CTA source images were retrieved and anonymized from the picture archiving and communication system and transferred to University of California, Los Angeles for reconstruction of CFD models.

CT protocol
All CT examinations were performed on a 64-slice CT scanner (Lightspeed VCT, GE Healthcare, US), including non-contrast CT scan of the whole brain and CTA of intracranial arteries. The non-contrast CT scan was performed in axial mode, covering the skull base to vertex region, and obtained at 120 kV 320 mA and 1.0 sec rotation. CTA was performed in helical mode with no tilting, covering the skull base to the level of lateral ventricles, and obtained at 120 kV 550 mA and 0.4 sec rotation. Intravenous contrast (70 ml Omnipaque 300, 3–3.5 ml/s) was injected via the antecubital vein using a power injector. Axial CTA images were reconstructed at 0.625 mm intervals and stored as source images for further image analysis.

CFD simulations of hemodynamics
The scientific basis of evaluating hemodynamics of ICAS lesions, such as the trans-stenotic pressure gradient, using simulated models constructed out of standard CTA source images, was that the hemodynamic features of such lesions could be calculated via the CFD technique by applying several assumptions on the three-dimensional (3D) vessel geometry obtained from CTA source images. CFD simulations of hemodynamics were performed through the following procedures. Firstly, the location of the target arterial segment was visually identified and delineated with a region-of-interest on CTA images. The region-of-interest was then segmented using a gradient-driven level set method [14] to extract the vascular volume. Centerlines were then computed from selected inlet and outlet points placed at the extreme points of the vessel. The diameter of the vessel along the centerline was derived using the Voronoi method which allowed a 3D geometry of the vessel to be constructed. A mesh of the 3D surface was then created using ANSYS ICEM-CFD (ANSYS, Inc.), composed of approximately 500,000 tetrahedral cells. Blood flow simulation was then performed on this mesh using ANSYS CFX software. It was assumed that blood was an incompressible Newtonian fluid with a constant viscosity of 0.004 kg·m^{-1}·s^{-1} and could be governed by the Navier–Stokes equations [15]. It was also assumed that blood has a density of 1060 kg/m^3. The boundary conditions placed on this simulation was one that assumed rigid, non-compliant walls with no-slip flow conditions. The inlet boundary condition was set to be 120 mmHg while the outlet velocity was prescribed as 60 cm/s. As it has been assumed that the vessel is non-compliant, the velocity downstream can be assumed to also follow ideal pipe-flow and thus physiological velocities. The simulation results were post-processed in ANSYS CFX-post (ANSYS, Inc.), for extraction of flow parameters, for instance, velocity, pressure, wall shear and shear strain rates (Figure 1).

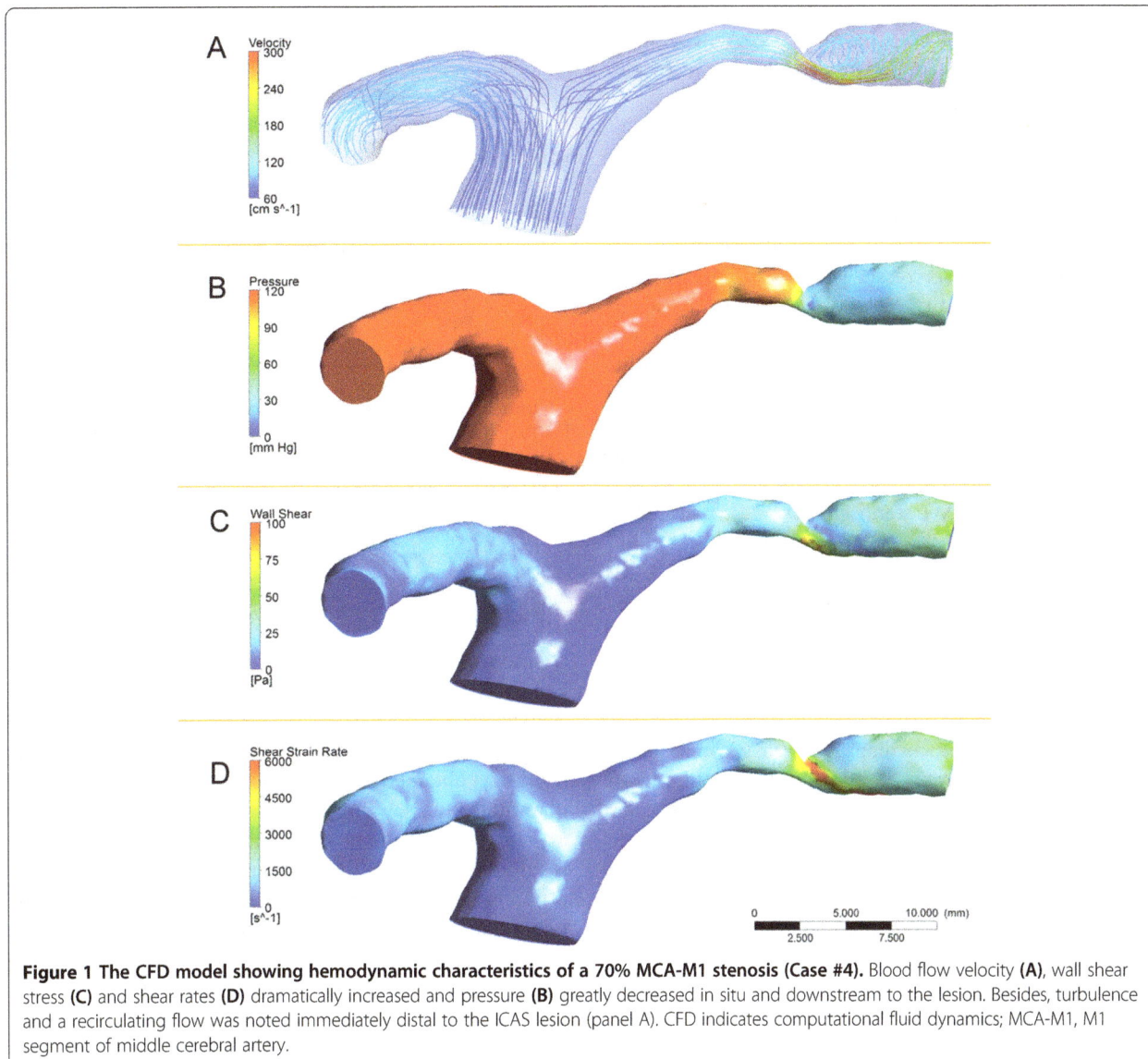

Figure 1 The CFD model showing hemodynamic characteristics of a 70% MCA-M1 stenosis (Case #4). Blood flow velocity **(A)**, wall shear stress **(C)** and shear rates **(D)** dramatically increased and pressure **(B)** greatly decreased in situ and downstream to the lesion. Besides, turbulence and a recirculating flow was noted immediately distal to the ICAS lesion (panel A). CFD indicates computational fluid dynamics; MCA-M1, M1 segment of middle cerebral artery.

Generation of mesh, simulation of blood flow and post-processing of simulation results were run on a Cray CX1 cluster (Cray Inc.).

Measurement of anatomic characteristics of ICAS

Proximal normal vessel diameter, anatomic severity, and length of the stenoses were measured on reconstructed 3D models. Anatomic severity of ICAS was measured according to the WASID criteria [13]. Length of a lesion was defined as the distance between the first normal diameters distal and proximal to the stenosis.

Evaluation of hemodynamic impact of ICAS

Evaluation of the CFD models was also performed in ANSYS CFX-post (ANSYS, Inc.). Hemodynamic impact of ICAS was evaluated by using 2 indices in the present study, which were PR and pressure gradient (PG) across the lesion. Pressures were measured at the 1st normal diameters distal and proximal to the lesion, for which spherical volumes-of-interest with the same radius of the vessel were selected within the vessel domain to get the mean pressure value. PR was defined as the distal to proximal pressure ratio, and PG (mmHg/cm) was defined as pressure drop across the ICAS divided by length of the lesion. Since this was a preliminary study, and that there had been no data about the cut-point value of PR to define a hemodynamically significant ICAS, we used the same cut-point of PR (0.80) as is used in the cardiac field for FFR [16], with a PR less than or equal to 0.80 considered hemodynamically significant in the present study.

Statistical analysis

Descriptive statistics were used in the current study to describe demographics of patients recruited and imaging characteristics of the symptomatic ICAS lesions.

Results

Among the 10 patients recruited in this study, the CTA source images of 9 subjects (median age was 62, and 7 were males) were successfully processed to CFD models. In the other one case, vessel geometry of the arterial segment containing the ICAS lesion failed to be extracted from the CTA source images due to poor image quality. The reconstructed CFD models could quantitatively depict hemodynamic environment at the stenosis. Blood flow velocity, wall shear stress and shear rates increased and pressure decreased in situ and downstream to a stenosis. Figure 1 shows hemodynamic characteristics of a 70% MCA-M1 stenosis (Case #4), revealed by the CFD model.

Among the 9 cases processed, 7 were MCA-M1 lesions, and the other 2 were ICA and BA lesions, respectively. Four cases were 70-99% stenoses. Patient demographics, anatomic characteristics of ICAS, and other parameters and indices measured and calculated from the CFD models are shown in Table 1. The median PR was 0.58 and the median PG was 93 mmHg/cm. Four anatomically severe and 1 anatomically moderate stenoses were considered hemodynamically significant (PR ≤0.80) in the current study. Besides, PRs and PGs varied in cases with similar percentages of stenoses (Table 1 and Figure 2). For instance, Case #5, #6 and #7, with similar anatomic severity of stenoses (around 80%) in MCA-M1 but different lesion lengths and proximal vessel diameters, greatly differed in hemodynamic severities as assessed via CFD models (Table 1). The pressure maps of Case #6 and #7 are shown in Figure 2, with PGs of 300 and 5,382 mmHg/cm, respectively.

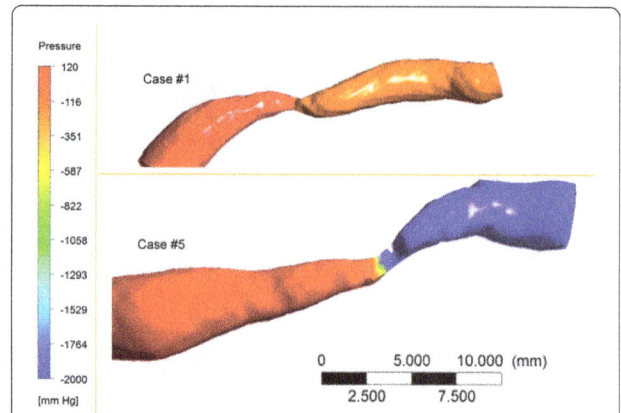

Figure 2 Pressure maps of Case #6 and #7. Both cases were around 80% stenoses of MCA-M1 but with different lengths (double-headed arrows) and proximal vessel diameters. Hemodynamic severities of the two cases differed in terms of PR and PG. The PRs were −1.30 and −75.70, respectively. And PGs were 300 and 5,382 mmHg/cm, respectively. MCA-M1 indicates M1 segment of middle cerebral artery; PR, pressure ratio; PG, pressure gradient.

Discussion

This was a feasibility study. Despite of the small sample size, we demonstrated the feasibility of simulating blood flow across ICAS lesions by CFD modeling based on routinely obtained CTA images, and the feasibility of quantitatively analyzing the hemodynamic characteristics of such lesions on the CFD models. Besides, the study results implied that the severity of luminal stenosis probably was not the only indicator to determine the hemodynamic impact of symptomatic ICAS lesions, which reinforced the urgent need for a more comprehensive paradigm for clinical evaluation of such lesions, to replace, or at least improve, the current unreasonable and misleading method of defining the significance of such lesions only based on the percentage of stenosis.

Table 1 Patient demographics and ICAS characteristics*

Patient #	Gender	Age	ICAS			Proximal vessel diameter (mm)	Proximal pressure (mmHg)	Distal pressure (mmHg)	Pressure ratio	Pressure gradient (mmHg/cm)
			Location	Anatomic severity (%)	Length (mm)					
1	M	44	MCA-M1	50	20	3.5	118	104	0.88	7
2	M	68	MCA-M1	51	11	2.7	118	107	0.91	10
3	M	51	MCA-M1	53	13	2.9	119	102	0.86	13
4	M	61	MCA-M1	70	10	2.7	120	29	0.24	93
5	F	74	MCA-M1	78	14	3.0	119	−184	−1.55	223
6	F	65	MCA-M1	79	9	2.5	120	−156	−1.30	300
7	M	62	MCA-M1	80	17	3.5	117	−8,847	−75.70	5,382
8	M	69	ICA distal	50	10	4.2	120	118	0.98	2
9	M	50	BA	62	5	3.4	116	67	0.58	98

*Patients are listed in the table by the lesion location and sequentially arranged according to the degree of luminal stenosis (%) of the lesions.
ICAS indicates intracranial atherosclerotic stenosis; MCA-M1, M1 segment of middle cerebral artery; ICA, internal carotid artery; BA, basilar artery.

Patients with symptomatic ICAS are at high risk of recurrent ischemic stroke, despite of medical and/or interventional treatment [17-19]. However, commonly used noninvasive imaging modalities have been found of relatively low positive predictive values for diagnosis of 50-99% intracranial stenosis, compared with digital subtract angiography (DSA) [20,21]. Moreover, the percentage of stenosis itself, even when diagnosed by DSA, was not the only factor that might be able to affect downstream hemodynamics in the case of ICAS. Irregularity and eccentricity of the lesion, which in many cases is influenced by the plaque compositions, as well as the collateral status, may also affect the hemodynamic impact of an ICAS lesion [22]. This may partly explain why patients with ICAS of moderate luminal stenosis would also be at risk of SIT [22,23]. Therefore, we aimed to evaluate hemodynamic impact of ICAS via reconstructed CFD models in the present study, which was found feasible using routinely obtained CTA source images, so that this single noninvasive imaging modality could provide much more information of ICAS beyond the anatomic severity of luminal stenosis.

Although biplane DSA images could also be used to reconstruct CFD models of ICAS [24], and that CTA may not be as accurate as DSA to depict the vessel geometry in ICAS [21], we assumed that CTA images would be a better source for CFD modeling of ICAS lesions from both the technical and clinical points of view. On one hand, CTA source images, with its three-dimensional nature, yield a better source for CFD modeling than biplane DSA images, from the technical angle. On the other hand, as a noninvasive imaging modality, CTA is more commonly used and easier to be obtained in clinical practice than DSA, which permits studies with relatively large sample sizes in the future. In addition, although the noninvasive time-of-flight MR angiography can also provide three-dimensional geometry of the cerebral vessels of interest as CTA does, vessel geometry obtained from CTA is more accurate than that from MR angiography, especially in cases with extremely low distal flow beyond the ICAS lesion when MR angiography could overestimate the degree of stenosis.

Hemodynamic impact of ICAS was assessed using PR in our study, paralleled to FFR in the cardiac field, with lower PR indicating more significantly decreased downstream flow. To our knowledge, there had been no data about the cut-point of simulated PR to define a hemodynamically significant ICAS. However, for coronary artery disease, virtual FFR based on CFD models of coronary lesions had been found to be closely correlated with FFR measured under induced hyperemia during percutaneous coronary angiography (correlation coefficient r =0.84), and to be able to accurately identify lesions with FFR <0.80 as mentioned above [10]. Thus for this pilot study, we used the same cut-point of PR (0.80) as is currently used in the cardiac field for invasively measured FFR and virtual FFR [10,16]. But in future studies, we will explore an optimal cut-point of PR to dichotomize ICAS lesions by the hemodynamic impact, for instance, by comparing PR values against brain perfusion results such as quantitative arterial spin labeling MR perfusion imaging. According to the results, distal pressures and PRs of ICAS lesions were in minus values in some cases. This was one of the limitations of CFD modeling in the current study that is further discussed below, and also one of the reasons that we also used another index, PG, to quantify the hemodynamic severity of ICAS.

In the measurement of invasive FFR for coronary artery disease, use of vasodilator could decrease the microcirculatory resistance, magnify the function of existing collaterals, and hence induce hyperemia, under which circumstance the hemodynamic impact of the lesion could be accurately evaluated in most cases [25]. However, it has also been recognized that the invasive FFR might not be reliable in cases with microvascular damage, in which cases maximal hyperemia could not be achieved [10]. In a latest study as mentioned above utilizing the CFD modeling technique to obtain virtual FFR of coronary lesions, generic downstream boundary conditions, including the microvascular resistance and compliance values, were developed and applied to the arterial outlet(s) with a Windkessel model [10,26]. The virtual FFR obtained in this way, not affected by the status of microcirculation and without the need of simulating hyperemic conditions, was proved of substantial consistency with invasively measured FFR, with an average absolute error of ±0.06 [10]. Therefore, virtual fractional flow of arterial stenosis based on vessel geometry and generic boundary conditions is potentially reliable in defining the hemodynamic significance of the lesion. In the current study, we did not take into account the effects of distal microvascular resistance and the collaterals in the CFD models of ICAS lesions, which needs to be addressed in future studies, probably by referring to the method for obtaining virtual FFR for coronary lesions as discussed above.

Fractional flow across ICAS, in terms of PR and PG in our study, was not exclusively determined by percentage of the stenosis. Other morphological characteristics of an ICAS lesion might also impact on the hemodynamic environment in situ and downstream, for instance, length of the lesion as implied by this study, though we did not do any statistical analysis to confirm the speculation concerning the relationships between the lesion length and the hemodynamic impact of an ICAS due to the small sample size, as well as the irregularity and eccentricity of the stenosis that were not yet investigated in the current study. To date, few data existed on relationships between morphology and hemodynamics of ICAS, but length of carotid plaque and patent ICA vessel diameter, besides degree of stenosis, were found to be significantly related to ipsilateral intracranial blood flow in studies of carotid stenosis [27]. Based on vessel geometry and therefore harboring all morphological information of a lesion, simulated CFD blood flow models could comprehensively reflect effects of morphological factors on hemodynamic characteristics of ICAS. Since risk of stroke recurrence could be altered by blood flow hemodynamics in patients with symptomatic ICAS, evaluation of CFD models, instead of using anatomic severity of luminal stenosis as almost the only imaging indicator, might play a role in risk stratification of these patients. In addition, evaluating the hemodynamic parameters embedded within the CFD models of symptomatic ICAS lesions, such as PR, PG, flow velocity, wall shear stress and shear strain rates, may be useful to embrace a better understanding of the effects of hemodynamics on diverse pathomechanisms of ICAS-related ischemic stroke, which are currently understudied.

The most important limitation of the present study was that CFD models were simplified and only based on geometry of short vessel segments containing the stenoses, trimming off artery branches and meanwhile ignoring effects of collaterals and other factors that may affect hemodynamics of the lesion. This may be part of the reasons for the minus downstream pressure values as detected in the CFD models of some cases. Besides, the prescribed outflow velocity may also partly contribute to the unrealistic minus pressures in some of the CFD models. In future studies, the following measures could be explored to improve the realistic accuracy of the simulated CFD models: covering longer vessel segments in the CFD models, at least long enough for post-stenotic blood flow to restore laminar flow; and assigning personalized pressures and flow velocities at the inlet and outlet that could be of higher physiological significance, for instance, flow velocities distal to an ICAS lesion at a major intracranial artery detected by transcranial Doppler. Moreover, unlike carotid arteries, intracranial arteries have plenty of braches and perforators, which could alter the hemodynamics of blood flow in a major intracranial artery. Therefore, including main adjacent branches and perforators in the CFD models of ICAS lesions in future studies, as what is currently done for CFD modeling of coronary lesions [9,28], could further optimize the realistic accuracy of the simulating results. Also, it would further enhance the clinical relevance of CFD blood flow simulation of symptomatic ICAS by considering the effects of distal microvascular resistance and collateral status, which might also facilitate better understanding of mechanisms of collateral recruitment in the presence of symptomatic ICAS. In addition, another limitation of the current study lay in that simulated pressure gradients were not validated against direct, invasive measures, or compared with indirect measures with other noninvasive methods, which will also be addressed in future studies.

Apart from the above measures to improve the CFD models of ICAS lesions, meanwhile we also need to balance the complexity and accuracy of the models with its generalizability in clinical studies. Simplified modeling would be less time-consuming for each patient involved and probably more generalizable for large clinical studies in the future, but at the meantime the consequent inaccuracy of simulated hemodynamic environment may compromise its clinical perspective. Thus, achieving an acceptable balance between the realistic accuracy and the generalizability of CFD modeling of symptomatic ICAS lesions is important for this technique to ultimately be of clinical significance and utility in the assessment of such lesions.

Conclusions

This pilot study demonstrated the feasibility to quantitatively assess hemodynamic impact of ICAS using CFD models reconstructed from routinely obtained CTA. A vast number of studies are required to evaluate the ultimate value of this technique, to seek improvement in the realistic accuracy and the generalizability of CFD modeling of ICAS, and to explore the role of specific hemodynamic characteristics from CFD models in risk stratification of patients with symptomatic ICAS.

Competing interests
The authors declare that they have no competing interests.

Authors' contributions
XL contributed to study design, data collection, analysis and interpretation, and manuscript preparation; FS, AKF, MJ and HLI contributed to image processing and computational modeling; YS and TL contributed to data collection and interpretation; LL and EF contributed to study design and manuscript preparation; KSW and DSL contributed to study design, data analysis and interpretation, and manuscript preparation. All authors read and approved the final manuscript.

Author details
[1]Department of Medicine and Therapeutics, the Chinese University of Hong Kong, Prince of Wales Hospital, Shatin, Hong Kong SAR, China. [2]UCLA Stroke Center, University of California, CA 90095 Los Angeles, USA. [3]Department of Neurology, Beijing Tiantan Hospital, Capital Medical University, Beijing 100050 China. [4]Department of Neurology, Tufts University, Boston MA 02111, USA. [5]UCLA Department of Neurology, Neuroscience Research Building, Suite 225, Los Angeles, CA 90095-7334, USA.

References
1. Wong LKS: **Global burden of intracranial atherosclerosis.** *Int J Stroke* 2006, 1:158–159.
2. Qureshi AI, Feldmann E, Gomez CR, Johnston SC, Kasner SE, Quick DC, Rasmussen PA, Suri MF, Taylor RA, Zaidat OO: **Intracranial atherosclerotic disease: an update.** *Ann Neurol* 2009, 66:730–738.
3. Saba L, Anzidei M, Piga M, Ciolina F, Mannelli L, Catalano C, Suri JS, Raz E: **Multi-modal CT scanning in the evaluation of cerebrovascular disease patients.** *Cardiovasc Diagn Ther* 2014, 4:245–262.

4.   Kasner SE, Chimowitz MI, Lynn MJ, Howlett-Smith H, Stern BJ, Hertzberg VS, Frankel MR, Levine SR, Chaturvedi S, Benesch CG, Sila CA, Jovin TG, Romano JG, Cloft HJ, for the Warfarin Aspirin Symptomatic Intracranial Disease (WASID) Trial Investigators: **Predictors of ischemic stroke in the territory of a symptomatic intracranial arterial stenosis.** *Circulation* 2006, **113**:555–563.

5.   Wang Y, Liu L, Wang Y, Soo Y, Pu Y, Wong KS: **A multicenter study of the prevalence and outcomes of intracranial large artery atherosclerosis among stroke and TIA patients in China [abstract].** *Stroke* 2012, **43**:A120.

6.   Liebeskind DS, Cotsonis GA, Saver JL, Lynn MJ, Turan TN, Cloft HJ, Chimowitz MI: **Collaterals dramatically alter stroke risk in intracranial atherosclerosis.** *Ann Neurol* 2011, **69**:963–974.

7.   Liebeskind DS, Cotsonis GA, Lynn MJ, Cloft HJ, Fiorella DJ, Derdeyn CP, Chimowitz MI, on behalf of the SAMMPRIS Investigators: **Collaterals determine risk of early territorial stroke and hemorrhage in the SAMMPRIS trial.** *Stroke* 2012, **43**:A124.

8.   Min JK, Koo BK, Erglis A, Doh JH, Daniels DV, Jegere S, Kim HS, Dunning AM, DeFrance T, Lansky A, Leipsic J: **Usefulness of noninvasive fractional flow reserve computed from coronary computed tomographic angiograms for intermediate stenoses confirmed by quantitative coronary angiography.** *Am J Cardiol* 2012, **110**:971–976.

9.   Koo BK, Erglis A, Doh JH, Daniels DV, Jegere S, Kim HS, Dunning A, DeFrance T, Lansky A, Leipsic J, Min JK: **Diagnosis of ischemia-causing coronary stenoses by noninvasive fractional flow reserve computed from coronary computed tomographic angiograms: results from the prospective multicenter DISCOVER-FLOW (Diagnosis of Ischemia-Causing Stenoses Obtained Via Noninvasive Fractional Flow Reserve) study.** *J Am Coll Cardiol* 2011, **58**:1989–1997.

10.   Morris PD, Ryan D, Morton AC, Lycett R, Lawford PV, Hose DR, Gunn JP: **Virtual fractional flow reserve from coronary angiography: modeling the significance of coronary lesions: results from the VIRTU-1 (VIRTUal Fractional Flow Reserve From Coronary Angiography) study.** *JACC Cardiovasc Interv* 2013, **6**:149–157.

11.   Schirmer CM, Malek AM: **Prediction of complex flow patterns in intracranial atherosclerotic disease using computational fluid dynamics.** *Neurosurgery* 2007, **61**:842–852.

12.   Liebeskind DS, Fong A, Scalzo F, Derdeyn CP, Fiorella DJ, Cloft HJ, Chimowitz MI, Feldmann E: **SAMMPRIS angiography discloses hemodynamic effects of intracranial stenosis: computational fluid dynamics of fractional flow.** *Stroke* 2013, **44**:A156.

13.   Samuels OB, Joseph GJ, Lynn MJ, Smith HA, Chimowitz MZ: **A standardized method for measuring intracranial arterial stenosis.** *AJNR Am J Neuroradiol* 2000, **21**:643–646.

14.   Antiga L, Piccinelli M, Botti L, Ene-Iordache B, Remuzzi A, Steinman DA: **An image-based modeling framework for patient-specific computational hemodynamics.** *Med Biol Eng Comput* 2008, **46**:1097–1112.

15.   Batchelor GK: *An Introduction to Fluid Dynamics.* Cambridge: Cambridge University Press; 1967.

16.   Min JK, Berman DS, Budoff MJ, Jaffer FA, Leipsic J, Leon MB, Mancini GBJ, Mauri L, Schwartz RS, Shaw LJ: **Rationale and design of the DeFACTO (Determination of Fractional Flow Reserve by Anatomic Computed Tomographic AngiOgraphy) study.** *J Cardiovas Comput Tomogr* 2011, **5**:301–309.

17.   Chimowitz MI, Lynn MJ, Howlett-Smith H, Stern BJ, Hertzberg VS, Frankel MR, Levine SR, Chaturvedi S, Kasner SE, Benesch CG, Sila CA, Jovin TG, Romano JG: **Comparison of warfarin and aspirin for symptomatic intracranial arterial stenosis.** *N Engl J Med* 2005, **352**:1305–1316.

18.   Chimowitz MI, Lynn MJ, Derdeyn CP, Turan TN, Fiorella D, Lane BF, Janis LS, Lutsep HL, Barnwell SL, Waters MF, Hoh BL, Hourihane JM, Levy EI, Alexandrov AV, Harrigan MR, Chiu D, Klucznik RP, Clark JM, McDougall CG, Johnson MD, Pride GL, Jr., Torbey MT, Zaidat OO, Rumboldt Z, Cloft HJ: **Stenting versus aggressive medical therapy for intracranial arterial stenosis.** *N Engl J Med* 2011, **365**:993–1003.

19.   Weber R, Kraywinkel K, Diener HC, Weimar C, German Stroke Study C: **Symptomatic intracranial atherosclerotic stenoses: prevalence and prognosis in patients with acute cerebral ischemia.** *Cerebrovasc Dis* 2010, **30**:188–193.

20.   Liebeskind DS, Kosinski AS, Saver JL, Feldmann E, for the SONIA Investigators: **CT angiography in the Stroke Outcomes and Neuroimaging of Intracranial Atherosclerosis (SONIA) study [abstract].** *Stroke* 2007, **32**:477.

21.   Feldmann E, Wilterdink JL, Kosinski A, Lynn M, Chimowitz MI, Sarafin J, Smith HH, Nichols F, Rogg J, Cloft HJ, Wechsler L, Saver J, Levine SR, Tegeler C, Adams R, Sloan M, the SONIA Trial Investigators: **The Stroke Outcomes and Neuroimaging of Intracranial Atherosclerosis (SONIA) trial.** *Neurology* 2007, **68**:2099–2106.

22.   Leng X, Wong KS, Liebeskind DS: **Evaluating intracranial atherosclerosis rather than intracranial stenosis.** *Stroke* 2014, **45**:645–651.

23.   Liebeskind DS, Cotsonis GA, Saver JL, Lynn MJ, Cloft HJ, Chimowitz MI, Warfarin-Aspirin Symptomatic Intracranial Disease Investigators: **Collateral circulation in symptomatic intracranial atherosclerosis.** *J Cereb Blood Flow Metab* 2011, **31**:1293–1301.

24.   Scalzo F, Hao Q, Walczak AM, Hu X, Hoi Y, Hoffmann KR, Liebeskind DS: **Computational hemodynamics in intracranial vessels reconstructed from biplane angiograms.** In *Advances in Visual Computing, Part III*, Volume 37. Edited by Bebis G, Boyle R, Parvin B, Koracin D, Chung R, Hammound R, Hussain M, Kar-Han T, Crawfis R, Thalmann D, Kao D, Avila L. Berlin Heidelberg: Springer; 2010:359–367. Lecture Notes in Computer Science.

25.   De Bruyne B, Sarma J: **Fractional flow reserve: a review.** *Heart* 2008, **94**:949–959.

26.   Westerhof N, Lankhaar JW, Westerhof BE: **The arterial Windkessel.** *Med Biol Eng Comput* 2009, **47**:131–141.

27.   Douglas AF, Christopher S, Amankulor N, Din R, Poullis M, Amin-Hanjani S, Ghogawala Z: **Extracranial carotid plaque length and parent vessel diameter significantly affect baseline ipsilateral intracranial blood flow.** *Neurosurgery* 2011, **69**:767–773.

28.   Min JK, Leipsic J, Pencina MJ, Berman DS, Koo BK, van Mieghem C, Erglis A, Lin FY, Dunning AM, Apruzzese P, Budoff MJ, Cole JH, Jaffer FA, Leon MB, Malpeso J, Mancini GB, Park SJ, Schwartz RS, Shaw LJ, Mauri L: **Diagnostic accuracy of fractional flow reserve from anatomic CT angiography.** *JAMA* 2012, **308**:1237–1245.

2

Imaging of cerebral aneurysms: a clinical perspective

Nam K. Yoon[1], Scott McNally[2], Philipp Taussky[1] and Min S. Park[1*]

Abstract

Neuroimaging is a critical element in evaluating and treating patients with cerebral aneurysms. Each neuroimaging technique has unique strengths, weaknesses, and current developments. In this review, we discuss the utility of two primary noninvasive radiological techniques—computed tomography angiography (CTA) and magnetic resonance angiography (MRA)—as well as of digital subtraction angiography (DSA) for evaluation of cerebral aneurysms. These techniques allow comprehensive evaluation of aneurysm size, location, rupture status, and other imaging characteristics that guide clinicians to make appropriate and timely treatment recommendations.

Keywords: Cerebral aneurysm, Neuroimaging, Computed tomography, Magnetic resonance imaging, Digital subtraction angiography

Background

Subarachnoid hemorrhage from rupture of an intracranial aneurysm is a devastating condition associated with approximately 50 % overall mortality and high survivor morbidity despite advances in treatment [1]. Although population studies have estimated the overall prevalence of intracranial aneurysms to be 3.2 % [2], the overall incidence of subarachnoid hemorrhage secondary to aneurysmal rupture in a population study spanning 21 countries was relatively low at approximately 9 per 100,000 persons per year, although rates differed by country (e.g., Japan and Finland had the highest rates at 22.7 and 19.7, respectively) [3].

The International Study of Unruptured Incidental Aneurysms (ISUIA) demonstrated that the location and size of incidentally found, unruptured cerebral aneurysms were predictive of risk of future rupture [4]. Aneurysms that have already ruptured have a much higher risk of re-hemorrhage [5, 6]. Additionally, the angiomorphology of the aneurysm has also been posited to influence future hemorrhage risk factors, such as irregular domes [7, 8], daughter sacs [9], and low wall shear stress [10]. Thus, it is critically important to accurately characterize aneurysmal morphology to guide treatment, making neuroimaging a critical element in evaluating and treating patients with cerebral aneurysms. Each neuroimaging technique has unique strengths, weaknesses, and current developments. Three major imaging methods are used for neuroimaging of cerebral aneurysms: computed tomography angiography, magnetic resonance angiography, and digital subtraction angiography. In this article, the authors review and compare imaging modalities used to evaluate intracranial aneurysms with particular focus on how each affects surgical or endovascular management.

Computed tomography and CT angiography
Evaluation of subarachnoid hemorrhage

A non-contrast-enhanced CT scan is commonly used as the first-line imaging modality for evaluating subarachnoid hemorrhage (Fig. 1a). This technology is rapid, inexpensive, and widely available. In the acute setting, the higher attenuation of hemorrhage compared with surrounding parenchyma allows 100 % sensitivity of subarachnoid hemorrhage if performed within the first six hours [11]. Additionally, the distribution of the hemorrhage can often predict the location of the underlying aneurysm, and CTs can determine the presence of intraventricular hemorrhage and degree of hydrocephalus, which can have significant impact on prognosis and treatment (Fig. 1a).

* Correspondence: neuropub@hsc.utah.edu
[1]Department of Neurosurgery, Clinical Neurosciences Center, University of Utah, Salt Lake City, Utah, USA
Full list of author information is available at the end of the article

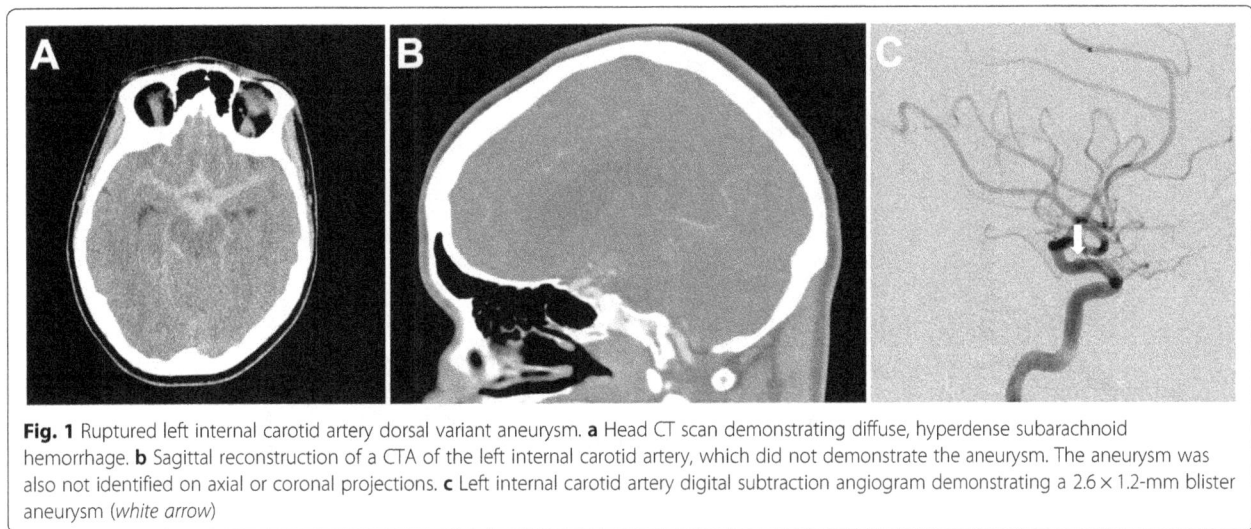

Fig. 1 Ruptured left internal carotid artery dorsal variant aneurysm. **a** Head CT scan demonstrating diffuse, hyperdense subarachnoid hemorrhage. **b** Sagittal reconstruction of a CTA of the left internal carotid artery, which did not demonstrate the aneurysm. The aneurysm was also not identified on axial or coronal projections. **c** Left internal carotid artery digital subtraction angiogram demonstrating a 2.6 × 1.2-mm blister aneurysm (*white arrow*)

Although CT is an excellent modality for evaluating acute subarachnoid hemorrhage, in the subacute setting, from six hours to one week after hemorrhage, the ability to detect subarachnoid hemorrhage with CT drops dramatically because of the brain's normal degradation of hemorrhagic blood products. An older study investigated the ability to detect subarachnoid hemorrhage of varying chronicity on CT and found 100 % sensitivity within two days, but sensitivity dropped to 85 % after five days, 50 % after one week, and 30 % after two weeks [12, 13]. A more recent study with newer technology also demonstrated difficulty detecting subacute and chronic subarachnoid hemorrhage, with only 36.4 % sensitivity after five days [14]. Thus, if a patient presents several days after ictus, a negative non-contrast CT is commonly supplemented with a lumbar puncture to evaluate for xanthochromia. Alternatively, CT angiography (CTA) has also been used to increase the detection rate of ruptured cerebral aneurysms in instances where there is a high index of clinical suspicion and a negative non-contrast CT. McCormack et al. [15] reported that a negative non-contrast CT followed by a negative CT angiogram carries a post-test probability of 99.43 % of being negative for aneurysmal subarachnoid hemorrhage. The investigators argued that a lumbar puncture in this setting would carry a less than 1 % probability of detecting subarachnoid hemorrhage and that patients should be informed of the low probability when lumbar puncture is offered.

Detection of cerebral aneurysm

CTA is performed on multi-detector helical CT scanners that allow multi-planar reformats, sub-millimeter slice thickness, and 3D reconstructions (Fig. 2a, b). Several investigators have demonstrated that current multi-detector scanners have a spatial resolution that can reliably diagnose aneurysms greater than 4 mm with nearly 100 % sensitivity [16–18]. A meta-analysis that surveyed studies performed on 64-slice CT scanners with sub-millimeter resolution used for detection of cerebral aneurysms showed a pooled 97 % sensitivity rate for all aneurysm sizes [19]. For aneurysms 3 mm and smaller, however, early CT technology has been shown to be inadequate, with sensitivity numbers as low as 84 % from four-channel multi-row detector CT scanners (Fig. 1b) [20]. Studies with recent technology have shown more promising results, with up to 99.6 % sensitivity on 16-slice CT scanners [21]. Xing et al. [17] demonstrated an even higher sensitivity for small aneurysms on a 64-slice CT scanner than conventional non-rotational digital subtraction angiography; however, Wang et al. [22] demonstrated an 81.8 % sensitivity for aneurysms smaller than 3 mm when performed on a 320-slice CT.

Current developments

As CT technology continues to advance with increasingly higher numbers of detectors, scans can be performed more quickly with thinner collimation, higher resolution, and better contrast bolus timing. Further increases in spatial resolution will likely allow greater sensitivity in detecting smaller aneurysms and small associated branch vessels. Time-resolved CTA, or 4D-CTA, is a technique that can evaluate the flow dynamics of aneurysms by obtaining multiple acquisitions of a region of interest for a period of time. It has the ability to separate different blood flow phases and can identify aneurysms previously difficult to distinguish from surrounding vessels, such as in the case of intranidal aneurysms associated with arteriovenous malformations [23]. Additionally, specific features now discernible on electrocardiogram-gated 4D-CTA can detect aneurysm

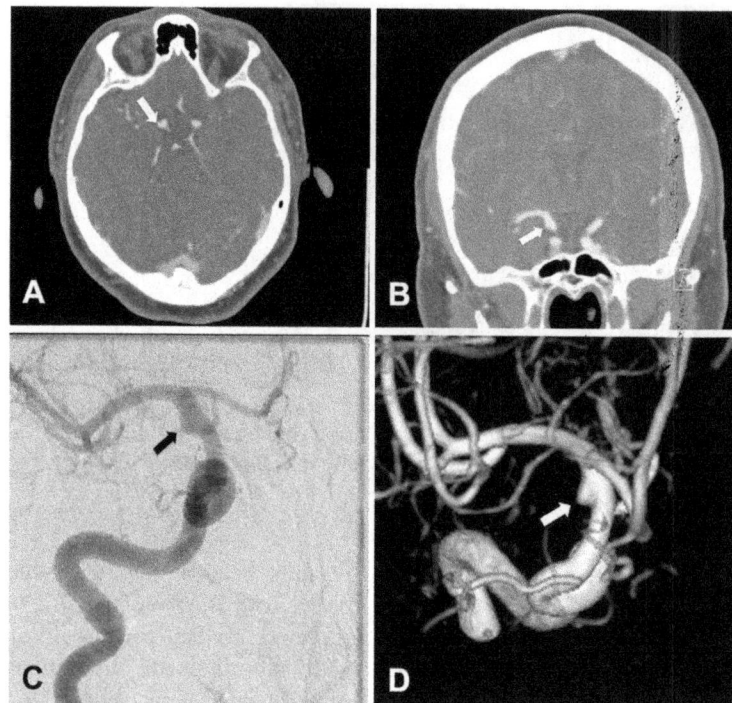

Fig. 2 Unruptured right internal carotid artery aneurysm. **a** Axial CT angiogram demonstrating 3-mm blister aneurysm (*arrow*). **b** Coronal CT angiogram reconstruction of the aneurysm (*arrow*). **c** Right internal carotid artery digital subtraction angiogram of the blister aneurysm (*arrow*). **d** 3D reconstruction during diagnostic cerebral angiogram of the aneurysm (*arrow*)

pulsations with the cardiac cycle and are currently being investigated for higher risk of growth and rupture [24]. Another recent development involves the use of computational fluid dynamics, which seeks to simulate blood flow within the aneurysm to calculate variables that would presumably correlate with rupture risk such as aneurysmal wall shear stress and peak wall tension. These simulations are subject to a wide range of mathematical assumptions and there has yet to be a consensus methodology for predicting rupture [25]. Certainly, computational fluid dynamics offers significant promise in the future to assist with the management of cerebral aneurysms.

Magnetic resonance imaging and MR angiography

Evaluation of subarachnoid hemorrhage

The use of MRI for evaluation of cerebral aneurysms is continually and rapidly evolving. MRI has advantages over CTA in that it does not use ionizing radiation and offers the ability to obtain images without the need for administration of intravenous contrast agents. Fluid-attenuated inversion recovery (FLAIR) sequences produce strong T2 weighting while suppressing the cerebro-spinal fluid (CSF) signal and can be particularly useful for detecting subarachnoid hemorrhage, especially in the subacute period. In a study of patients with acute and subacute subarachnoid hemorrhage, da Rocha et al. [26] demonstrated a 100 % sensitivity for detection of subarachnoid hemorrhage with FLAIR compared with a 66 % sensitivity on CT. Gradient-echo T2*-weighted imaging was found to be superior to FLAIR for detection of subarachnoid hemorrhage of even older age [14]. However, because of the higher cost and longer acquisition times, MRI is not considered the initial diagnostic test of choice and is usually reserved for patients with a high pre-test probability of aneurysmal subarachnoid hemorrhage and a negative initial work-up with CT scans and/or cerebral angiography. It has the added benefit of screening for other pathologies that may present with similar symptoms, some of which may also produce hyperintense sulcal signal on FLAIR such as meningitis, meningeal carcinomatosis, leptomeningeal metastasis, subdural hematoma, adjacent neoplasms, and dural venous thrombosis.

MRI/MRA aneurysm detection

The use of time-of-flight (TOF) sequences on MRA eliminates the need for administration of contrast agents, which may be contraindicated in patients with renal failure or contrast allergy (Fig. 3a, b and Fig. 4). A meta-analysis of MRA studies for evaluating aneurysms demonstrated that contrast-enhanced MRA (CE-MRA) and TOF had similar sensitivity for the

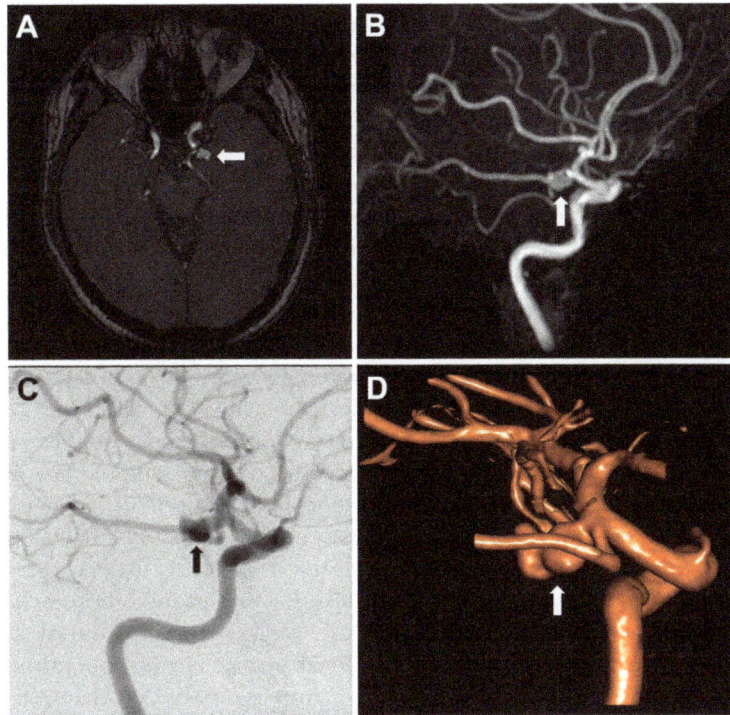

Fig. 3 Unruptured 8×4-mm left posterior communicating artery aneurysm. **a** 3D TOF MRA demonstrating irregular 8-mm aneurysm (*arrow*). **b** 3D MRA reconstruction of the aneurysm (*arrow*). **c** Left internal carotid artery digital subtraction angiogram of the aneurysm (*arrow*). **d** 3D reconstruction during diagnostic cerebral angiogram of the posterior communicating artery aneurysm (*arrow*)

detection of aneurysms [27]. CE-MRA, however, was found to be superior to TOF sequences because of its ability to eliminate flow-related artifacts and spin saturation [28]. Although CE-MRA had a lower spatial resolution compared with CT angiography (0.7 × 0.7 × 0.8 versus 0.35 × 0.35 × 0.8 mm), the images were qualitatively graded to be comparable with similar diagnostic results (Fig. 4) [29]. Small branch vessels were also reportedly better visualized on 3 T MRA

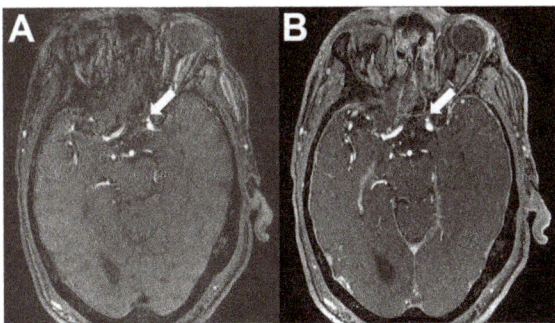

Fig. 4 MRA scan of aneurysms. **a** Axial TOF MRA demonstrates a left ophthalmic artery aneurysm (*arrow*). Although it avoids the use of contrast, the longer acquisition time introduces some motion artifact. **b** Contrast-enhanced axial MRA in the same patient with less motion artifact of the aneurysm (*arrow*)

over CTA, because of the lack of venous contrast contamination and in spite of lower spatial resolution [30]. Despite these findings, MRA is generally not the diagnostic test of choice for the evaluation of cerebral aneurysms in the acute setting and is reserved as a screening test or for follow-up, where avoiding repeated ionizing radiation and/or contrast nephropathy is important.

As MRA technology continues to improve, spatial resolution and sensitivity to smaller aneurysms is also expected to improve. With current sequences, the spatial resolution at 1.5 T is often as low as 1 mm [31], whereas at 3 T the spatial resolution can be as low as 0.6–0.7 mm while preserving the signal-to-noise ratio [32]. Radiologists also unanimously report significantly better visualization of aneurysms at 3 T. A meta-analysis by Sailer et al. [27] that evaluated the sensitivity of MRA for detection of cerebral aneurysms found a trend towards significance in better detection of smaller aneurysms on 3 T versus 1.5 T scanners ($p = 0.054$). This study reported a pooled sensitivity of 1.5 T and 3 T scanners of approximately 95 % for all aneurysms. Although the above study showed that 90 % of aneurysms that were missed were smaller than 5 mm in size, the pooled sensitivity for detecting aneurysms smaller than 3 mm was still 86 %.

Future developments

Although ISUIA argued that aneurysms smaller than 7 mm have very low rates of hemorrhage [4], the majority of ruptured aneurysms tend to be small [33]. There is a current unmet need to identify signs of high rupture risk in these small aneurysms. The pathophysiology of aneurysm growth, wall thinning, and rupture involves multiple histologic changes including endothelial disruption, collagen loss, and inflammatory cell migration [34]. Current imaging cannot detect these changes, but contrast agents could permeate through the disrupted endothelium into the aneurysm wall or even the surrounding CSF. Researchers have recently developed black-blood T1-weighted MRI sequences that help identify rupture site in patients with aneurysmal subarachnoid hemorrhage by demonstrating the inflamed, enhancing wall of the recently ruptured aneurysm. These techniques can identify the causative rupture site in patients with multiple intracranial aneurysms, allowing for more accurate and timely treatment [35].

Aneurysmal wall enhancement correlates with previous rupture, with some enhancement (strong or weak) identified in 98.4 % of ruptured aneurysms and no enhancement identified in 81.9 % of unruptured aneurysms [36]. Aneurysm wall permeability can also be quantified using dynamic contrast-enhanced (DCE)-MRI and the perfusion parameter K^{trans}, which is a size-independent predictor of rupture risk [37]. Additional imaging protocols are being developed to help further characterize aneurysms and identify characteristics associated with rupture risk. High-field-strength 7 T MRI scanners have an extremely high signal-to-noise ratio, allowing the spatial resolution needed to detect variations in aneurysm wall thickness, which may be a marker of rupture risk [38]. Other protocols can define aneurysmal wall motion abnormalities associated with higher risk of rupture [39]. Another advanced imaging technique combines MRA with postprocessing algorithms from computational fluid dynamics to create 4D flow modeling [40, 41]. Time-resolved MRA, or 4D MRA, directly measures flow velocities and shear stresses within an aneurysm [42]. This may allow for the identification of the inflow zone of aneurysms and may guide endovascular treatment [43, 44].

Digital subtraction angiography

Digital subtraction angiography (DSA) is typically performed using femoral catheterization with a biplane unit with rotational/3-dimensional capabilities. The catheter is guided to each of the major cerebral arteries, and iodinated contrast is injected while obtaining various 2D views, with rotational angiography used to create a 3-dimensional model of the vessels.

Considered the reference standard for evaluating intracranial aneurysms, DSA has high spatial resolution to identify aneurysms that may be missed on CTA or MRA (Figs. 1, 2 and 3). It also has the temporal resolution to separately evaluate the arterial, capillary, and venous phases of the injection. Similar to CTA, DSA requires the use of ionizing radiation and iodinated contrast. In addition, this procedure is invasive and requires operator expertise to guide the catheter to the major intracranial vessels while minimizing the risk of stroke, vascular injury, femoral artery occlusion, or retroperitoneal hematoma. A review of eight prospective and seven retrospective studies to determine the complication rate of DSA for evaluation of carotid stenosis demonstrated a mortality rate of 0.06 % and a rate of permanent neurologic deficit from stroke of 1 % [45]. Another study showed greater re-hemorrhage rates when DSA was used to evaluate ruptured aneurysms within the first six hours post ictus [46]; however, as these are operator-dependent procedures, overall risks may be related to operator expertise, with reports of complication rates of DSA for various indications below 0.3 % [47].

In addition to conventional DSA, 3-dimensional rotational angiography (3DRA) further increases the sensitivity of small aneurysms less than 3 mm in size (Figs. 1 and 2). van Rooij et al. [48] demonstrated that the addition of 3DRA identified 94 additional aneurysms in the evaluation of 350 target aneurysms initially screened by CTA/MRA. The mean size of these additional aneurysms was 3.54 mm, with the smallest detected aneurysm at 0.5 mm. Twenty-seven of these 94 aneurysms (mean size 1.94 mm) were even missed on DSA without 3DRA. Compared with 64- and 256-detector-row CTA, 3DRA is superior in detecting aneurysms 3 mm and smaller [49] and should be used when CT and/or MRI fails to demonstrate an aneurysm in the setting of spontaneous subarachnoid hemorrhage. Even when DSA fails to demonstrate an aneurysm in the setting of spontaneous subarachnoid hemorrhage, delayed repeat imaging is indicated. One literature review identified 37 aneurysms out of 368 angiography-negative subarachnoid hemorrhage patients on delayed, repeat DSA from one to six weeks after their initial study [50]. The higher resolution of DSA also allows for better neck characterization to guide endovascular versus open surgical treatment and better visualization of associated branch vessels [30].

Conclusion

It is important to accurately determine the size, morphology, location, and rupture status of a cerebral aneurysm and/or to identify specific imaging characteristics that may portend a higher risk of rupture so that potential treatment can be guided more accurately. While CT, MRI, and DSA are excellent tools at our disposal to identify subarachnoid hemorrhage and cerebral aneurysms, future advances will likely allow for faster, safer, and more accurate identification of cerebral aneurysms.

Competing interests

The authors declare that they have no competing interests.

Authors' contributions

All authors read and approved the final manuscript.

Author details

[1]Department of Neurosurgery, Clinical Neurosciences Center, University of Utah, Salt Lake City, Utah, USA. [2]Department of Radiology, University of Utah Health Care, Salt Lake City, Utah, USA.

References

1. Hop JW, Rinkel GJ, Algra A, van Gijn J. Case-fatality rates and functional outcome after subarachnoid hemorrhage: a systematic review. Stroke. 1997;28:660–4.
2. Vlak MH, Algra A, Brandenburg R, Rinkel GJ. Prevalence of unruptured intracranial aneurysms, with emphasis on sex, age, comorbidity, country, and time period: a systematic review and meta-analysis. Lancet Neurol. 2011;10:626–36.
3. de Rooij NK, Linn FH, van der Plas JA, Algra A, Rinkel GJ. Incidence of subarachnoid haemorrhage: a systematic review with emphasis on region, age, gender and time trends. J Neurol Neurosurg Psychiatry. 2007;78:1365–72.
4. Wiebers DO, Whisnant JP, Huston 3rd J, Meissner I, Brown Jr RD, Piepgras DG, et al. Unruptured intracranial aneurysms: natural history, clinical outcome, and risks of surgical and endovascular treatment. Lancet. 2003;362:103–10.
5. Winn HR, Richardson AE, Jane JA. The long-term prognosis in untreated cerebral aneurysms: I. The incidence of late hemorrhage in cerebral aneurysm: a 10-year evaluation of 364 patients. Ann Neurol. 1977;1:358–70.
6. Eskesen V, Rosenorn J, Schmidt K. The impact of rebleeding on the life time probabilities of different outcomes in patients with ruptured intracranial aneurysms. A theoretical evaluation. Acta Neurochir (Wien). 1988;95:99–101.
7. Raghavan ML, Ma B, Harbaugh RE. Quantified aneurysm shape and rupture risk. J Neurosurg. 2005;102:355–62.
8. Dhar S, Tremmel M, Mocco J, Kim M, Yamamoto J, Siddiqui AH, et al. Morphology parameters for intracranial aneurysm rupture risk assessment. Neurosurgery. 2008;63:185–96. discussion 196-197.
9. UCAS Japan Investigators. The natural course of unruptured cerebral aneurysms in a Japanese cohort. N Engl J Med. 2012;366:2474–82.
10. Boussel L, Rayz V, McCulloch C, Martin A, Acevedo-Bolton G, Lawton M, et al. Aneurysm growth occurs at region of low wall shear stress: patient-specific correlation of hemodynamics and growth in a longitudinal study. Stroke. 2008;39:2997–3002.
11. Boesiger BM, Shiber JR. Subarachnoid hemorrhage diagnosis by computed tomography and lumbar puncture: are fifth generation CT scanners better at identifying subarachnoid hemorrhage? J Emerg Med. 2005;29:23–7.
12. Perry JJ, Stiell IG, Sivilotti ML, Bullard MJ, Emond M, Symington C, et al. Sensitivity of computed tomography performed within six hours of onset of headache for diagnosis of subarachnoid haemorrhage: prospective cohort study. BMJ. 2011;343:d4277.
13. van Gijn J, van Dongen KJ. The time course of aneurysmal haemorrhage on computed tomograms. Neuroradiology. 1982;23:153–6.
14. Yuan MK, Lai PH, Chen JY, Hsu SS, Liang HL, Yeh LR, et al. Detection of subarachnoid hemorrhage at acute and subacute/chronic stages: comparison of four magnetic resonance imaging pulse sequences and computed tomography. J Chin Med Assoc. 2005;68:131–7.
15. McCormack RF, Hutson A. Can computed tomography angiography of the brain replace lumbar puncture in the evaluation of acute-onset headache after a negative noncontrast cranial computed tomography scan? Acad Emerg Med. 2010;17:444–51.
16. Uysal E, Yanbuloglu B, Erturk M, Kilinc BM, Basak M. Spiral CT angiography in diagnosis of cerebral aneurysms of cases with acute subarachnoid hemorrhage. Diagn Interv Radiol. 2005;11:77–82.
17. Xing W, Chen W, Sheng J, Peng Y, Lu J, Wu X, et al. Sixty-four-row multislice computed tomographic angiography in the diagnosis and characterization of intracranial aneurysms: comparison with 3D rotational angiography. World Neurosurg. 2011;76:105–13.
18. McKinney AM, Palmer CS, Truwit CL, Karagulle A, Teksam M. Detection of aneurysms by 64-section multidetector CT angiography in patients acutely suspected of having an intracranial aneurysm and comparison with digital subtraction and 3D rotational angiography. AJNR Am J Neuroradiol. 2008;29:594–602.
19. Guo W, He XY, Li XF, Qian DX, Yan JQ, Bu DL, et al. Meta-analysis of diagnostic significance of sixty-four-row multi-section computed tomography angiography and three-dimensional digital subtraction angiography in patients with cerebral artery aneurysm. J Neurol Sci. 2014;346:197–203.
20. Teksam M, McKinney A, Casey S, Asis M, Kieffer S, Truwit CL. Multi-section CT angiography for detection of cerebral aneurysms. AJNR Am J Neuroradiol. 2004;25:1485–92.
21. Prestigiacomo CJ, Sabit A, He W, Jethwa P, Gandhi C, Russin J. Three dimensional CT angiography versus digital subtraction angiography in the detection of intracranial aneurysms in subarachnoid hemorrhage. J Neurointerv Surg. 2010;2:385–9.
22. Wang H, Li W, He H, Luo L, Chen C, Guo Y. 320-detector row CT angiography for detection and evaluation of intracranial aneurysms: comparison with conventional digital subtraction angiography. Clin Radiol. 2013;68:e15–20.
23. Chandran A, Radon M, Biswas S, Das K, Puthuran M, Nahser H: Novel use of 4D-CTA in imaging of intranidal aneurysms in an acutely ruptured arteriovenous malformation: is this the way forward? J Neurointerv Surg. (in press).
24. Hayakawa M, Tanaka T, Sadato A, Adachi K, Ito K, Hattori N, et al. Detection of pulsation in unruptured cerebral aneurysms by ECG-gated 3D-CT angiography (4D-CTA) with 320-row area detector CT (ADCT) and follow-up evaluation results: assessment based on heart rate at the time of scanning. Clin Neuroradiol. 2014;24:145–50.
25. Berg P, Roloff C, Beuing O, Voss S, Sugiyama S, Aristokleous N, et al. The Computational Fluid Dynamics Rupture Challenge 2013-Phase II: Variability of hemodynamic simulations in two intracranial aneurysms. J Biomech Eng. 2015;137:121008.
26. da Rocha AJ, da Silva CJ, Gama HP, Baccin CE, Braga FT, de Araújo Cesare F, et al. Comparison of magnetic resonance imaging sequences with computed tomography to detect low-grade subarachnoid hemorrhage: Role of fluid-attenuated inversion recovery sequence. J Comput Assist Tomogr. 2006;30:295–303.
27. Sailer AM, Wagemans BA, Nelemans PJ, de Graaf R, van Zwam WH. Diagnosing intracranial aneurysms with MR angiography: systematic review and meta-analysis. Stroke. 2014;45:119–26.
28. Nael K, Villablanca JP, Saleh R, Pope W, Nael A, Laub G, et al. Contrast-enhanced MR angiography at 3 T in the evaluation of intracranial aneurysms: a comparison with time-of-flight MR angiography. AJNR Am J Neuroradiol. 2006;27:2118–21.
29. Nael K, Villablanca JP, Mossaz L, Pope W, Juncosa A, Laub G, et al. 3-T contrast-enhanced MR angiography in evaluation of suspected intracranial aneurysm: comparison with MDCT angiography. AJR Am J Roentgenol. 2008;190:389–95.
30. Goto M, Kunimatsu A, Shojima M, Mori H, Abe O, Aoki S, et al. Depiction of branch vessels arising from intracranial aneurysm sacs: Time-of-flight MR angiography versus CT angiography. Clin Neurol Neurosurg. 2014;126:177–84.
31. Schellinger PD, Richter G, Kohrmann M, Dorfler A. Noninvasive angiography (magnetic resonance and computed tomography) in the diagnosis of ischemic cerebrovascular disease. Techniques and clinical applications. Cerebrovasc Dis. 2007;24 Suppl 1:16–23.
32. Bernstein MA, Huston 3rd J, Lin C, Gibbs GF, Felmlee JP. High-resolution intracranial and cervical MRA at 3.0 T: technical considerations and initial experience. Magn Reson Med. 2001;46:955–62.
33. Forget Jr TR, Benitez R, Veznedaroglu E, Sharan A, Mitchell W, Silva M, et al. A review of size and location of ruptured intracranial aneurysms. Neurosurgery. 2001;49:1322–5. discussion 1325-1326.
34. Frosen J, Piippo A, Paetau A, Kangasniemi M, Niemela M, Hernesniemi J, et al. Remodeling of saccular cerebral artery aneurysm wall is associated with rupture: histological analysis of 24 unruptured and 42 ruptured cases. Stroke. 2004;35:2287–93.
35. Matouk CC, Mandell DM, Gunel M, Bulsara KR, Malhotra A, Hebert R, et al. Vessel wall magnetic resonance imaging identifies the site of rupture in patients with multiple intracranial aneurysms: proof of principle. Neurosurgery. 2013;72:492–6. discussion 496.
36. Nagahata S, Nagahata M, Obara M, Kondo R, Minagawa N, Sato S, et al. Wall enhancement of the intracranial aneurysms revealed by magnetic

resonance vessel wall imaging using three-dimensional turbo spin-echo sequence with motion-sensitized driven-equilibrium: A sign of ruptured aneurysm? Clin Neuroradiol. (in press).

37. Vakil P, Ansari SA, Cantrell CG, Eddleman CS, Dehkordi FH, Vranic J, et al. Quantifying intracranial aneurysm wall permeability for risk assessment using dynamic contrast-enhanced MRI: A pilot study. AJNR Am J Neuroradiol. 2015;36:953–9.

38. Kleinloog R, Korkmaz E, Zwanenburg JJ, Kuijf HJ, Visser F, Blankena R, et al. Visualization of the aneurysm wall: a 7.0-tesla magnetic resonance imaging study. Neurosurgery. 2014;75:614–22. discussion 622.

39. Vanrossomme AE, Eker OF, Thiran JP, Courbebaisse GP, Zouaoui Boudjeltia K. Intracranial aneurysms: Wall motion analysis for prediction of rupture. AJNR Am J Neuroradiol. 2015;36:1796–1802.

40. Cebral JR, Vazquez M, Sforza DM, Houzeaux G, Tateshima S, Scrivano E, et al. Analysis of hemodynamics and wall mechanics at sites of cerebral aneurysm rupture. J Neurointerv Surg. 2015;7:530–6.

41. Schnell S, Ansari SA, Vakil P, Wasielewski M, Carr ML, Hurley MC, et al. Three-dimensional hemodynamics in intracranial aneurysms: influence of size and morphology. J Magn Reson Imaging. 2014;39:120–31.

42. Boussel L, Rayz V, Martin A, Acevedo-Bolton G, Lawton MT, Higashida R, et al. Phase-contrast magnetic resonance imaging measurements in intracranial aneurysms in vivo of flow patterns, velocity fields, and wall shear stress: comparison with computational fluid dynamics. Magn Reson Med. 2009;61:409–17.

43. Schneiders JJ, Marquering HA, van Ooij P, van den Berg R, Nederveen AJ, Verbaan D, et al. Additional value of intra-aneurysmal hemodynamics in discriminating ruptured versus unruptured intracranial aneurysms. AJNR Am J Neuroradiol. 2015;36:1920–6.

44. Futami K, Sano H, Misaki K, Nakada M, Ueda F, Hamada J. Identification of the inflow zone of unruptured cerebral aneurysms: comparison of 4D flow MRI and 3D TOF MRA data. AJNR Am J Neuroradiol. 2014;35:1363–70.

45. Hankey GJ, Warlow CP, Sellar RJ. Cerebral angiographic risk in mild cerebrovascular disease. Stroke. 1990;21:209–22.

46. Inagawa T, Kamiya K, Ogasawara H, Yano T. Rebleeding of ruptured intracranial aneurysms in the acute stage. Surg Neurol. 1987;28:93–9.

47. Fifi JT, Meyers PM, Lavine SD, Cox V, Silverberg L, Mangla S, et al. Complications of modern diagnostic cerebral angiography in an academic medical center. J Vasc Interv Radiol. 2009;20:442–7.

48. van Rooij WJ, Sprengers ME, de Gast AN, Peluso JP, Sluzewski M. 3D rotational angiography: the new gold standard in the detection of additional intracranial aneurysms. AJNR Am J Neuroradiol. 2008;29:976–9.

49. Bechan RS, van Rooij SB, Sprengers ME, Peluso JP, Sluzewski M, Majoie CB, et al. CT angiography versus 3D rotational angiography in patients with subarachnoid hemorrhage. Neuroradiology. 2015;57:1239–46.

50. Bakker NA, Groen RJ, Foumani M, Uyttenboogaart M, Eshghi OS, Metzemaekers JD, et al. Repeat digital subtraction angiography after a negative baseline assessment in nonperimesencephalic subarachnoid hemorrhage: a pooled data meta-analysis. J Neurosurg. 2014;120:99–103.

3

Accuracy of gadoteridol enhanced MR-angiography in the evaluation of carotid artery stenosis

Fulvio Zaccagna[1], Beatrice Sacconi[1], Luca Saba[2], Isabella Ceravolo[1], Andrea Fiorelli[1], Iacopo Carbone[1], Alessandro Napoli[1], Michele Anzidei[1*] and Carlo Catalano[1]

Abstract

Background: To compare image quality and diagnostic performance of Gadoteridol-enhanced MR angiography (MRA) with Gadobutrol-enhanced MRA in the evaluation of carotid artery stenosis.

Methods: MRA was performed in 30 patients with carotid stenosis diagnosed at DUS. Patients were randomly assigned to group A (Gadobutrol-enhanced MRA) or group B (Gadoteridol-enhanced MRA). All examinations were performed with a 3T MR system. Image quality was assessed qualitatively by a 3-grade scale and quantitatively with SNR measurements. Diagnostic performance in the assessment of stenosis, plaque length and morphology was evaluated in the two MRA groups by accuracy calculation and RoC curves analysis using CTA as reference standard. Statistically significant differences in SNR and quality scale were evaluated by the Independent-Samples T Test and Mann–Whitney test, while the Z-statistics was used to compare diagnostic accuracy in the two groups.

Results: Image quality was graded adequate to excellent for both GBCAs, without significant differences ($p = 0.165$). SNR values were not significantly different in group B (Gadoteridol-enhanced MRA) as compared to group A (Gadobutrol-enhanced MRA) (89.32 ± 70.4 vs 81.09 ± 28.38; $p = 0.635$). Diagnostic accuracy was 94 % for the evaluation of stenosis degree and 94 % for the identification of ulcerated plaques in group A, while it was 93 % for the evaluation of stenosis degree and 76 % for the identification of ulcerated plaques in group B, without statistically significant differences ($p = 0.936$).

Conclusion: No significant difference in terms of image quality and diagnostic accuracy was observed between Gadoteridol-enhanced MRA and Gadobutrol-enhanced MRA in patients undergoing evaluation of carotid stenosis.

Background

Ischemic stroke is estimated to be responsible for 10 % of all deaths worldwide. It is the second cause of mortality in western countries and the leading cause of mortality in China and Japan [1]. Atherosclerotic disease of the extracranial internal carotid arteries can be recognized as the cause of stroke at least in 25–30 % of patients [1]. Over the last decade, CT-angiography (CTA) and MR-angiography (MRA) have attained a cardinal role in the imaging of carotid arteries thanks to their increasing diagnostic reliability [2–5]. Since the introduction of contrast-enhanced MRA, several gadolinium-based contrast agents (GBCA) have been tested and implemented in clinical practice [6–9], ranging from standard interstitial molecules to high relaxivity and blood-pool agents [4, 9, 10]. Currently, however, there is no common consensus as to which contrast medium should be used for MRA. Gadoteridol (ProHance®, Bracco) is a macrocyclic gadolinium chelate with a recognized low-rate of adverse side effects. Moreover, it is the sole agent approved for high-dose administration (0.3 mmol/kg) due in part to its high stability and thus lower potential for toxicity from long-term heavy metal deposition [11, 12]. Despite the inherent safety of Gadoteridol, only a few studies have evaluated the performance of this contrast medium in MRA [13–16].

* Correspondence: michele.anzidei@gmail.com
[1]Department of Radiological, Oncological and Anatomopathological Sciences, Sapienza – University of Rome, Viale Regina Elena 324, 00161 Rome, Italy
Full list of author information is available at the end of the article

The purpose of this study was to prospectively compare the image quality and diagnostic performance of Gadoteridol enhanced MRA with that of Gadobutrol (Gadovist®, Bayer) enhanced MRA in the evaluation of carotid artery stenosis, using CTA as reference standard.

Methods
Patient population
Between November 2013 and February 2015, 30 consecutive patients (19 men, 11 women; mean age 71.96 ± 7.6, age range 51–76 years) with confirmed internal carotid artery (ICA) stenosis were enrolled. Institutional Review Board (IRB) (Sapienza - University of Rome) and patient informed consent were obtained. For a patient to be included confirmation of at least one of the following criteria was needed:

1. Doppler-ultrasonography (DUS) showing a hemodynamically significant stenosis of the internal carotid artery (PSV 125 cm/s);
2. Ultrasound examination showing a stenosis of >30 % according to NASCET criteria [17];
3. Ultrasound examination showing a heterogeneous plaque, irregular surface, intra-plaque hemorrhage or ulceration;

Patients with a general contraindication to MRA/CTA examination and/or with a known allergy to contrast agents and/or laboratory signs of renal failure were excluded from the study.

Imaging technique
Patients were randomly assigned to group A or B, undergoing MRA after the administration of 0.1 mmol/kg Gadobutrol (0.1 mL/kg) and 0.1 mmol/kg Gadoteridol (0.2 ml/kg), respectively; randomization was performed according to a 2:1 ratio with 2/3 of patients undergoing Gadoteridol enhanced MRA.

All examinations were performed on a 3T system (Discovery MR750, GE Healthcare, Milwaukee-WIS, USA; with peak gradient strength 50 mT/m, peak slew rate 200 mT/m/ms, HD Neurovascular Array configuration 8-channel, 12-element) with the same technical parameters (T1-weighted 3D SPGRE sequence, TR 4.8 ms, TE 1.8, FA 25°, thickness 0.8 mm, matrix 418 × 418) in both groups. A contrast agent bolus was administered with an automatic injector at a rate of 1 ml/s through an 18-gauge cannula placed in the antecubital vein of the right arm, followed by 15 ml of saline solution. The optimal delay between injection and MRA acquisition was visually evaluated by the bolus tracking technique. CTA was performed on a 128-MDCT scanner (Somatom Definition, Siemens Medical System Erlangen, Germany) using a dual-energy protocol (80 kV and 140 kV, 200 mAs,

pitch 0.8, slice-thickness 1 mm, recon increment 0.9 mm, matrix 512×512). The optimal delay between contrast administration and scan was evaluated with the bolus-tracking technique, with a region of interest (ROI) placed at the level of the aortic arch and automatic scan triggering with enhancement threshold set at 150 HU. The acquisition was performed after administration of 50 ml of nonionic iodinated contrast material (Iomeprol 400 mgI/ml, Iomeron 400, Bracco, Milan, Italy), followed by the injection of 30 ml of saline solution at a rate of 4 ml/s with the use of a dual-head injector.

Image analysis
An independent observer (B.S. with 8 years of experience in cardiovascular imaging), blinded to the contrast agent used, assessed the quality of all MRA datasets using a 3-point scale (poor: inhomogeneous vessel enhancement, poor intraluminal signal and wall delineation; adequate: homogenous vessel enhancement, sufficient intraluminal signal and wall delineation, motion artifacts that did not impair measurements; excellent: homogenous vessel enhancement, high intraluminal signal, precise wall delineation, no motion artifacts). Quantitative measurements of signal-to-noise ratio (SNR; signal Intensity in the vessel/Standard Deviation (SD) outside the body) were also performed on each dataset by the same observer. More in detail, in each case a vessel ROI was placed in the terminal common carotid artery just proximal to carotid bifurcation, whereas the background-ROIs were obtained for 3 different images, in ghosts-free areas. Two readers (F.Z. with 9 years' experience and M.A. with 13 years' experience in MRA of the carotid arteries), who were blinded to the contrast agent used, independently evaluated MRA datasets for the presence and degree of steno-occlusive disease (according to NASCET criteria) and plaque characteristics. All image sets were presented in random order to each reader. An independent reader (I.C. with 18 years' experience in cardiovascular imaging) evaluated the stenosis degree and plaque characteristics on CTA images.

Statistical analysis
Statistical analysis was performed using dedicated software (STATA SE 12 for Macintosh; Stata Corporation; College Station, Texas, USA). The normality of each continuous variable group was tested using the Kolmogorov-Smirnov Z test. Continuous data are described as the mean value ± Standard Deviation [95 % confidence interval] or [minimum – maximum] as appropriate; categorical data are expressed as number (percentage). The Mann–Whitney test was applied to determine significant differences in image quality between the two contrast agents. CTA was used as the reference standard for ROC curve analysis and to calculate sensitivity, specificity, positive predictive value (PPV), negative predictive value (NPV) and

Table 1 Table shows demographic and clinical characteristics of the groups; categorical data are expressed as number (percentage), continuous data are described as the mean value ± Standard Deviation [95 % confidence interval] or [minimum – maximum] as appropriate

	Gadoteridol ($n = 21$)	Gadobutrol ($n = 9$)	p
Sex, male	14 (66.7 %)	5 (55.6 %)	0.57
Age, years	73.38 ± 6.4 [61–85]	68.56 ± 9.3 [51–81]	0.11
Weight, kg	71.29 ± 10.9 [53–92]	71.78 ± 11.4 [57–96]	0.91

Differences between the groups were tested using the unpaired t-test and the Mann–Whitney according to the nature of examined data

accuracy for stenosis degree and plaque morphology (i.e. plaque ulceration or surface irregularity); a stenosis of 70 % was used as threshold level for stenosis degree. Areas under the curve (AUC) were compared using the Z-statistic to determine differences in diagnostic performance between the two contrast agents [18]. Pearson's correlation coefficient was used to assess performance in the evaluation of plaque length. Agreement between the two readers was tested using Cohen's kappa test and was deemed poor for kappa values of 0.21–0.40, fair for values of 0.41–0.60, good for values of 0.61–0.80 and excellent for values of 0.81–1.00 [19]. SNR values were compared using the Independent-Samples T Test. A p value < 0.05 was considered as statistically significant for all tests used.

Results

MRA and CTA examinations were successfully performed in all patients, without any adverse reaction related to gadolinium- or iodine-based contrast agent administration. 18 carotid arteries were evaluated in the 9 patients in group A (Gadobutrol-enhanced MRA) and 42 carotid arteries were evaluated in the 21 patients in group B

(Gadoteridol-enhanced MRA) (Table 1). The average contrast agent volume administered was 7.3 ± 1.2 ml [6–10] in group A and 14 ± 1.9 ml [11–18] in group B.

The quality of MRA examination was deemed excellent in 4/9 (44.4 %), adequate in 4/9 (44.4 %) and poor in 1/9 (11.1 %) of cases in group A (Gadobutrol-enhanced MRA) and excellent in 15/21 (71.4 %), adequate in 5/21 (23.8 %) and poor in 1/21 (4.8 %) of cases in group B (Gadoteridol-enhanced MRA), without significant differences (Mann–Whitney test's $p = 0.165$). The mean SNR values were 81.09 ± 28.38 [33.03–151.36] in group A and 89.32 ± 70.4 [28.3–277.5] in group B, without significant differences (independent-Samples T Test $p = 0.635$) (Fig. 1).

Diagnostic accuracy in the evaluation of vessel stenosis was 0.94 in group A and 0.93 in group B (sensitivity, specificity, PPV and NPV are reported in Table 2). ROC curve analysis (Fig. 2a and b) demonstrated an AUC of 0.974 ± 0.028 [95 % c.i. 0.814–1.0] in group A and 0.969 ± 0.018 [95 % c.i. 0.874–0.999] in group B, without significant differences in the assessment of vessel stenosis (z-statistic $p = 0.936$).

Diagnostic accuracy in the evaluation of plaque morphology was 0.94 in group A and 0.76 in group B (sensitivity, specificity, PPV and NPV are reported in Table 3). ROC curve analysis (Fig. 2c and d) demonstrated an AUC of 0.954 ± 0.045 [95 % c.i. 0.727–0.98] in group A and 0.813 ± 0.058 [95 % c.i. 0.658–0.913] in group B, without significant differences in the assessment of vessel stenosis (z-statistic $p = 0.155$).

The average plaque length was 12.94 ± 6.23 mm [6–20] in group A and 11.9 ± 7.4 mm [4–25] in group B. Pearson's correlation coefficient revealed a good correlation between MRA and CTA both for Gadoteridol ($r = 0.784$; $p = 0.000$) and Gadobutrol ($r = 0.751$; $p = 0.000$).

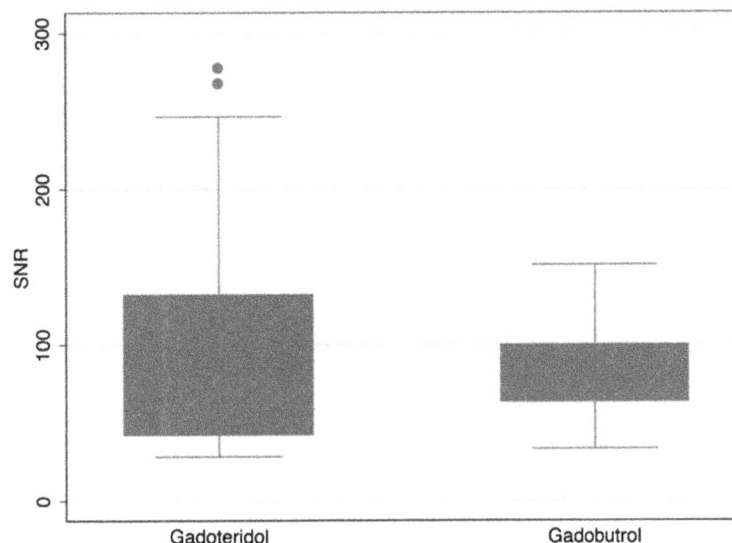

Fig. 1 Figure shows the box plot relative Signal-to-noise ratio according to contrast agents

Table 2 Table shows accuracy, sensibility, specificity, Positive Predictive Value (PPV) and Negative Predictive Value (NPV) of Gadoteridol-enhanced MRA and Gadobutrol-enhanced MRA in determining stenosis degree

	Gadoteridol ($n = 42$)	Gadobutrol ($n = 18$)
Accuracy	0.93 (39/42)	0.94 (17/18)
Sensibility	1 (10/10)	0.86 (6/7)
Specificity	0.91 (29/32)	1 (11/11)
PPV	0.77 (10/13)	1 (6/6)
NPV	1 (29/29)	0.92 (11/12)

Cohen's kappa revealed excellent agreement in stenosis degree evaluation between the two readers ($k = 0.861$) and good agreement in morphology detection ($k = 0.733$) and length determination ($k = 0.722$).

Discussion

Very few studies have compared Gadoteridol and Gadobutrol for clinical applications [20, 21]. In our study no significant differences emerge in terms of image quality and diagnostic accuracy between Gadoteridol-enhanced and Gadobutrol-enhanced carotid MRA. Several properties of contrast agents (molecular structure and size, interaction with blood components, concentration) may affect R1 relaxivity and thus influence vascular enhancement, image quality and diagnostic performance in MRA. It has often been claimed that Gadobutrol offers superior image quality in vascular and extravascular applications because of its higher gadolinium concentration (1 M) in the marketed vial as compared with standard contrast agents (0.5 M); however, the clinically approved dose of Gadobutrol is not different from that of other extracellular contrast agents (0.1 mmol/kg bodyweight) and, since it belongs to the extracellular class of contrast agents, its relaxivity at standard clinical doses is not affected by the higher concentration [22]. In line with these observations, our results demonstrate that Gadoteridol-enhanced carotid MRA is not inferior to Gadobutrol-enhanced carotid MRA in terms of image quality and diagnostic accuracy. Moreover, the two contrast agents were substantially equivalent in the

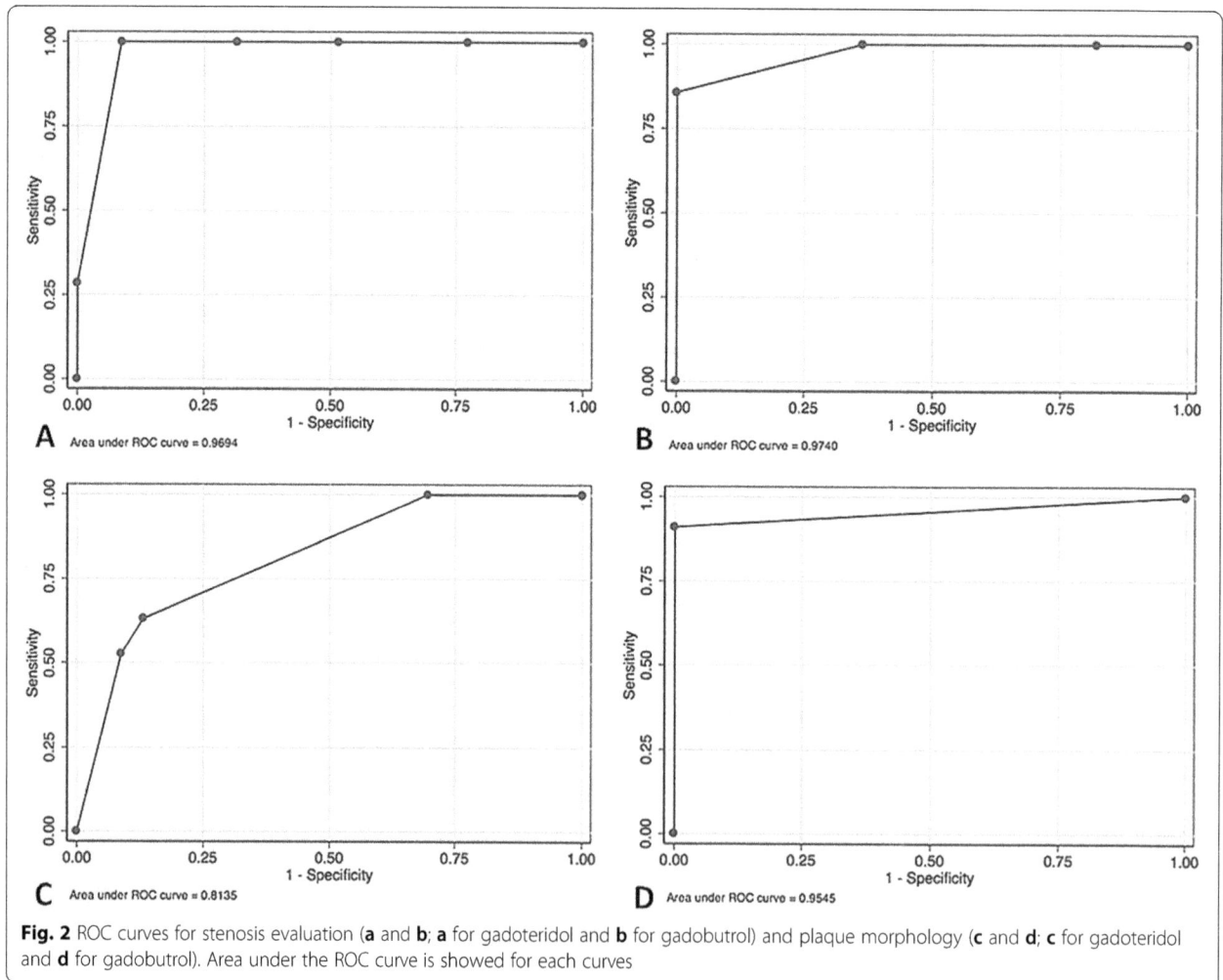

Fig. 2 ROC curves for stenosis evaluation (**a** and **b**; **a** for gadoteridol and **b** for gadobutrol) and plaque morphology (**c** and **d**; **c** for gadoteridol and **d** for gadobutrol). Area under the ROC curve is showed for each curves

Table 3 Table shows accuracy, sensibility, specificity, Positive Predictive Value (PPV) and Negative Predictive Value (NPV) of Gadoteridol-enhanced MRA and Gadobutrol-enhanced MRA in plaque morphology evaluation

	Gadoteridol (n = 42)	Gadobutrol (n = 18)
Accuracy	0.76 (22/42)	0.94 (17/18)
Sensibility	0.63 (12/19)	0.91 (10/11)
Specificity	0.87 (20/23)	1 (7/7)
PPV	0.8 (12/15)	1 (10/10)
NPV	0.74 (20/27)	0.875 (7/8)

evaluation of stenosis degree, plaque morphology and length (Figs. 3 and 4). As regards the evaluation of image quality, our results for both subjective assessment and quantitative measurements of SNR, succeed in demonstrating the absence of statistically significant differences in the two groups of patients ($p = 0.635$). It should be noted that high field (3T) scanners, as used in our study, may affect image quality by influencing gadolinium relaxivity and enhancement generated on T1-weighted sequences after intravenous injection in a slightly different manner to that at 1.5T, at which the majority of contrast agent comparisons have been performed. In particular, at increasing magnetic field strengths gadolinium R1 relaxivity tends to decrease, hence one might expect a parallel deterioration of image contrast in MRA; however, the increased SNR achieved at higher magnetic field, as well as the improved background suppression due to the higher T1 of extravascular tissues, leads to an overall increase of vascular enhancement after contrast agent injection [22]. Even if the relaxivity of both Gadoteridol and Gadobutrol is negatively affected by the increased field strength, the resulting difference remains similar to what has been reported at 1.5T, with a difference that is not sufficient to significantly influence intravascular enhancement and SNR [6, 23, 24].

The implications of this study for routine practice may be relevant in terms of cost and convenience, since Gadoteridol is less expensive (around 80 euros per single dose vial) in comparison with Gadobutrol (around 130 euros per single dose vial). Moreover Gadoteridol is the sole agent approved for high-dose administration (0.3 mmol/kg), due in part to its high stability and lower potential for toxicity from long-term heavy metal

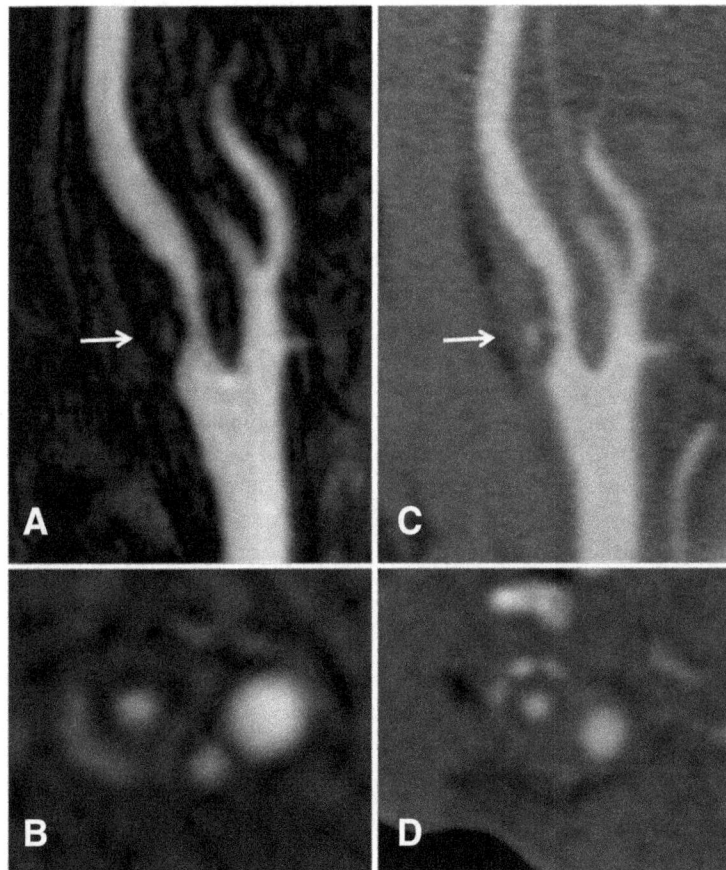

Fig. 3 85-year-old male with tight stenosis of right internal carotid artery (arrow). **a** and **b** CE-MRA images acquired after 0.2 ml/kg of Gadoteridol, **c** and **d** CTA images. CE-MRA demonstrates a ulcerated plaque causing 60 % stenosis of right internal carotid artery; CTA confirms the findings of CE-MRA. Vessel delineation on CE-MRA images was deemed as sharp as on CTA images

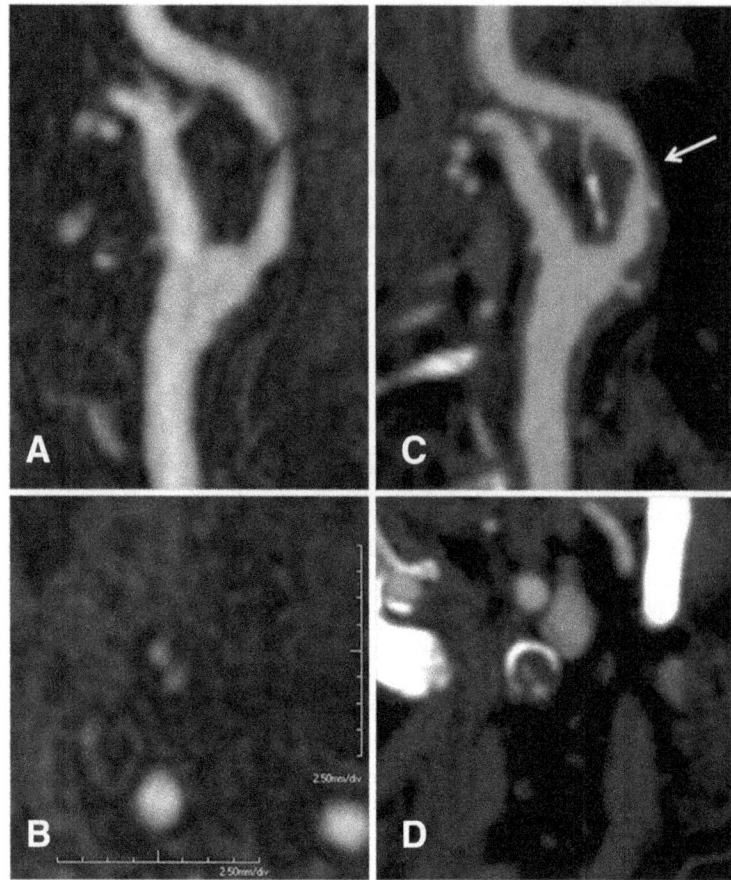

Fig. 4 73-year-old-male referred for carotid imaging to guide revascularization of symptomatic stenosis. **a** and **b** CE-MRA images, **c** and **d** CTA images. Images show an atherosclerotic plaque arising from left carotid arteries bifurcation and involving the proximal segment of internal carotid artery (arrow). Although sagittal-reformatted CE-MRA fails to show residual lumen, axial CE-MRA images demonstrated a severe (90 %) stenosis of left internal carotid artery; CTA confirmed the severe stenosis as well as the absence of ulceration

deposition [10, 11]; this may represent an additional advantage at lower magnetic fields [25]. Furthermore, the adverse effects of Gadoteridol are reported to be very infrequent; it contains a cyclic nonionic chelate and has a high thermodynamic stability constant (23.8) and a long dissociation half-life (3 h). It's inclusion in the group of agents considered to be at low risk for Nephrogenic Systemic Fibrosis is probably related to these properties [26].

It should be noted that this study has some relevant limitations, the most important being the small sample size; however an extended study with a larger patient population is currently ongoing. In addition, digital subtraction angiography was not available for comparison in our series, since just a minority of patients with clinically significant stenosis underwent stenting procedures while the others were treated with endarterectomy without angiography. However, it should be noted that CTA has been shown to be a valid alternative to DSA as reference standard in comparative studies and, in daily clinical practice, it is currently used as the modality of choice for carotid imaging [27, 28]. Another relevant limitation

is represented by the inter-individual design of the study; however, this was due to ethical reasons since patients with significant disease are referred for treatment rather than a second contrast-enhanced MRA exam. The final limitation concerns the different sizes of the two patient groups; however, unequal randomization has been reported to be an accepted strategy in clinical trials to gain greater experience when comparing a new treatment to a reference standard, hence we adopted this randomization due to the lack of data on Gadobutrol-enhanced carotid MRA (in this regard it is also worth noting that the statistical power of a 1:1 allocation is 0.95 while the statistical power of a 2:1 ratio is 0.925, with a negligible difference).

Conclusions

In conclusion, from our study, similar results of Gadoteridol-enhanced MRA compared with Gadobutrol-enhanced MRA were observed, both in terms of image quality and diagnostic accuracy, in patients undergoing evaluation of carotid stenosis.

Competing interests

The authors declare that they have no competing interests.

Authors' contributions

SFZ conceived the original study design, carried out the MR examinations, drafted the manuscript, read and approved the final manuscript. BS contributed to the study design, carried out the literature review, drafted the manuscript, read and approved the final manuscript. LS carried out the statistical analysis, drafted the manuscript, read and approved the final manuscript. IC carried out the patients' enrollment, drafted the manuscript, read and approved the final manuscript. AF carried out the MR examinations, drafted the manuscript, read and approved the final manuscript. IC contributed to the study design, drafted the manuscript, read and approved the final manuscript. AN contributed to the study design, drafted the manuscript, read and approved the final manuscript. MA contributed to the study design, carried out the literature review, drafted the manuscript, read andapproved the final manuscript.CC contributed to the study design, drafted the manuscript, read and approved the final manuscript.

Author details

[1]Department of Radiological, Oncological and Anatomopathological Sciences, Sapienza – University of Rome, Viale Regina Elena 324, 00161 Rome, Italy. [2]Department of Radiology, Azienda Ospedaliero Universitaria (A.O.U.), di Cagliari-Polo di Monserrato, Italy.

References

1. Hasso AN, Stringer WA, Brown KD. Cerebral ischemia and infarction. Neuroimaging Clin N Am. 1994;4(4):733–52.
2. Saba L, Mallarini G. Comparison between quantification methods of carotid artery stenosis and computed tomographic angiography. J Comput Assis Tomograf. 2010;34(3):421–30.
3. Clevert DA, Johnson T, Michaely H, Jung EM, Flach PM, Strautz TI, et al. High-grade stenoses of the internal carotid artery: comparison of high-resolution contrast enhanced 3D MRA, duplex sonography and power Doppler imaging. Eur J Radiol. 2006;60(3):379–86.
4. Anzidei M, Napoli A, Marincola BC, Nofroni I, Geiger D, Zaccagna F, et al. Gadofosveset-enhanced MR angiography of carotid arteries: does steady-state imaging improve accuracy of first-pass imaging? Comparison with selective digital subtraction angiography. Radiology. 2009;251(2):457–66.
5. Altaf N, Daniels L, Morgan PS, Auer D, MacSweeney ST, Moody AR, et al. Detection of intraplaque hemorrhage by magnetic resonance imaging in symptomatic patients with mild to moderate carotid stenosis predicts recurrent neurological events. J Vasc Surg. 2008;47(2):337–42.
6. Xing X, Zeng X, Li X, Zhao Q, Kirchin MA, Pirovano G, et al. Contrast-enhanced MR angiography: does a higher relaxivity MR contrast agent permit a reduction of the dose administered for routine vascular imaging applications? Radiol Med. 2015;120(2):239–50.
7. Anzalone N, Scotti R, Vezzulli P. High relaxivity contrast agents in MR angiography of the carotid arteries. Eur Radiol. 2006;16 Suppl 7:M27–34.
8. Goyen M, Debatin JF. Gadobenate dimeglumine (MultiHance) for magnetic resonance angiography: review of the literature. Eur Radiol. 2003;13 Suppl 3:N19–27.
9. Amarteifio E, Essig M, Böckler D, Attigah N, Schuster L, Demirel S. Comparison of gadofosveset (Vasovist®) with gadobenate dimeglumine (Multihance®)-enhanced MR angiography for high-grade carotid artery stenosis. J Neuroradiol. 2014;42(4):236–44.
10. Aime S, Caravan P. Biodistribution of gadolinium-based contrast agents, including gadolinium deposition. J Magn Reson Imaging. 2009;30(6):1259–67.
11. Runge VM, Wells JW. Update: safety, new applications, new MR agents. Top Magn Reson Imaging. 1995;7(3):181–95.
12. Shellock FG, Kanal E. Safety of magnetic resonance imaging contrast agents. J Magn Reson Imaging. 1999;10(3):477–84.
13. Hathout GM, Duh MJ, El-Saden SM. Accuracy of contrast-enhanced MR angiography in predicting angiographic stenosis of the internal carotid artery: linear regression analysis. AJNR Am J Neuroradiol. 2003;24(9):1747–56.
14. Froger CL, Duijm LE, Liem YS, Tielbeek AV, Donkers-van Rossum AB, Douwes-Draaijer P, et al. Stenosis detection with MR angiography and digital subtraction angiography in dysfunctional hemodialysis access fistulas and grafts. Radiology. 2005;234(1):284–91.
15. Hood MN, Ho VB, Foo TK, Marcos HB, Hess SL, Choyke PL. High-resolution gadolinium-enhanced 3D MRA of the infrapopliteal arteries. Lessons for improving bolus-chase peripheral MRA. Magn Reson Imaging. 2002;20(7):543–9.
16. Bremerich J, Colet JM, Giovenzana GB, Aime S, Scheffler K, Laurent S, et al. Slow clearance gadolinium-based extracellular and intravascular contrast media for three-dimensional MR angiography. J Magn Reson Imaging. 2001;13(4):588–93.
17. North American Symptomatic Carotid Endarterectomy Trial Collaborators. Beneficial effect of carotid endarterectomy in symptomatic patients with high-grade carotid stenosis. North American Symptomatic Carotid Endarterectomy Trial Collaborators. N Engl J Med. 1991;325(7):445–53.
18. Hanley JA, McNeil BJ. The meaning and use of the area under a Receiver Operating Characteristic (ROC) curve. Radiology. 1982;143:29–36.
19. Landis JR, Koch GG. The measurement of observer agreement for categorical data. Biometrics. 1977;33(1):159–74.
20. Maravilla KR, Smith MP, Vymazal J, Goyal M, Herman M, Baima JJ, et al. Are there differences between macrocyclic gadolinium contrast agents for brain tumor imaging? Results of a multicenter intraindividual crossover comparison of gadobutrol with gadoteridol (the TRUTH study). AJNR Am J Neuroradiol. 2015;36(1):14–23.
21. Koenig M, Schulte-Altedorneburg G, Piontek M, Hentsch A, Spangenberg P, Schwenke C, et al. Intra-individual, randomised comparison of the MRI contrast agents gadobutrol versus gadoteridol in patients with primary and secondary brain tumours, evaluated in a blinded read. Eur Radiol. 2013;23(12):3287–95.
22. Shen Y, Goerner FL, Snyder C, Morelli JN, Hao D, Hu D, et al. T1 relaxivities of gadoliniumbased magnetic resonance contrast agents in human whole blood at 1.5, 3, and 7 T. Invest Radiol. 2015;50(5):330–8.
23. Hagberg GE, Scheffler K. Effect of r1 and r2 relaxivity of gadolinium-based contrast agents on the T1-weighted MR signal at increasing magnetic field strengths. Contrast Media Mol Imaging. 2013;8(6):456–65.
24. Salvolini U, Scarabino T. High Field Brain MRI: Use in Clinical Practice. 1st ed. Berlin Heidelberg: Springer; 2006.
25. Rinck PA, Muller RN. Field strength and dose dependence of contrast enhancement by Gadolinium- based MR contrast agents. Eur Radiol. 1999;9:998–1004.
26. Reilly RF. Risk for nephrogenic systemic fibrosis with gadoteridol (ProHance) in patients who are on long-term hemodialysis. Clin J Am Soc Nephrol. 2008;3(3):747–51.
27. Anderson GB, Ashforth R, Steinke DE, Ferdinandy R, Findlay JM. CT Angiography for the Detection and Characterization of Carotid Artery Bifurcation Disease. Stroke. 2000;31:2168–74.
28. Herzig R, Burval S, Krupka B, Vlachovà I, Urbanek K, Mares J. Comparison of ultrasonography, CT angiography and digital subtraction angiography in severe carotid stenoses. Eur J Neurol. 2004;11(11):774–81.

4

Review on treatment of craniocervical soft tissues arterovenous malformations and hemangiomas

Pierleone Lucatelli[1], Beatrice Sacconi[1,2]*, Michele Anzidei[1], Mario Bezzi[1] and Carlo Catalano[1]

Abstract

Vascular malformations include several vascular abnormalities, congenital in most cases, classified according to their dynamic flow characteristics into high-flow and low-flow abnormalities; both types are commonly located in the head and neck region. Imaging modalities such as Echocolor-Doppler, CT, and MRI can be employed in the evaluation of vascular malformations' in order to describe their size, flow velocity, flow direction, and relationship with the surrounding structures, and, even more important, to differentiate between different types of malformations, since treatment modalities differ depending on their nature (low- vs high-flow).

Keywords: Vascular malformations, Low-flow vascular malformations, High-flow vascular malformations, Arterovenous malformation, Sclerotherapy

Background

The term "vascular malformations" includes a large number of vascular abnormalities, originally classified in 1982 by Mulliken & Glowacki [1]; a modified version proposed in 1992 by Mulliken & Young is currently the widely used classification to differentiate these malformations in clinical and radiological practice [2] (Fig. 1).

Vascular malformations are congenital in most cases, although not always evident. They usually develop during childhood, increase their dimension following the child growth and show no spontaneous regression. Their growth can be exacerbated during puberty or pregnancy due to hormonal changes, or as a result of thrombosis, infection or trauma. Unlike other vascular abnormalities, they can have an infiltrative behavior, involving multiple tissue planes [3].

Vascular malformations are classified according to their dynamic flow characteristics into high-flow (arteriovenous malformations [AVM] and arteriovenous fistulas [AVFs]) and low-flow abnormalities (venous, lymphatic, capillary, capillary-venous, and capillary-

* Correspondence: beatrice.sacconi@fastwebnet.it
[1]Department of Radiological, Oncological and Anatomopathological Sciences – Radiology, 'Sapienza' University of Rome, Viale Regina Elena 324, 00161 Rome, Italy
[2]Center for Life Nano Science@Sapienza, Istituto Italiano di Tecnologia, Rome, Italy

lymphatic-venous); the differential diagnosis between these two groups plays a very important role in the patient management, since malformations with different hemodynamic characteristics follow different treatment pathways [4].

Both high- and low-flow vascular malformation are commonly located in the head and neck region, with the venous and lymphatic malformations ones being located in this region in up to 40 and 80 % of cases respectively, especially in the posterior cervical triangle [5]. AVM and congenital AVF are also frequently localized in the craniocervical region [6, 7].

Our purpose is to provide a comprehensive review on management of cranio-cervical vascular malformations, with a special focus on imaging and treatment and their strong interdependency; more in detail, we want to describe the different treatment strategies, and the imaging findings that the radiologists should report before treatment and during the post-procedural follow-up.

Review

General features

Low-flow vascular malformations

They are usually classified into venous, lymphatic, capillary and mixed abnormalities. A venous malformation generally consists of small and large dysplastic thin-walled

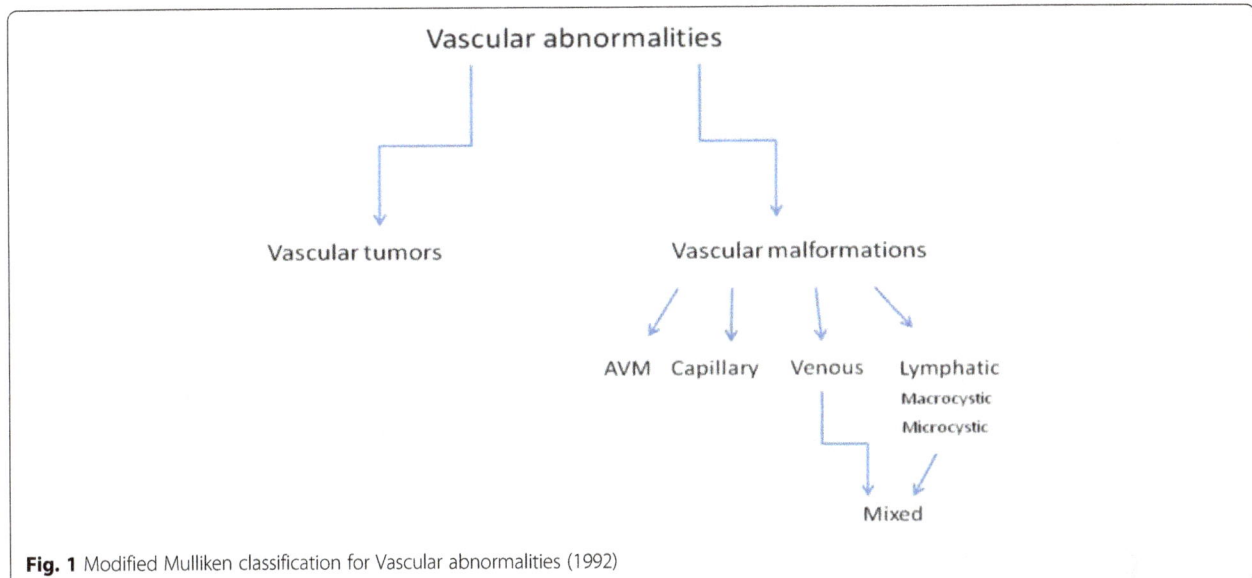

Fig. 1 Modified Mulliken classification for Vascular abnormalities (1992)

venous channels with variable amounts of hamartomatous stroma, thrombi, and phleboliths, and appearing as a blue, soft, non compressible, non pulsatile mass [8]. Lymphatic malformations composed of chyle-filled cysts lined with endothelium and can be divided into microcystic (multiple cysts smaller than 2 mm) and macrocystic types (larger cysts) [3]. Capillary malformations are areas of congenital ectasia of thin-walled small vessels of the skin typically confined to the dermis or mucous membranes and appearing as cutaneous red discoloration; they might also be the hallmark of complex anomalies such as Klippel-Trenaunay, Sturge-Weber, and Parkes Weber syndromes [7]. Venous, lymphatic and capillary components can be combined in mixed low-flow malformations.

High-flow vascular malformations
AVFs are composed by a single vascular channel between an artery and a vein, while AVMs consist of feeding arteries, draining veins, and a nidus formed by multiple dysplastic vascular channels connecting arteries and veins, with absence of a normal capillary bed, usually resulting in an ill-defined mass.

Imaging features
Multiple imaging modalities should be employed in the evaluation of vascular malformations' characteristics, such as size, flow velocity, flow direction, relationship with the surrounding structures and lesion's appearance and content. US and Echo-Color Doppler usually represent the first imaging techniques to be used, at least in case of superficial vascular lesions, allowing a real-time visualization of arterial and venous flows and flow velocities' measurement. Conventional radiography plays a limited role, being especially useful in evaluating bone

(bone erosion or sclerosis, periosteal reaction, and pathologic fracture). Multidetector Computed Tomography (MDCT) permits to evaluate the enhancement pattern of the lesion, thanks to its high temporal resolution, and the presence of thrombosis or calcification. Magnetic Resonance Imaging (MRI) is currently the most valuable modality for the classification of vascular anomalies, allowing to define the extension of vascular lesions and their anatomic relationship to adjacent structures without radiation exposure. Since a functional analysis of the involved vessels is required for treatment planning, the use of Dynamic time-resolved MR angiography has become mandatory (TRICKs, GE or, TWIST, Siemens). These sequences allow the acquisition of images with high temporal and spatial resolution, enabling a clear separation of the arterial inflow from venous drainage and the detection of early venous shunting, and providing information about the contrast material arrival time and the flow direction [5, 9].

Low-flow vascular malformations
In MRI diagnosis of a low-flow malformation is based on the absence of flow voids on SE images and lack of arterial/early venous enhancement on post-contrast sequences; low-flow malformations, especially venous malformations typically show slow gradual filling with contrast material [7, 10]. In case of hemorrhage or thrombosis, signal heterogeneity can be observed on T1-weighted images, whereas the best sign for identification of a venous malformation is the presence of phleboliths [7]. Delayed contrast-enhanced sequence may demonstrate connections between the malformation and the deep venous system, which can be useful during treatment planning, since it can increase the risk of deep venous thrombosis [3]. Lymphatic malformations

are usually seen as lobulated, septated masses with high signal intensity on T2-weighted sequences, usually with no post-contrast enhancement in case of microcystic variants and rim and septal enhancement in case of macrocystic lesions. Imaging findings of mixed Malformation may be non-distinguishable from those of venous malformations [3].

High-flow vascular malformations

MR imaging findings of high-flow malformations include high-flow enlarged feeding arteries and draining veins, appearing as flow voids on SE images or high-signal-intensity foci on GRE images, usually as a poorly defined mass. The dynamic enhancement of the AVM is generally well assessed by using time-resolved dynamic 3D MR angiography, with a contrast material rise time of 5–10 s, tipically showing arterial feeders and early venous filling of the lesion [5, 8, 10, 11].

Treatment

When planning the treatment of any vascular malformations it should be remembered that treatment must be multidisciplinary involving several specialist such as plastic surgeon, vascular surgeon, interventional radiologist and dermatologist. Usually treatment indication is patient's complaint due to the lesion localization (unaesthetic) or for functional (cramps due to stealing syndrome) or loco-regional reason (compression of vital structure). Complete eradication of the pathology is rarely achieved after the first procedure; multiple treatment sessions are usually needed,

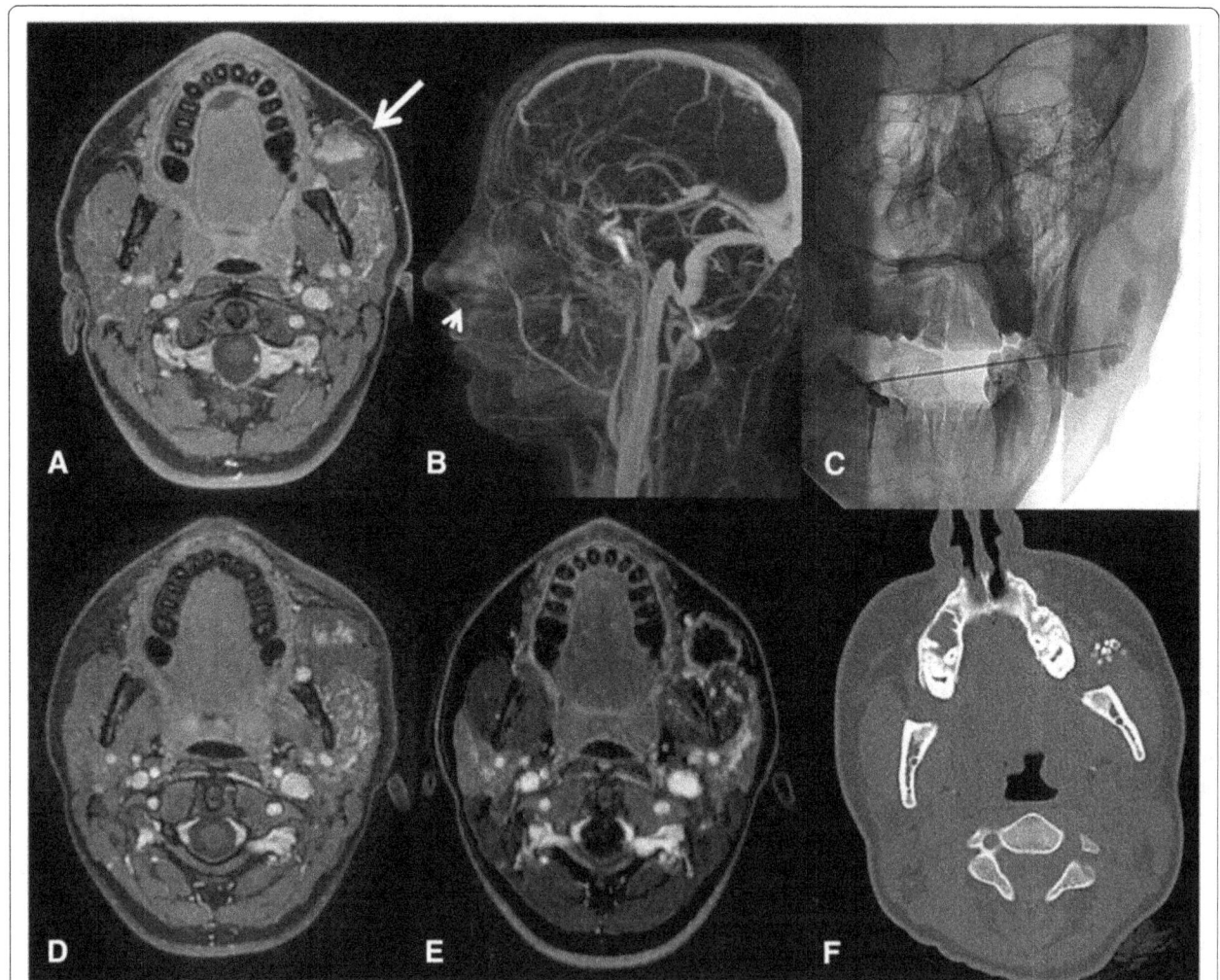

Fig. 2 29-year old female presenting with a venous malformation of the left malar region. **a** Post-contrast T1-weighted sequence shows partial filling of the lesion with contrast material; (**b**) TRICKs sequence (MIP) mainly shows the venous drainage into the facial vein; (**c**) DSA images showing the procedure of percutaneous sclerotherapy; (**d**) At post-treatment follow up the lesion shows a reduced enhancement on post-contrast T1-weighted images; (**e**) Follow-up after a new sclerotherapy session: the lesion does not show any central filling, with a peripheral hyperenhancement due to reactive hyperemia (post-contrast T1-weighted images, subtraction tecnique); (**f**) Late post-treatment follow-up with CT: the lesion has markedly reduced in size and shows internal calcified foci, probably related to residual phleboliths

even due to the natural tendency of treated vascular malformations to recur. The aim of the treatment is to destroy the nidus of the malformation. Depending on its nature (low- or high-flow) treatment modalities differ [4, 8, 9, 12].

Low-flow malformation

Low flow malformations are treated percutaneously only if not surgically removable. Due to their usual localization within deep muscles, major surgery is needed to dissected the entire nidus. Percutaneous route is preferred if the nidus is reachable. The nidus is punctured under US guidance or with blind technique (if clinically evident) with a 21 G butterfly needle. Prior to flebography esecution, direct back flow from the nidus should be obtained by gently moving forward or withdrawing the needle tip. Then digital subtraction angiography should be performed in order to observe the anatomy of the nidus and its venous drainage. Careful evaluation of the amount of contrast media needed to opacify the nidus is required in order to identify the correct amount of embolic agent to be injected afterwards. Embolization can be performed only

if no direct flow to a drainage vein is seen. Otherwise, needle repositioning is mandatory. The procedure varies depending on the embolic agent employed (atossisclerol vs alchool) after deepening of the analgesia level. Atossisclerol mousse requires less volume in comparison with liquid alcohol, resulting in a moderate pro-thrombotic effect. Alchool provokes immediate thrombosis and edema in the injected vessel by inducing protein denaturation, being more painful than atossisclerol. Antibiotic prophylaxis and corticosteroids in the immediate post-procedural stay are suggested [4, 8, 9, 12] (Fig. 2).

High-flow malformation

Different approaches are needed to treat an high flow vascular malformation. Treatment options are trans-arterial, trans-venous, or a combination of these with percutaneous embolization. The aim of the treatment is always to obtain exclusion of the nidus. Pre-procedural dynamic MRI helps in choosing the best treatment modality to be used. Arterial approach is usually performed via femoral approach with selective catheterization of the nidus feeder. Microcatethers

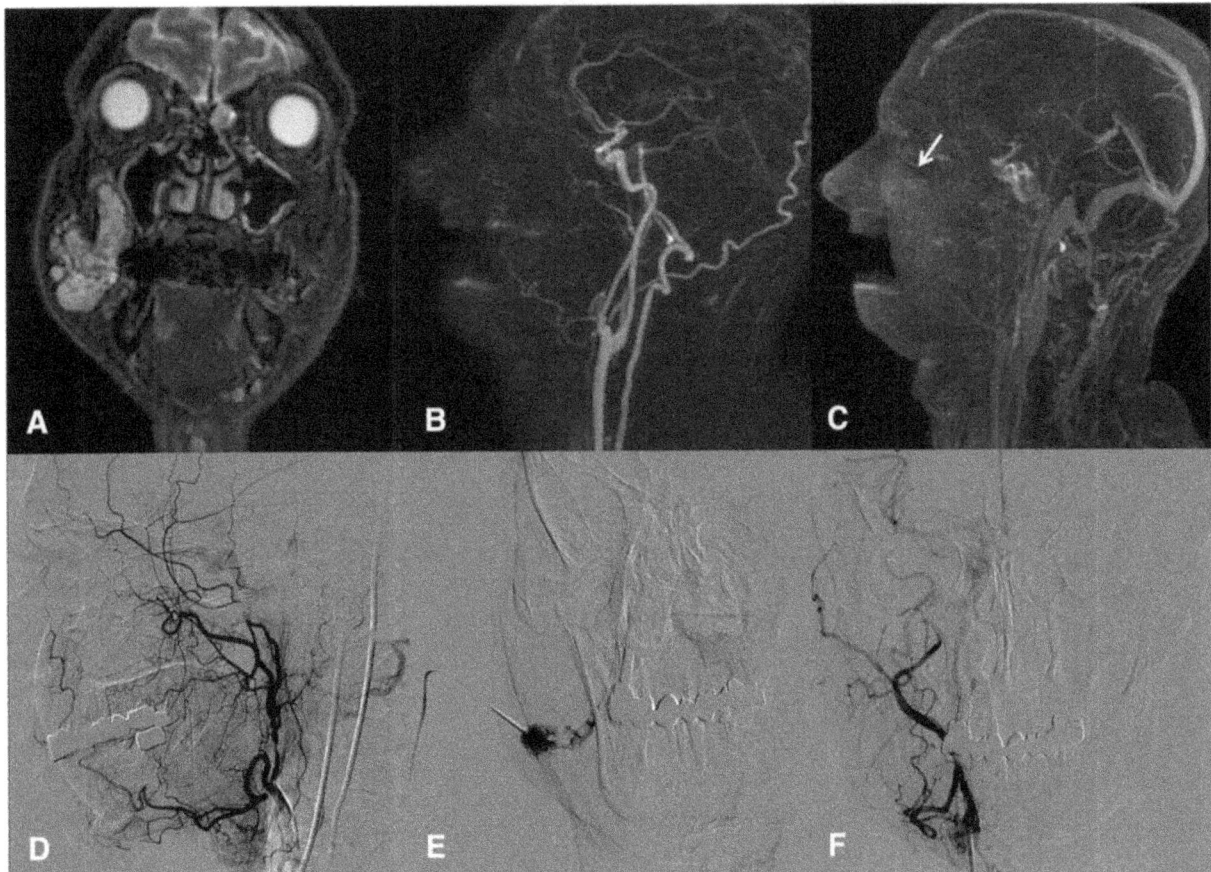

Fig. 3 38 year-old male, with a vascular malformation of the right malar region; (**a**) Coronal fat-suppressed T2-weighted sequence showing a large T2-hyperintense lesion of the malar region; (**b, c**) TRICKS sequence showing the very poor arterial component of the lesion and its gradual filling with contrast material; (**d**) DSA performed before the sclerotherapy procedure; (**e**) Percutaneous sclerotherapy (**f**) The malformation was subsequently treated with chemoembolization

are required in order to perfom superselective embolization with either glue, foam, particles or coils. Transvenous route is employed when a too fast venous drainage could impair embolic agent deposition within the nidus, thus leading to non target embolization. Occlusion compliant ballons, derived from neuro-intervention procedures, can be used. Percutaneous adjunctive embolization could be needed in case partial opacification or visualization of the nidus are obtained during transvenous/transarterial embolization [4, 8, 9, 12] (Fig. 3).

Post-procedural imaging

US and MRI are the most useful techniques to assess treatment results and to plan the long-term management strategy [9, 12]. Imaging technique employed during the

follow-up does not differ from the preoperative one in terms of MRI protocol and technical aspects. There is no consensus on timing for the first imaging evaluation after the procedure in literature; at our Institution, post treatment imaging follow-up timeline is usually scheduled within 3 months after the treatment and therefore with longer time interval. However, it is worthy to mention that follow-up timeline could be modified in case of symptoms recurrence.

Treatment-related complications could be minor or major according to the impairment caused to the patient. Minor complications include simple swelling of the treated region, hematoma, partial nidus thrombosis, venous outflow thrombosis. Usually minor complications do not require longer hospitalization time nor adjunctive care. Major complications are usually dependent on treatment modality

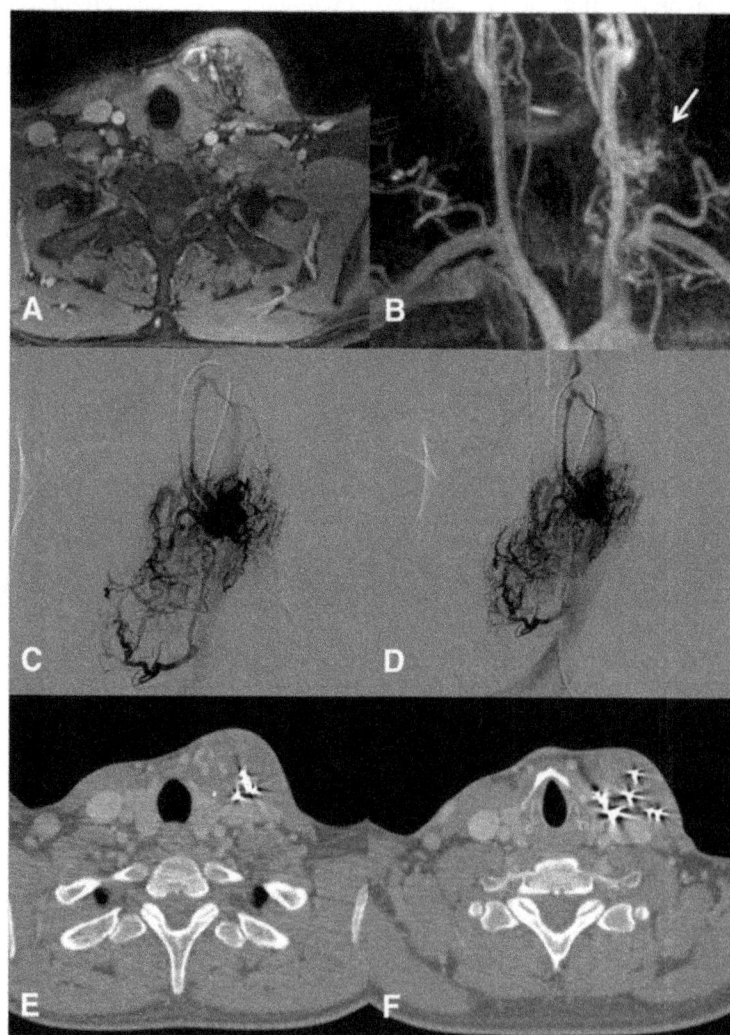

Fig. 4 34 year-old male, with an arterovenous malformation of the left aspect of the anterior cervical region; (**a**) Post-contrast T1-weighted sequence shows a large lesion characterized by heterogeneous enhancement; (**b**) TRICKS sequence (MIP) showing the arterial feeders, mainly represented by branches of the tireocervical trunk; (**c, d**) DSA images during the procedure showing the arterial component and the venous drainage of the lesion; (**e, f**) Post-treatment CT images shows coils and residual post-contrast enhancement in the medial aspect of the lesion

(percutaneous/ endovascular/ combined), on the agent employed (glue, foam, alcohol, coils) and on the district (cranio-facial being the more dangerous). Skin ulceration could be the effect of a not perfect involved injection of embolic agent within the nidus but in the surrounding subcutaneous fat, or to a non target embolization. Nerve paresis is usually due to non target embolization or either compression by swelling of the embolized site and concomitant nerve compression [7–9].

Low-flow malformation

Ethanol causes almost instantaneous denudation of endothelium with severe inflammatory reaction and thrombosis [7]. Then fibrosis develops and the lesion progressively shrinks. In order to accurately evaluate the therapeutic response after sclerotherapy, the transient inflammatory response needs to be resolved [13]. At MRI, venous malformations after sclerotherapy demonstrate an early high signal intensity related to the inflammatory reaction, associated with no enhancement in the central portion of the treated lesion and peripheral hyperenhancement due to reactive hyperemia [13]. After few months the enhancement usually disappears and a central scar appears as a dark area on both T1-and T2-weighted images; a progressive shrinkage of the malformation is frequently observed [13, 14].

High-flow malformation

Since any incomplete treatment may stimulate the lesion's growth and the recruitment of new arterial feeders, the treatment strategy must be planned with the aim of achieving a complete eradication of the nidus [7]. After transarterial embolization, thrombosis of the vascular malformation should be seen; MR angiography may show decreased/absent shunting and reduced/absent venous system's opacification. Any residual component of the malformation must be treated in a second stage. In some cases, Doppler US can be particularly useful during the follow-up, especially in case of ferromagnetic coils have been used; in these cases coils produce artifacts at MRI and MDCT which can hinder an optimal post-procedural evaluation of the malformation [13] (Fig. 4).

Conclusions

Head and neck region represents one of the most common location for both high- and low-flow vascular malformations, observed in this region in up to 40 and 80 % of cases respectively, especially in the posterior cervical triangle. An accurate pre-procedural depiction of the malformation is mandatory in order to differentiate between high- and low-flow abnormalities and therefore to guide therapeutic decisions; imaging plays an addition role also in the post-procedural follow-up of the treated lesions.

Abbreviations
AVM: arteriovenous malformations; AVF: arteriovenous fistulas; MRI: magnetic resonance imaging; MDCT: multidetector computed tomography.

Competing interests
The authors declare that they have no competing interests.

Authors' contributions
PL, BS: draft editing, literature review, clinical data collection, evaluation of the mri scan (preoperative and post-treatment).MA: draft revision and acceptance, evaluation of the mri scan (preoperative and post-treatment).MB,CC: draft guarantor. All authors read and approved the final manuscript.

References
1. Mulliken JB, Glowacki J. Hemangiomas and vascular malformations in infants and children: a classification based on endothelial characteristics. Plast Reconstr Surg. 1982;69:412e20.
2. Jackson IT, Carreño R, Potparic Z, Hussain K. Hemangiomas, vascular malformations, and lymphovenous malformations: classification and methods of treatment. Plast Reconstr Surg. 1993;91(7):1216–30.
3. Moukaddam H, Pollak J, Haims AH. MRI characteristics and classification of peripheral vascular malformations and tumors. Skeletal Radiol. 2009;38(6):535–47.
4. McCafferty IJ, Jones RG. Imaging and management of vascular malformations. Clinical Radiology. 2011;66:1208e1218.
5. Dubois J, Alison M. Vascular anomalies: what a radiologist needs to know. Pediatr Radiol. 2010;40(6):895–905.
6. Navarro OM, Laffan EE, Ngan BY. Pediatric soft-tissue tumors and pseudotumors: MR imaging features with pathologic correlation. I. Imaging approach, pseudotumors, vascular lesions, and adipocytic tumors. RadioGraphics. 2009;29(3):887–906.
7. Ernemann U, Kramer U, Miller S, Bisdas S, Rebmann H, Breuninger H, et al. Current concepts in the classification, diagnosis and treatment of vascular anomalies. Eur J Radiol. 2010;75(1):2–11.
8. Dubois J, Soulez G, Oliva VL, Berthiaume MJ, Lapierre C, Therasse E. Soft-tissue venous malformations in adult patients: imaging and therapeutic issues. RadioGraphics. 2001;21(6):1519–31.
9. Hyodoh H, Hori M, Akiba H, Tamakawa M, Hyodoh K, Hareyama M. Peripheral vascular malformations: imaging, treatment approaches, and therapeutic issues. RadioGraphics. 2005;25 suppl 1:S159–71.
10. Herborn CU, Goyen M, Lauenstein TC, Debatin JF, Ruehm SG, Kröger K. Comprehensive time-resolved MRI of peripheral vascular malformations. AJR Am J Roentgenol. 2003;181(3):729–35.
11. Anzidei M, Cavallo Marincola B, Napoli A, Saba L, Zaccagna F, Lucatelli P, et al. Low-dose contrast-enhanced time-resolved MR angiography at 3T: diagnostic accuracy for treatment planning and follow-up of vascular malformations. Clin Radiol. 2011;66(12):1181–92.
12. Lee BB, Do YS, Yakes W, Kim DI, Mattassi R, Hyon WS. Management of arteriovenous malformations: a multidisciplinary approach. J Vasc Surg. 2004;39(3):590–600.
13. Lucatelli P, Allegritti M, Fanelli F. Chapter 15: Vascular malformations. Catalano C, Anzidei M, Napoli A (eds). Cardiovascular CT and MR Imaging From Technique to Clinical Interpretation. 2013 (ISBN 978-88-470-2868-5).
14. Lucatelli P, Allegritti M, Fanelli F. Chapter 15: Arteriovenous Malformation. Catalano C, Anzidei M, Napoli A (eds). Cardiovascular CT and MR Imaging. 2013 (ISBN 978-88-470-2868-5).

5

Intracranial vessel wall imaging: current applications and clinical implications

Marinos Kontzialis[1] and Bruce A. Wasserman[2*]

Abstract

Conventional CT, MR, and digital subtraction angiography rely on the presence of luminal narrowing for the identification of vascular pathology offering limited insight into the offending pathophysiologic mechanism affecting the vessel. High-resolution MRI vessel wall imaging (VWI) has the potential to directly depict and characterize vessel wall pathology affecting the intracranial circulation increasing diagnostic accuracy for vasculopathies with similar angiographic findings.

Keywords: Vessel wall imaging, Black blood MRI, Intracranial, Vasculopathy, Intracranial stenosis, Atherosclerosis, MRI

Background

Blood flow and CSF suppression are essential for optimal vessel wall visualization in the intracranial circulation [1]. Intracranial VWI is especially challenging due to the small caliber and tortuosity of the intracranial vessels necessitating submillimeter spatial resolution and high field strength magnets [1–3]. Black blood MRI (BBMRI) sequences are designed to achieve blood flow suppression and have historically utilized 2-dimensional (2D) pre- and postcontrast T1- or proton-weighted sequences to characterize the vessel wall [1, 3]. The 2D sequences are prone to partial volume artifacts, which are accentuated by the tortuosity and small size of intracranial vessels [2]. Three-dimensional (3D) sequences have more recently become achievable and have the advantage of a large field of view, which allows substantial coverage in a single acquisition in a clinically acceptable scan time obviating the need for prospective slice placement, and isotropic resolution, which allows post hoc reconstruction along the short and long axis of vessels minimizing overestimation of wall thickness (Fig. 1) [2].

Specific vessel wall characteristics that are sought on VWI include vessel wall thickening (smooth, irregular, circumferential, concentric, eccentric), signal, and enhancement [4]. A short axis view perpendicular to an intracranial vessel is best for evaluation of vessel wall

* Correspondence: bwasser@jhmi.edu
[2]The Russell H. Morgan Department of Radiology and Radiological Sciences, Johns Hopkins University School of Medicine, 600 North Wolfe Street, Baltimore, MD 21287, USA
Full list of author information is available at the end of the article

thickening and pattern of enhancement (Fig. 1b). In this text we review the major current applications of BBMRI in the intracranial circulation.

Atherosclerosis

The hallmark of atherosclerosis on BBMRI is the heterogeneity of the thickened vessel wall due to various plaque components, which may include lipid core, fibrous cap, intraplaque hemorrhage [5], calcifications, and enhancement (Figs. 1, 2, 3 and 4) [1, 6]. These components are better demonstrated in the extracranial circulation due to the larger vessel size, and current MRI techniques cannot characterize consistently individual intracranial atherosclerotic disease (ICAD) components [3, 6]. Nevertheless, plaque features detected by BBMRI, such as enhancement and hemorrhage, have been shown to relate to downstream strokes (Figs. 1, 2, 3 and 4) [5–7]. Furthermore, BBMRI can detect small atherosclerotic plaques in vessels that are not yet stenosed even in advanced atherosclerosis due to remodeling [1, 8]. Subtle atherosclerotic changes, including wall thickening and positive remodeling, have been observed in non-stenotic arteries in stroke patients when compared with controls [9, 10]. Atherosclerotic changes identified on BBMRI in non-stenotic intracranial arteries appear to be the most significant risk factor for white matter hyperintensities [11].

Atherosclerotic plaques in the intracranial circulation tend to present as eccentric and usually irregular wall thickening with or without luminal stenosis and variable enhancement (Figs. 1, 2, 3 and 4) [3, 6, 7, 12]. When

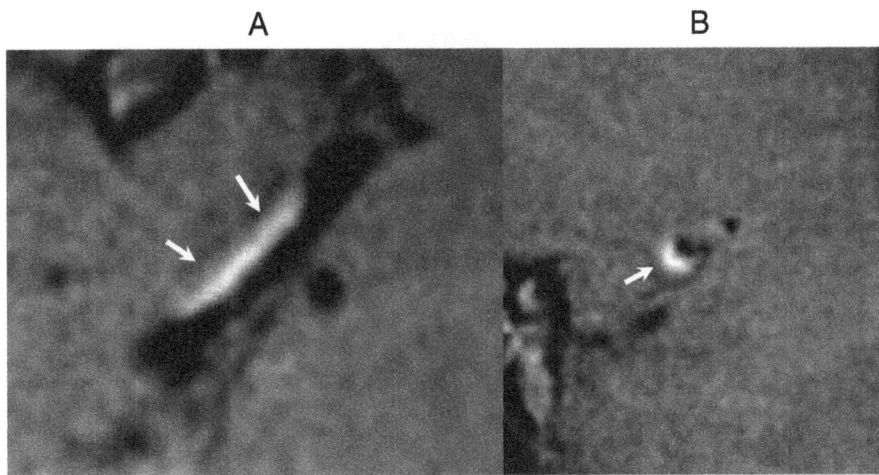

Fig. 1 Utility of 3D BBMRI. Postcontrast 3D BBMRI images (acquired resolution, 0.52 mm isotropic) of the left middle cerebral artery (MCA) M1 segment in a 48 year old man with hypertension, diabetes, and coronary artery disease who presented with acute on subacute left MCA territory infarctions. Long axis (**a**) and short axis (**b**) reconstructions demonstrate eccentric thickening and intense enhancement of the M1 segment vessel wall (*arrows*)

compared with reversible cerebral vasoconstriction syndrome (RCVS) and vasculitic lesions, ICAD lesions are significantly more likely to have eccentric wall involvement [3], and can demonstrate lesional T2 hyperintensity presumably corresponding to the fibrous cap (80 % sensitivity), which presents as a T2 juxtaluminal hyperintense band occasionally overlying a T2 hypointense component, the lipid core [12]. T2 hyperintensities and heterogeneous signal are reportedly absent in vasculitis and RCVS [12]. Luminal narrowing can be identified with conventional angiographic studies, and the goal of VWI is the definite characterization of a focal stenotic lesion as athrosclerosis,

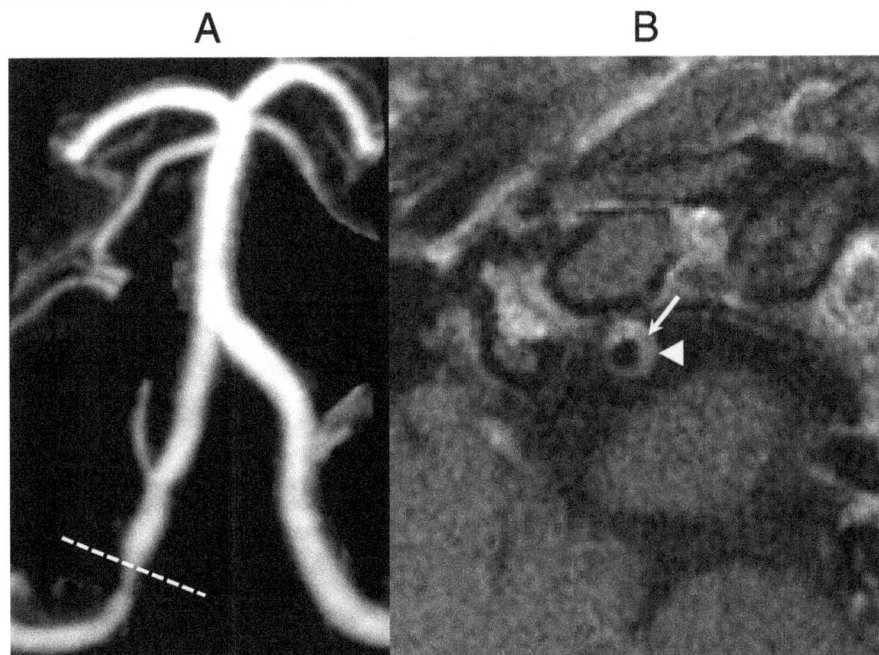

Fig. 2 Maximum intensity reconstruction (MIP) from a contrast-enhanced MRA (**a**) and postcontrast 2D BBMRI (**b**) images through a right vertebral artery plaque in a 49 year old woman with multifocal intracranial arterial narrowing presenting with an acute distal anterior cerebral artery infarction., The 2D BBMRI slice (**b**), positioned through focal narrowing of the proximal V4 segment of the right vertebral artery (**a**, line), demonstrates eccentric wall thickening and enhancement (*arrowhead*) with central hypointesity (*arrow*) representing a partially calcified core. BBMRI was achieved using double inversion recovery with the inversion time set to the null point of blood

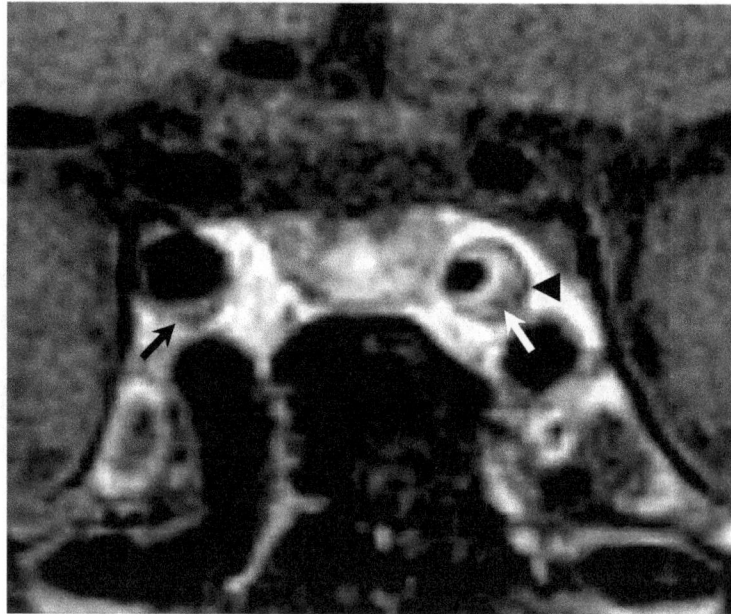

Fig. 3 Imaging through the cavernous carotid arteries of a 56 year old HIV positive man with type 1 diabetes who presented with acute left MCA territory infarcts. Postcontrast 3D BBMRI through the short axes of the juxtasellar cavernous ICA segments demonstrates eccentric wall enhancement and thickening on the left compatible with atherosclerotic plaque with a hypointense rim (*arrowhead*) that is highlighted by surrounding venous enhancement and compatible with calcifcation. A hypoenhancing focus (*white arrow*) within the enhancing, thickened wall suggests a lipid core. A small atherosclerotic plaque with minimal enhancement is seen on the right (*black arrow*)

the discrimination of active and stable plaques, and the demonstration of nonstenotic atherosclerotic burden. In a recent study, atherosclerotic plaques involving the basilar artery were more frequently identified on BBMRI than on time-of-flight MRA [13].

Plaque enhancement can be used to identify lesions responsible for cerebrovascular ischemic events (Fig. 1). Plaque enhancement could represent inflammation and/ or neovascularization and a more strongly enhancing intracranial plaque more likely represents the culprit lesion for an ischemic event [6, 7, 14]. Enhancement in an ICAD lesion that causes more than 50 % stenosis has been shown to be associated with its likelihood to have caused a recent ischemic event, and this is independent of plaque thickness [6]. Strong plaque enhancement has been observed in the vessel supplying the stroke

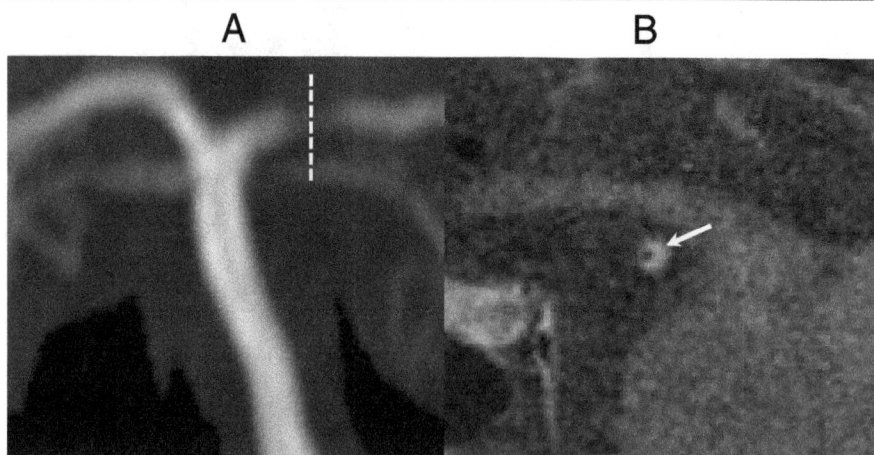

Fig. 4 Imaging of the basilar artery terminal branches in a 55 year old man with acute medial bithalamic infarctions. 3D time-of-flight MRA MIP image through the distal basilar artery shows a focal high grade stenosis of the left posterior cerebral artery (PCA) P1 segment. 2D postcontrast BBMRI image (**b**) oriented through the short axis of the stenosed vessel (**a**, line) demonstrates circumferential eccentric wall thickening and enhancement (*arrow*) compatible with an atherosclerotic plaque

territory within 4 weeks of the ischemic insult, and the enhancement decreased following the ictus [6, 15]. Plaque enhancement might serve as a more precise marker of stroke risk than luminal stenosis, enabling risk stratification in low-grade or even angiographically occult lesions [6]. Qiao et al. observed a lack of contrast enhancement only in nonculprit plaques [6]. This suggests that BBMRI can identify stable plaques with lack of enhancement, which might not need aggressive treatment [6], though a prospective study is needed to validate plaque enhancement as a predictor of future events.

The effects of intracranial thromboembolism and recanalization have been described in a small number of patients, and include smooth concentric wall thickening and enhancement at the site of recent arterial occlusion, which is more common in patients who received mechanical thrombectomy than in patients treated with medical therapy alone [16]. This pattern of enhancement following thrombectomy is reminiscent of and could be potentially confused with central nervous system (CNS) vasculitis if the patient's history is unknown. BBMRI also has been used for the identification of eccentric atherosclerotic plaques in the basilar artery and their relationship to the ostia of the major side branches before basilar artery stenting to minimize procedural complications [17].

Vasculitis

CNS vasculitis represents inflammation of intracranial blood vessels [18]. CNS vasculitis is rare and represents a group of diseases with various underlying mechanisms that affect vessels of different sizes and are characterized by non-atheromatous inflammation and necrosis of the arterial wall [14]. Conventional angiographic findings of vasculitis when present include multifocal luminal irregularities and stenosis, which are nonspecific and cannot reliably differentiate vasculitis from atherosclerosis and RCVS. In contrast to intracranial atherosclerosis, wall thickening and enhancement in vasculitis tends to be homogeneous, circumferential and concentric. However, there is overlap with ICAD, and ICAD lesions can present with circumferential vessel wall involvement, and vasculitic lesions can demonstrate eccentric enhancement [3, 7, 12, 14, 19]. Hyperintense T2 signal has been shown to be absent in vasculitic lesions, and a concentric enhancing lesion with hyperintense or heterogeneous T2 signal is more likely ICAD [12]. In our clinical experience, vasculitic enhancement and inflammation can occasionally extend beyond the vessel wall to involve the adjacent perivascular space and/or brain parenchyma (Fig. 5). We hypothesize that this periadventitial enhancement might represent a specific pattern of involvement in vasculitis. Finally, 3D black blood sequences can be used for intraoperative navigation to target individual vascular branches to increase diagnostic yield when biopsy is contemplated in suspected cases of vasculitis.

Reversible cerebral vasoconstriction syndrome

RCVS is a noninflammatory disorder of arterial tone regulation, which results in multifocal segmental narrowing of cerebral arteries that resolves spontaneously within 3 months [14, 20]. The main differential consideration is vasculitis especially when there are overlapping clinical features; and discrimination between the two

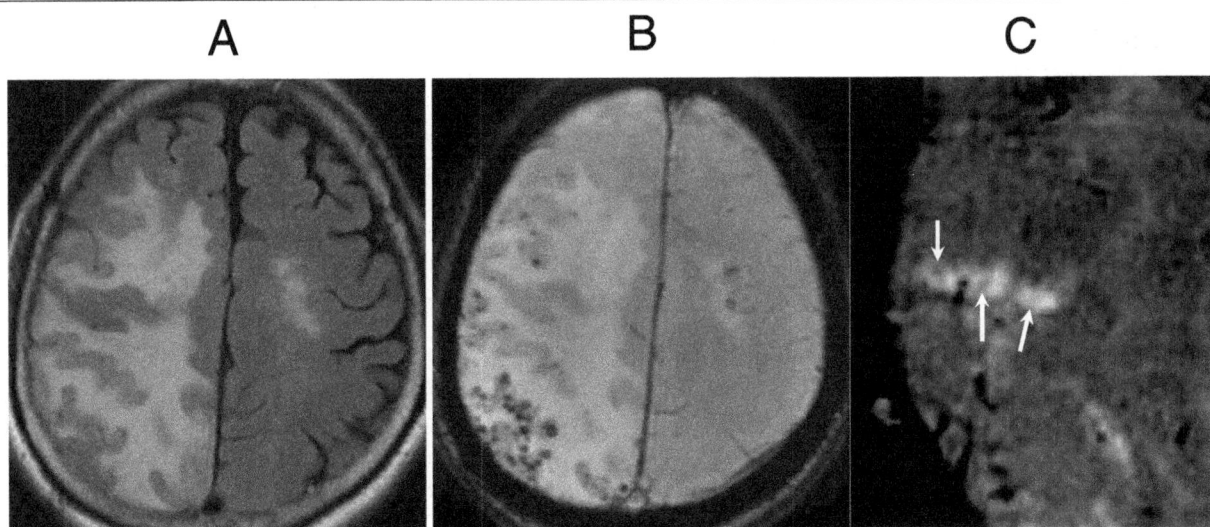

Fig. 5 Brain imaging in a 79 year old man with biopsy confirmed amyloid-β-related angiitis. Extensive confluent T2 FLAIR hyperintense vasogenic edema (**a**) and multiple punctate cortical foci of susceptibility (**b**) are seen in the right frontal and parietal lobes. Axial postcontrast 3D BBMRI (**c**) demonstrates 3 small cortical arteries with patent central hypointense lumen (*arrows*), and extensive circumferential wall enhancement, which appears to extend into the adjacent perivascular brain parenchyma compatible with vasculitis

conditions is important because vasculitis is treated with steroids, which can be harmful in RCVS [4, 20, 21]. Angiographic imaging fails to distinguish the two conditions due to nonspecific luminal narrowing in both [19]. A pilot VWI study that assessed consecutive cases with multifocal segmental narrowing on angiographic imaging demonstrated vessel wall thickening and enhancement in CNS vasculitis and cocaine vasculopathy, and minimal to no enhancement in RCVS [20]. Cocaine vasculopathy creates vasospasm, but unlike RCVS it results in arterial wall inflammation on histopathologic evaluation [22]. A larger study recruited 13 vasculitis and 13 RCVS patients [19]. Twelve out of 13 vasculitis patients had wall thickening and enhancement. The enhancement involved a short segment and was concentric in 9 patients and eccentric in 3 [19]. In RCVS, 10 patients had diffuse uniform wall thickening continuous throughout the entire wall of the diseased vessel likely due to smooth muscle contraction [20], and only 4 patients had mild vessel wall enhancement [19]. Wall enhancement in RCVS was less intense compared to CNS vasculitis with early resolution within 3 months when present [19]. These results suggest that BBMRI is helpful in the differentiation of RCVS from CNS vasculitis.

Aneurysm

A pilot study in 5 patients with aneurysmal subarachnoid hemorrhage demonstrated thick vessel wall enhancement in all ruptured aneurysms, and absent enhancement in the unruptured aneurysms [23]. In a larger study that included 117 patients, there was strong aneurysmal wall enhancement in 73.8 % of ruptured versus 4.8 % of unruptured aneurysms [24]. The authors concluded that in patients with multiple aneurysms and subarachnoid hemorrhage the presence of aneurysmal wall enhancement will likely identify the ruptured lesion [23, 24]. However, it is important to note that these are retrospective investigations and the enhancement could be a consequence of the rupture. In surgically treated aneurysms with partial wall enhancement, the enhancement corresponded to the point of rupture during surgery, which might be helpful in treatment planning [24].

In another study that included 87 patients with 108 aneurysms, circumferential aneurysmal wall enhancement was more frequently seen in unstable than in stable aneurysms (87 % versus 28.5 %, respectively) [25]. The unstable aneurysm group included ruptured aneurysms, aneurysms with change in morphology, and symptomatic aneurysms [25]. Identification of aneurysm wall enhancement could correspond to vasa vasorum formation and inflammatory activity, and it may relate to the aneurysm's risk of rupture [14, 24, 25]. A prospective study could confirm the role of VWI in the non-invasive follow-up of unruptured aneurysms [25].

Moyamoya disease

Moyamoya disease (MMD) is an idiopathic disorder causing progressive narrowing of the distal intracranial internal carotid arteries (ICAs) and the proximal circle of Willis vessels, and is characterized by the development of hypertrophied lenticulostriate branches. MMD and ICAD are both more prevalent in Asians, and differentiation between the two conditions is important because of different treatment strategies (revascularization surgery in MMD versus aggressive medical treatment in ICAD) [26]. Prior reports have suggested that MMD is characterized by little to no wall enhancement, and that this could differentiate it from radiation-induced arteritis, which presents with concentric enhancement, or an ICAD lesion that presents with eccentric enhancement [3, 27, 28]. More recent studies have described concentric enhancement in symptomatic and asymptomatic MMD patients affecting the distal ICAs, which could correspond to intimal hyperplasia pathologically [1, 26, 29]. Ryoo et al. suggested that concentric wall enhancement in bilateral distal ICAs and shrinkage of the middle cerebral arteries in MMD can distinguish it from ICAD, which presents with focal eccentric enhancement on BBMRI [26]. Additional studies are needed to further investigate the appearance of MMD using optimized BBMRI imaging and clarify whether a noninvasive diagnosis can be made.

Dissection

Dissection represents blood tracking into the vessel wall through an intimal tear. BBMRI findings suggestive of dissection include eccentric wall thickening with T1 hyperintense signal representing intramural hematoma, the identification of a false lumen, and eccentric wall enhancement, which might imply involvement by vasa vasorum [3, 14, 30]. However, the hyperintense T1 vessel wall signal is not specific for dissection since it could represent intraplaque hemorrhage in an ICAD lesion [3, 5], and studies have yet to validate these imaging features given the general lack of intracranial vessel specimens for comparison [3].

Conclusions

VWI is a rapidly growing and evolving area of clinical and research interest that holds promise to improve diagnostic accuracy for intracranial vasculopathies. VWI enables direct visualization of offending vessel wall pathology, which wouldn't be detectable on conventional imaging unless it resulted in luminal narrowing. Specific vessel wall thickening and enhancement patterns have been described in several conditions with similar angiographic findings enabling discrimination of these diseases that was not previously possible. VWI appears to allow for assessment of atherosclerotic burden and for risk stratification of individual ICAD lesions with potential to influence treatment decisions. Further prospective studies are needed to better define the role of VWI in predicting risk from intracranial vasculopathies and determining the best management approach.

Abbreviations
2D: 2-dimensional; 3D: 3-dimensional; BBMRI: Black blood MRI; CNS: central nervous system; ICA: internal carotid artery; ICAD: intracranial atherosclerotic disease; MCA: middle cerebral artery; MMD: Moyamoya disease; PCA: posterior cerebral artery; RCVS: reversible cerebral vasoconstriction syndrome; VWI: MRI vessel wall imaging.

Competing interests
BAW has a patent application pending (no. 13/922,111) for the 3D BBMRI technique used in Figures 1, 3 and 5.

Authors' contributions
Both authors contributed to, read, and approved the final manuscript.

Acknowledgements
BAW has received grant support from the National Heart, Lung, and Blood Institute (RO1HL105930-01A1).

Author details
[1]Department of Radiology, Rush University Medical Center, 1725 W. Harrison St., Chicago, IL 60612, USA. [2]The Russell H. Morgan Department of Radiology and Radiological Sciences, Johns Hopkins University School of Medicine, 600 North Wolfe Street, Baltimore, MD 21287, USA.

References
1. Dieleman N, van der Kolk AG, Zwanenburg JJ, Harteveld AA, Biessels GJ, Luijten PR, et al. Imaging intracranial vessel wall pathology with magnetic resonance imaging: current prospects and future directions. Circulation. 2014;130:192–201.
2. Qiao Y, Steinman DA, Qin Q, Etesami M, Schar M, Astor BC, et al. Intracranial arterial wall imaging using three-dimensional high isotropic resolution black blood MRI at 3.0 Tesla. J Magn Reson Imaging. 2011;34:22–30.
3. Swartz RH, Bhuta SS, Farb RI, Agid R, Willinsky RA, Terbrugge KG, et al. Intracranial arterial wall imaging using high-resolution 3-tesla contrast-enhanced MRI. Neurology. 2009;72:627–34.
4. Miller TR, Shivashankar R, Mossa-Basha M, Gandhi D. Reversible Cerebral Vasoconstriction Syndrome, Part 2: Diagnostic Work-Up, Imaging Evaluation, and Differential Diagnosis. AJNR Am J Neuroradiol. 2015;36:1580–8.
5. Turan TN, Bonilha L, Morgan PS, Adams RJ, Chimowitz MI. Intraplaque hemorrhage in symptomatic intracranial atherosclerotic disease. J Neuroimaging. 2011;21:e159–61.
6. Qiao Y, Zeiler SR, Mirbagheri S, Leigh R, Urrutia V, Wityk R, et al. Intracranial plaque enhancement in patients with cerebrovascular events on high-spatial-resolution MR images. Radiology. 2014;271:534–42.
7. Vergouwen MD, Silver FL, Mandell DM, Mikulis DJ, Swartz RH. Eccentric narrowing and enhancement of symptomatic middle cerebral artery stenoses in patients with recent ischemic stroke. Arch Neurol. 2011;68:338–42.
8. van der Kolk AG, Hendrikse J, Brundel M, Biessels GJ, Smit EJ, Visser F, et al. Multi-sequence whole-brain intracranial vessel wall imaging at 7.0 tesla. Eur Radiol. 2013;23:2996–3004.
9. Lee WJ, Choi HS, Jang J, Sung J, Kim TW, Koo J, et al. Non-stenotic intracranial arteries have atherosclerotic changes in acute ischemic stroke patients: a 3 T MRI study. Neuroradiology. 2015;57:1007–13.
10. de Havenon A, Yuan C, Tirschwell D, Hatsukami T, Anzai Y, Becker K, et al. Nonstenotic Culprit Plaque: The Utility of High-Resolution Vessel Wall MRI of Intracranial Vessels after Ischemic Stroke. Case Rep Radiol. 2015;2015:356582.
11. Kim TH, Choi JW, Roh HG, Moon WJ, Moon SG, Chun YI, et al. Atherosclerotic arterial wall change of non-stenotic intracracranial arteries on high-resolution MRI at 3.0 T: Correlation with cerebrovascular risk factors and white matter hyperintensity. Clin Neurol Neurosurg. 2014;126:1–6.
12. Mossa-Basha M, Hwang WD, De Havenon A, Hippe D, Balu N, Becker KJ, et al. Multicontrast high-resolution vessel wall magnetic resonance imaging and its value in differentiating intracranial vasculopathic processes. Stroke. 2015;46:1567–73.
13. Kim YS, Lim SH, Oh KW, Kim JY, Koh SH, Kim J, et al. The advantage of high-resolution MRI in evaluating basilar plaques: a comparison study with MRA. Atherosclerosis. 2012;224:411–6.
14. Portanova A, Hakakian N, Mikulis DJ, Virmani R, Abdalla WM, Wasserman BA. Intracranial vasa vasorum: insights and implications for imaging. Radiology. 2013;267:667–79.
15. Skarpathiotakis M, Mandell DM, Swartz RH, Tomlinson G, Mikulis DJ. Intracranial atherosclerotic plaque enhancement in patients with ischemic stroke. AJNR Am J Neuroradiol. 2013;34:299–304.
16. Power S, Matouk C, Casaubon LK, Silver FL, Krings T, Mikulis DJ, et al. Vessel wall magnetic resonance imaging in acute ischemic stroke: effects of embolism and mechanical thrombectomy on the arterial wall. Stroke. 2014;45:2330–4.
17. Jiang WJ, Yu W, Ma N, Du B, Lou X, Rasmussen PA. High resolution MRI guided endovascular intervention of basilar artery disease. J Neurointerv Surg. 2011;3:375–8.
18. Kuker W, Gaertner S, Nagele T, Dopfer C, Schoning M, Fiehler J, et al. Vessel wall contrast enhancement: a diagnostic sign of cerebral vasculitis. Cerebrovasc Dis. 2008;26:23–9.
19. Obusez EC, Hui F, Hajj-Ali RA, Cerejo R, Calabrese LH, Hammad T, et al. High-resolution MRI vessel wall imaging: spatial and temporal patterns of reversible cerebral vasoconstriction syndrome and central nervous system vasculitis. AJNR Am J Neuroradio. 2014;35:1527–32.
20. Mandell DM, Matouk CC, Farb RI, Krings T, Agid R, ter Brugge K, et al. Vessel wall MRI to differentiate between reversible cerebral vasoconstriction syndrome and central nervous system vasculitis: preliminary results. Stroke. 2012;43:860–2.
21. Miller TR, Shivashankar R, Mossa-Basha M, Gandhi D. Reversible Cerebral Vasoconstriction Syndrome, Part 1: Epidemiology, Pathogenesis, and Clinical Course. AJNR Am J Neuroradiol. 2015;36:1392–9.
22. Han JS, Mandell DM, Poublanc J, Mardimae A, Slessarev M, Jaigobin C, et al. BOLD-MRI cerebrovascular reactivity findings in cocaine-induced cerebral vasculitis. Nat Clin Pract Neurol. 2008;4:628–32.
23. Matouk CC, Mandell DM, Gunel M, Bulsara KR, Malhotra A, Hebert R, et al. Vessel wall magnetic resonance imaging identifies the site of rupture in patients with multiple intracranial aneurysms: proof of principle. Neurosurgery. 2013;72:492–6. discussion 496.
24. Nagahata S, Nagahata M, Obara M, Kondo R, Minagawa N, Sato S, et al. Wall Enhancement of the Intracranial Aneurysms Revealed by Magnetic Resonance Vessel Wall Imaging Using Three-Dimensional Turbo Spin-Echo Sequence with Motion-Sensitized Driven-Equilibrium: A Sign of Ruptured Aneurysm? Clinical neuroradiology 2014.
25. Edjlali M, Gentric JC, Regent-Rodriguez C, Trystram D, Hassen WB, Lion S, et al. Does aneurysmal wall enhancement on vessel wall MRI help to distinguish stable from unstable intracranial aneurysms? Stroke. 2014;45:3704–6.
26. Ryoo S, Cha J, Kim SJ, Choi JW, Ki CS, Kim KH, et al. High-resolution magnetic resonance wall imaging findings of Moyamoya disease. Stroke. 2014;45:2457–60.
27. Aoki S, Hayashi N, Abe O, Shirouzu I, Ishigame K, Okubo T, et al. Radiation-induced arteritis: thickened wall with prominent enhancement on cranial MR images report of five cases and comparison with 18 cases of Moyamoya disease. Radiology. 2002;223:683–8.
28. Kim JM, Jung KH, Sohn CH, Park J, Moon J, Han MH, et al. High-resolution MR technique can distinguish moyamoya disease from atherosclerotic occlusion. Neurology. 2013;80:775–6.
29. Kim YJ, Lee DH, Kwon JY, Kang DW, Suh DC, Kim JS, et al. High resolution MRI difference between moyamoya disease and intracranial atherosclerosis. Eur J Neurol. 2013;20:1311–8.
30. Mauermann ML, Phillips CD, Worrall BB. Intraplaque dissection of the basilar artery. Neurology. 2006;66:1544.

6

Imaging predictors of procedural and clinical outcome in endovascular acute stroke therapy

Nicholas A. Telischak* and Max Wintermark

Abstract

Acute stroke affects 795,000 people per year in the United States, and eighty-seven percent of these represent ischemic stroke. New level I evidence has created a need for consistent, effective and rapid triage of stroke patients to properly select those who will most benefit from endovascular stroke therapy. This review highlights anatomical factors and imaging signs that are prognostic with respect to stroke outcome and which could aid in the selection of patients that could most benefit from interventional stroke therapies, as well as exclude patients from therapy who are at a high risk of complication.

Keywords: Stroke, Endovascular stroke, Perfusion imaging, Clot characteristics, Blood brain permeability, Core infarct

Introduction

Acute stroke affects 795,000 people per year in the United States, and eighty-seven percent of these represent ischemic stroke. The prevalence of stroke is projected to increase 20.5 % by the year 2030, as a result of an aging population [1]. While intravenous tissue plasminogen activator (tPA) has been a mainstay of stroke therapy since its approval by the Food and Drug Administration in 1996, interventional treatment of stroke provides the best possible chance of a good clinical outcome when patients are appropriately selected, as has recently been borne out by a handful of randomized controlled trials [2–5]. While this wealth of new data is very exciting, predicting which patients will respond best to stroke therapy remains a challenge. In this review, we aim to highlight imaging findings prior to stroke therapy that may predict therapeutic and clinical success.

Clinical trials of endovascular treatment of stroke

Interventional treatment of stroke denotes any catheter-directed therapy and has progressed from intra-arterial administration of tPA to mechanical clot disruption with a microwire, the MERCI device, suction thrombectomy (e.g. Penumbra), and use of stent-retriever devices including Solitaire and TREVO. Initially the IMS III, SYNTHESIS expansion, and MR RESCUE trials failed to show a clinical benefit to interventional stroke. Lessons learned from

these trials have resulted in recent randomized controlled trials overwhelmingly favoring endovascular stroke therapy.

Intra-arterial thrombolysis was originally evaluated in a randomized-controlled trial using the drug pro-urokinase in the PROACT II trial, which showed 66 % recanalization in patients randomized to treatment, but also showed a relatively high rate of symptomatic intra-cranial hemorrhage. The clinical outcomes showed no difference in mortality between groups, and an absolute increase in favorable outcome of 15 % in the interventional group, corresponding to a number needed to treat of 7 [6]. The drug used in this trial, urokinase, was pulled by the FDA due to "significant deviations from Current Good Manufacturing Practices" [7].

The IMS III trial randomized 656 participants and showed similar rates of functional independence (mRS 0-2) of 40.8 % and 38.7 % in the endovascular and IV tPA groups, respectively, with a trend toward better outcomes in the endovascular group among patients with National Institute of Health Stroke Scale (NIHSS) >20 [8]. A strong criticism of this trial is that less than half of patients got a CTA resulting in 20 % of patients without a large vessel occlusion being randomized to the interventional arm. Standard dose IV tPA was not given to the majority of patients in the interventional arm. Due to the slow trial recruitment, there were many protocol iterations with many patients receiving interventional therapy with first-generation devices that do not have the same efficacy or safety profile as

* Correspondence: teli@stanford.edu
Department of Neuroradiology, S047 300 Pasteur Drive, Stanford, CA 94305, USA

Table 1 Modified Rankin Scale (mRS) for standardized evaluation of clinical outcome after stroke

Modified Rankin Scale (mRS)	Clinical Description
0	No symptoms.
1	No significant disability. Able to carry out all usual activities despite some symptoms.
2	Slight disability. Able to look after own affairs without assistance, but unable to carry out all previous activities.
3	Moderate disability. Requires some help, but able to walk unassisted.
4	Moderately severe disability. Unable to attend to own bodily needs without assistance. Unable to walk unassisted.
5	Severe disability. Requires constant nursing care and attention, bedridden, incontinent.
6	Dead.

today's stentrievers (40 % recanalization in IMS III versus 68 % -80 % recanalization with modern stentrievers) [8].

The SYNTHESIS expansion trial enrolled 362 patients with AIS to IV tPA within 4.5 h versus IA therapy within 6 h of symptom onset. No pre-procedural imaging was required (10 % of patients did not have a large vessel occlusion), nor was a lower boundary of NIHSS at presentation defined (nearly half of enrolled patients had NIHSS scores of 10 or less). Once randomized, 165 of 181 patients in the interventional arm received an endovascular procedure, and only 56 of these received mechanical thrombectomy. Additionally, the intervention arm received treatment one hour later on average compared to the IV arm. Success of revascularization was not reported. Despite lack of confirmation of a large vessel occlusion, withholding of IV tPA, and the delivery of IA tPA to patients without a vessel occlusion, there was no increase in death or intracranial hemorrhage compared to IV tPA. Not surprisingly given these shortcomings, the trial failed to show a benefit in 3 month mRS in the interventional arm [9].

The Mechanical Retrieval and Recanalization of Stroke Clots Using Embolectomy (MR RESCUE) Trial was a multi-center randomized trial comparing standard medical care to interventional stroke therapy in patients presenting within 8-h with a large vessel anterior circulation stroke. All patients received a perfusion MR or CT prior to randomization. Interventional stroke therapy was not superior to standard medical care, but this trial did show that patients with revascularization had improved 3-month mRS (3.2 versus 4.1) and lower median absolute infarct growth (9.0 mL vs. 73 mL) [10]. Importantly, MR RESCUE included first generation thrombectomy devices only, and

achieved a very low reperfusion rate (27 %) compared with modern trials [10].

Many lessons learned from the shortcomings of these trials have highlighted the attributes of an ideal candidate for stroke intervention: 1) A proximal vessel occlusion that can be reached by an endovascular approach, 2) a small area of core infarction, and 3) viable tissue at risk of infarction if reperfusion is not achieved, the ischemic "penumbra" [11]. This knowledge has resulted in a wealth of recent trials showing overwhelming benefit of endovascular stroke therapy beginning with the MR CLEAN trial from the Netherlands.

MR CLEAN enrolled 500 patients with a confirmed proximal arterial occlusion in the anterior cerebral circulation who could be treated intra-arterially within 6 h of symptom onset. The majority (89 %) of enrolled patients were treated with IV-tPA prior to endovascular therapy, and in the interventional arm four out of five patients (81.5 %) were treated with retrievable stent devices resulting in a good rate (58.7 %) of recanalization. Using modified Rankin scale shift at 90 days, the adjusted common odds ratio was 1.67 in favor of the intervention [2].

The REVASCAT trial was halted early citing loss of equipoise after the publication of the MR CLEAN results. REVASCAT randomized 206 patients with a proximal anterior circulation occlusion without a large infarct who could be treated within 8 h from symptom onset to medical therapy alone (IV tPA) or medical therapy and endovascular therapy with the Solitaire stent retriever. Ischemic core was estimated by ASPECTS, admitting patients only with ASPECTS of 6 to 10; NIHSS was at least 6 for admission into the trial. This trial showed benefit of endovascular stroke therapy, with a common odds ratio of 1.7 in the Rankin shift analysis in favor of endovascular therapy, and 15.5 % absolute difference in the proportion of patients who were functionally independent at 90 days (43.7 % vs. 28.2 %) [4].

The ESCAPE trial was halted early after an interim analysis was prompted by the MR CLEAN results. ESCAPE

Table 2 TICI Scoring for assessment of procedural success in acute stroke therapy

Grade	TICI Score
0	No Perfusion.
1	Antegrade reperfusion past the initial occlusion but limited distal branch filling with little or slow distal reperfusion.
2a	Antegrade reperfusion of less than half of the occluded target artery previously ischemic territory (e.g. 1 major MCA division and its territory).
2b	Antegrade reperfusion of more than half of the previously occluded target artery ischemic territory.
3	Complete antegrade reperfusion of the previously occluded target artery without visualized distal occlusion in all distal branches.

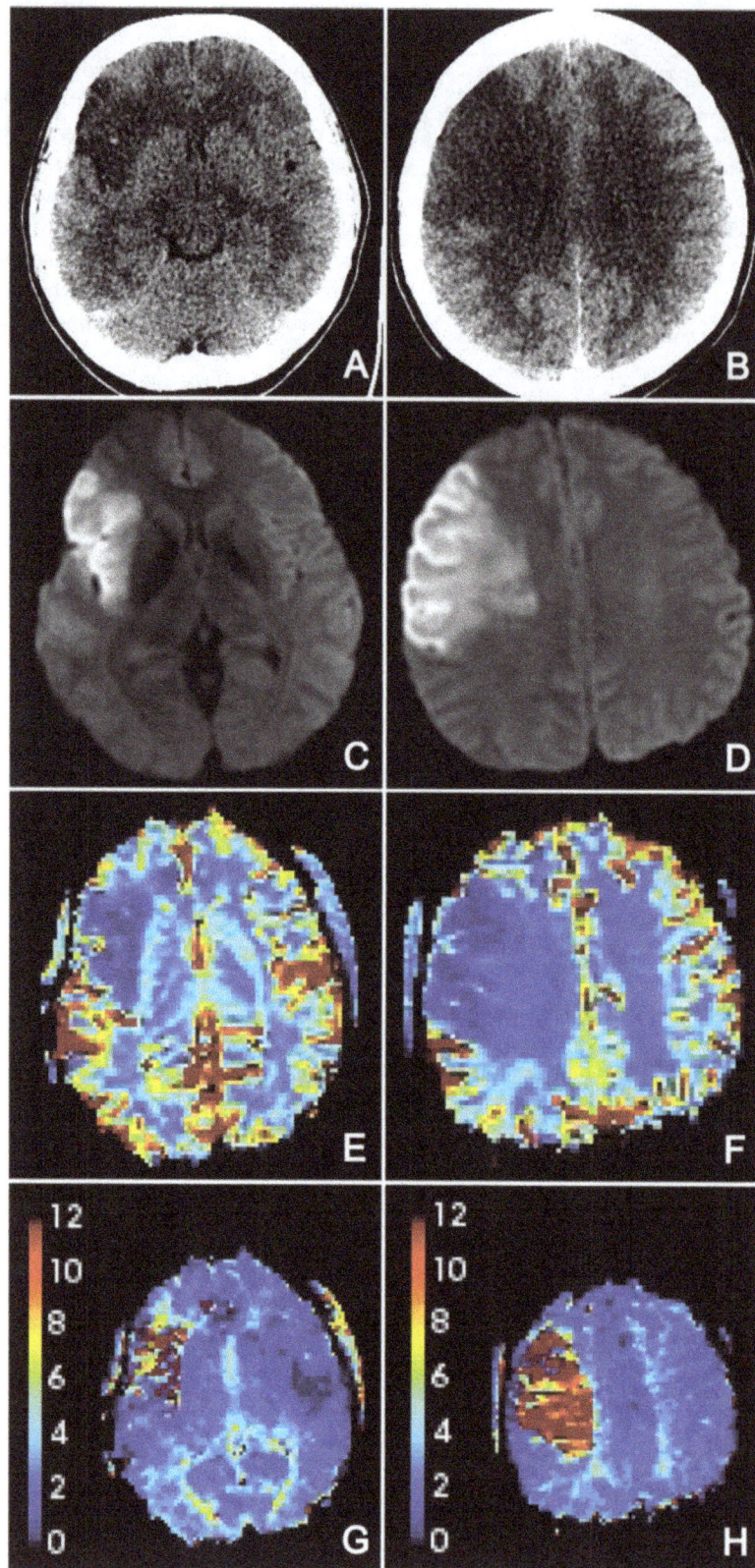

Fig. 1 (See legend on next page.)

Fig. 1 Large ischemic core in a 37-year-old female who awoke with right gaze preference and left sided-weakness. Axial non-contrast computed tomography (CT) images at the level of the basal ganglia (**a**) and through the centrum semiovale (**b**) show hypodensity and loss of grey-white differentiation of the right insular cortex, putamen, and right frontal grey matter. This is similarly shown by axial diffusion weighted images (**c,d**). Cerebral blood volume (CBV) map from the perfusion CT show decreased CBV corresponding to those territories consistent with a large core of completed infarct (**e, f**). The Tmax maps demonstrate a matched perfusion deficit (**g, h**)

recruited 316 patients with a proximal anterior circulation occlusion and randomized to standard of care with IV tPA vs. standard of care plus endovascular treatment with thrombectomy devices up to 12 h from symptom onset. Patients with large infarct (Alberta Stroke Program Early CT Score, ASPECTS < 6) or poor collaterals (<50 % filling of pial collaterals on CTA) were excluded. This study showed both an improvement in mRS at 90 days in the interventional arm of 53.0 % vs. 29.3 % as well as a decreased mortality in the interventional arm of 10.4 % vs. 19.0 % [5].

The EXTEND-IA trial was also stopped early once the results of MR CLEAN became available, after recruitment of 70 patients who were receiving IV tPA within 4.5 h from symptom onset to interventional treatment with the Solitaire stent-retriever device or to continuation of IV tPA alone. Eligible patients were selected with perfusion-CT and CT-angiogram to have a proximal anterior circulation arterial occlusion and an ischemic core of less than 70 mL. Compared with IV tPA alone, endovascular therapy resulted in a significantly higher probability of reperfusion (89 % vs. 34 %), and this translated to a significant clinical benefit with more patients in the interventional arm (71 % vs. 40 %) achieving functional independence (mRS 0-2) at 90 days [3].

The SWIFT PRIME study enrolled patients with a NIHSS > 8 resulting from a proximal anterior circulation arterial occlusion and utilized perfusion-CT with automated software to compute the volume of core infarct selecting patients with a core <50 cc (later modified to read baseline evidence of a moderate/large core as defined by ASPECTS < 6). Patients with a Tmax lesion of >100 cc were excluded (see malignant perfusion profile, below). The treatment window in SWIFT PRIME was 6 h. Again, this trial showed a benefit of endovascular therapy showing a number needed to treat of only 2.6 for an improved disability outcome, and of only 4 patients for one additional patient to be functionally independent at 90 days [12].

Beyond the proven clear benefit of endovascular stroke therapy, there are lessons to be learned. Three studies that showed the highest frequency of functional independence were the SWIFT PRIME (60 %), the ESCAPE trial (53 %) and the EXTEND IA trial (71 %). This likely reflects commonalities among these trials including fast time to endovascular therapies, exclusion of patients

with large core infarcts on the basis of advanced imaging, and higher rates of reperfusion in the endovascular arms. Advanced imaging clearly plays a role in patient selection for endovascular stroke therapy; the goal of this paper is to review predictive signs and measures of advanced imaging in acute stroke.

Outcome measures in endovascular stroke therapy

Outcome measures in endovascular acute stroke therapy may be graded with clinical metrics (e.g. mRS at 90 days) [13, 14], and with imaging metrics (e.g. TICI reperfusion score) [15]. These are well reviewed elsewhere and are summarized in Table 1 and Table 2.

There are numerous fixed clinical variables that impact the outcome of a stroke patient after reperfusion therapy, including presentation NIHSS, baseline functional status, time from stroke onset to reperfusion, patient age, patient comorbidities, etc. In this paper, we focus on imaging findings that can predict procedural success and clinical outcome.

Results: Imaging predictors of good outcomes in endovascular stroke therapy
Side of occlusion
The laterality of the stroke has a great effect on patient outcome, with dominant hemisphere strokes having a greater impact per volume of infarct than a non-dominant hemisphere stroke. In a study relating DWI lesion volume to poor outcome (mRS >2), the 95 % specificity lesion volume was 51.8 mL for the left hemisphere compared to 98.5 mL for right hemisphere involvement, indicating that non-dominant hemisphere strokes are better tolerated [16]. While some of this difference relates to an inherent bias of the NIHSS scoring towards dominant hemisphere stroke, it is clear that a dominant hemisphere infarct portends a worse prognosis.

Ischemic core estimation
The size of the completed infarct when a patient presents with a stroke represents irrecoverable damage and therefore more than success of recanalization sets the stage for how much recovery can be expected [17]. Ischemic core size is an independent predictor of outcome after stroke, whether measured by CT or DWI MR (Fig. 1) [18–21]. In a retrospective study, good outcome (mRS 0-2) occurred with average lesion volumes of 16.3 mL whereas the average lesion size in poor outcome (mRS >2) was 63.4 mL

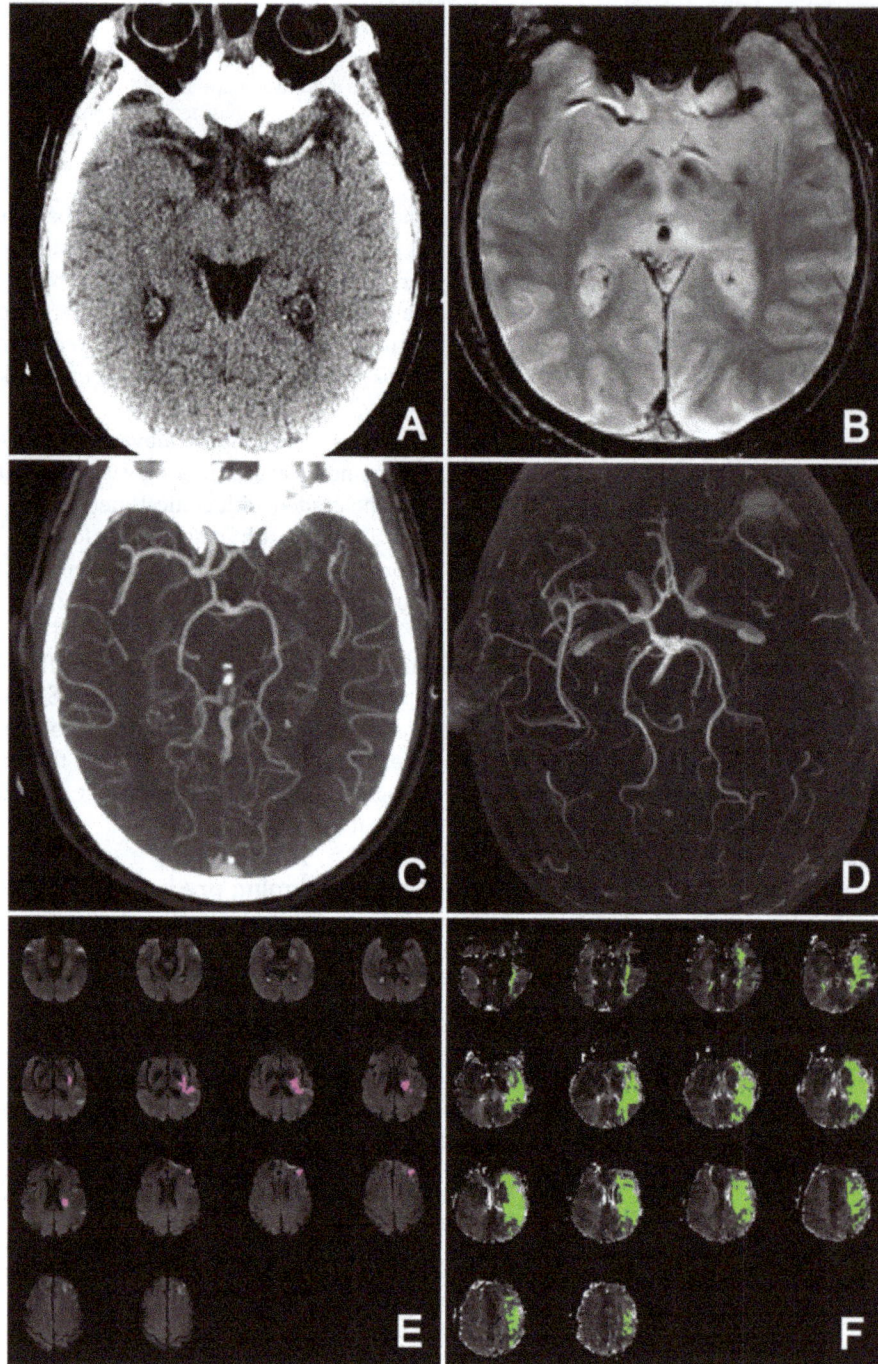

Fig. 2 Dense middle cerebral artery (MCA) sign with an ischemic penumbra in a 68-year-old male with acute stroke. Non-contrast computed tomography (CT) demonstrates a dense left MCA with long length of thrombus (**a**). This manifests "blooming" on gradient recalled echo (GRE, **b**) magnetic resonance imaging. CT angiography (CTA) shows a left carotid terminus occlusion extending into the left middle cerebral artery (**c**), with a better depiction of collaterals than can be seen on the time-of-flight magnetic resonance angiogram (MRA, **d**). Diffusion weighted MR image (DWI, **e**) and perfusion weighted MRI Tmax map with colorized overlay representing the infarcted core (pink, **e**) and the territory at risk (green, **f**), here showing a favorable perfusion pattern with a small ischemic core and large penumbra

again demonstrating the link between lesion size at presentation and outcome [16]. When measured by MRI at 48 h, the infarct volume is an independent predictor of outcome [18]. The estimation of ischemic core by DWI during acute stroke is highly correlative with final stroke volume, with normalization of brain tissue previously showing abnormal DWI signal ("DWI reversal") representing an unlikely event. When DWI reversal does occur it is not of sufficient size to meaningfully alter the degree of diffusion-perfusion mismatch [22].

Because MRI is difficult to obtain at many centers alternate methods have been devised to estimate ischemic core with CT. The Alberta Stroke Program Early CT Score (ASPECTS) divides the brain into 10 territories with points removed for loss of grey matter-white matter differentiation in each territory based on a non-contrast CT evaluation [23]. This score has been shown repeatedly to correlate with outcome; for instance when applied to the National Institute of Neurological Disorders and Stroke (NINDS) cohort, ASPECTS 8-10 group had a greater benefit from IV thrombolysis and a trend toward reduced mortality [24]. In the original study ASPECTS score of 7 or below demarcated good from poor outcomes [23]. The rate of change of ASPECTS score in patients transferred to a comprehensive stroke center having already undergone a CT scan at an outside hospital is likely a reflection of collateral perfusion and is also predictive of outcome [25].

Perfusion CT (PCT) imaging is used at many stroke centers to triage patients to appropriate therapy because it is fast to obtain and nearly universally available. The primary goal of perfusion imaging is to differentiate ischemic core from the penumbra [26]. Within an ischemic core both cerebral blood flow (CBF) and cerebral blood volume (CBV) are lowered; CBV is the most accurate predictor of the core infarct [27]. A trial investigating whether PCT can predict response to recanalization, Computed Tomography Perfusion to Predict Response to Recanalization in Ischemic Stroke Project (CRISP), is ongoing [28].

Clot location

The location of the occluded vessel has an effect both on success of revascularization but also on clinical outcomes. Large vessel occlusion, defined in one study as vertebral, basilar, internal carotid, proximal (M1 segment) middle cerebral and proximal (A1 segment) anterior cerebral artery occlusion, correlates to worse outcome. Specifically, the odds ratio for mortality is 4.5 and the odds ratio of good outcome (mRS ≤2) is 0.33 in patients with a large vessel occlusion compared to those without [29].

In patients treated with IV tPA, the rates of complete recanalization for ICA terminus, proximal MCA, and distal MCA are 5 %, 10 % and 22 %, respectively [30]. In the SWIFT trial, the ICA, M1 MCA, and M2 MCA made up 21 %, 66 %, and 10 %, respectively, of patients randomized to the Solitaire device with overall recanalization of 69 % as assessed by the core laboratory [31]. In TREVO2, rates of ICA, M1 and M2 enrollment were 16 %, 60 %, and 16 %, respectively, with overall recanalization (TICI ≥2) of 86 % [32]. More proximal occlusions are therefore much less likely to respond to IV compared to IA therapy. In the DEFUSE2 trial, using largely first-generation thrombectomy devices, ICA and MCA occlusions were revascularized with

similar success (61 % and 59 %, respectively) with similar proportions of good clinical outcome after revascularization of 65 % for ICA recanalization and 63 % for MCA recanalization [33].

Even when applied to the M1 segment, patients harboring proximal M1 segment MCA lesions are less likely to have a good functional outcome compared to distal M1 segment MCA lesions (8 % vs. 39 %), and are more likely to sustain a basal ganglia infarct comprising the internal capsule (83 % vs. 11 %) [34]. A similar study examined patient outcome based on location of hyperdense MCA sign, and showed improved clinical outcome in distal as compared with proximal sites of occlusion (85 % vs. 15 % mRS 0-2) [35].

Clot characteristics

Thrombus is most commonly the cause of ischemic stroke, but not every thrombus is the same. Thrombus subtype has been stratified into platelet-rich and red blood cell-rich varieties, and this distinction has been shown to have an effect on success of tPA and on interventional stroke therapy [36]. Surrogate markers of clot composition include density on non-contrast CT, and the degree of blooming artifact on GRE MR images (Fig. 2). Dense clots on CT and blooming clots on GRE MRI both imply a red blood cell predominant composition. Red cell predominant clots infer a favorable response to both IV and IA stroke therapies compared with clots of lower density or without GRE blooming artifact [37].

The length of thrombus, also described as clot burden, has been shown to predict likelihood of recanalization, as well as final stroke outcome. In one study, no thrombus exceeding 8-mm in length resulted in recanalization after treatment with IV tPA [38]. Another study in which 54 % of patients received IV tPA and the other 46 % received IV tPA plus IA therapy, recanalization was achieved 85 % of the time for thrombi <10 mm, 37.5 % for thrombi 10-20 mm, and in no cases for thrombi >20 mm, demonstrating that a longer thrombus is more resistant to both IV and IA therapies [39]. When a "clot burden" score is

Table 3 ASITN/SIR Collateral flow grading system

Grade 0	No collaterals visible to the ischemic site
Grade 1	Slow collaterals to the periphery of the ischemic site with persistence of some of the defect
Grade 2	Rapid collaterals to the periphery of ischemic site with persistence of some of the defect and to only a portion of the ischemic territory
Grade 3	Collaterals with slow but complete angiographic blood flow of the ischemic bed by the late venous phase
Grade 4	Complete and rapid collateral blood flow to the vascular bed in the entire ischemic territory by retrograde perfusion

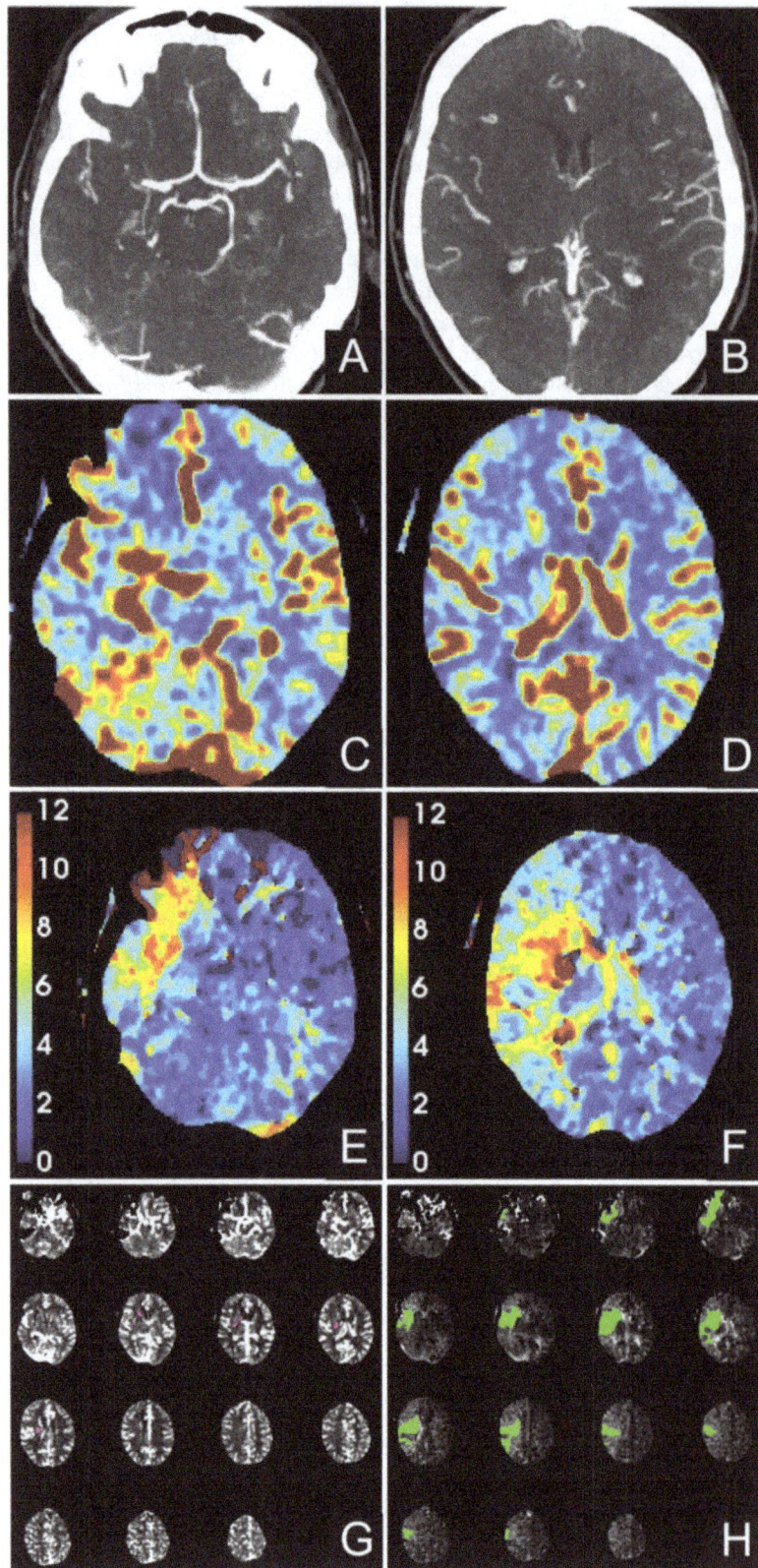

Fig. 3 (See legend on next page.)

(See figure on previous page.)
Fig. 3 Favorable collaterals in a 67-year-old with acute right MCA occlusion. Axial maximum intensity projection (MIP) of the CTA show a right M1 segment MCA occlusion (**a**) with excellent collateral filling of the affected territory (**a**, **b**). Correlative CTP shows no CBV evidence of a completed core infarct (**c**, **d**). A large ischemic penumbra is evident on the Tmax maps (**e**, **f**). Colorized threshold maps demonstrate a small region of core infarct (pink, **g**) with a relatively large territory at risk (green, **h**)

allocated for thrombotic occlusion of vascular territories, increasing clot burden is associated with both worse functional outcome as well as with larger final infarct as assessed by ASPECTS score [40]. Looking forward, imaging may serve as a tool to better define clot constituents and help guide treatment decisions based on probability of success for a given clot composition.

Collateral scoring

In ischemic stroke, neuronal loss occurs at an average rate of 1.9 million per minute [41]. While this number is grossly simplified, it speaks to the exquisite sensitivity of a neuron to oxygen debt. It therefore stands to reason that collateral flow is a critical factor in determining both the rate of stroke completion and the extent of involvement of the affected hemisphere. A recent review cited 63 different methods of assessing collateral flow, however the most commonly used method, developed by the American Society of Interventional and Therapeutic Neuroradiology (ASITN) and the Society of Interventional Radiology (SIR) is summarized in Table 3 [42].

High quality collaterals have been shown to be independent predictors of both favorable outcome and recanalization (Fig. 3) [43–46]. When applied to stroke, a malignant profile representing a complete lack of collateral vessels in the affected territory, is a discriminator of lesion volume >100 mL (itself a strong predictor of outcome), and of being functionally dependent (mRS ≥ 3) at 3 months [47].

Good collaterals are a strong predictor of recanalization; conversely patients with poor collaterals are less likely to achieve recanalization and more likely to have hemorrhagic transformation [48, 49]. In the ENDOSTROKE study, better collateral vessels (ASITN/SIR grades of 0 or 1, 2, and 3 or 4) were associated with higher reperfusion rates (21 %, 48 %, and 77 %), a higher proportion of infarcts smaller than one-third of the MCA territory (32 %, 48 %, and 69 %), and a higher proportion of good clinical outcome (11 %, 35 %, and 49 %) [50].

In the ESCAPE trial of endovascular stroke therapy, in addition to proof of small infarct core and proximal vessel occlusion, patients were selected on the basis of a moderate to good collateral score, which has also been shown to be an independent predictor of outcome after stroke [5, 51]. Good patient selection in this trial clearly contributed to the favorable treatment results, highlighting the value of collateral scoring.

Penumbra imaging

Estimate of the ischemic penumbra in acute stroke in relation to the core infarct is a critical piece of information when triaging candidates for interventional stroke therapy. While ischemic penumbra is present in 90 % to 100 % of patients with anterior circulation stroke in a three hour window, 75 % to 80 % continue to have some degree of penumbral tissue at 6 h [26]. Selecting patients with preserved tissue at risk prevents futile reperfusion of infarcted tissue and improves outcomes in stroke therapy [2–5]. Indeed, recent trials that selected patients for endovascular stroke therapy with perfusion imaging show the largest benefit [2, 3]. This estimate may be made clinically using the NIHSS as a surrogate marker of ischemia, but using PCT imaging adds specificity and reproducibility to this estimate (Fig. 4). Penumbral information as assessed by PCT provides information that cannot be inferred clinically, and is an independent predictor of stroke outcome. An important point with respect to perfusion imaging is a finding termed the malignant profile, which denotes a large lesion with markedly delayed perfusion as defined by a DWI core > 100 mL or a perfusion-weighted image lesion of 100 mL or more with Tmax delay of 8 s or more. The malignant profile is associated with poor outcome and a higher rate of symptomatic intracranial hemorrhage after interventional stroke therapy (Fig. 5) [52].

White matter injury

Diffusion tensor imaging (DTI) allows visualization of white matter tracts, the injury of which has prognostic value in acute stroke. For instance, the integrity of the corticospinal tract as assessed by MRI can predict the probability of motor recovery after corona radiata stroke [53–55]. In the acute stage, diffusion tractography predicted motor function at 90 days better than clinical scores [55].

Blood-brain barrier (BBB) permeability

Symptomatic intracranial hemorrhage is a complication of endovascular stroke therapy with an incidence ranging from 0-7.7 % in recent trials [2–5]. This can have important consequences for final outcome after endovascular stroke therapy and therefore it is important to have imaging metrics to prospectively exclude patients who are at a high risk of hemorrhage from endovascular therapies. The hyperintense acute reperfusion marker (HARM) is an early marker of BBB breakdown, observed as hyperintense signal seen

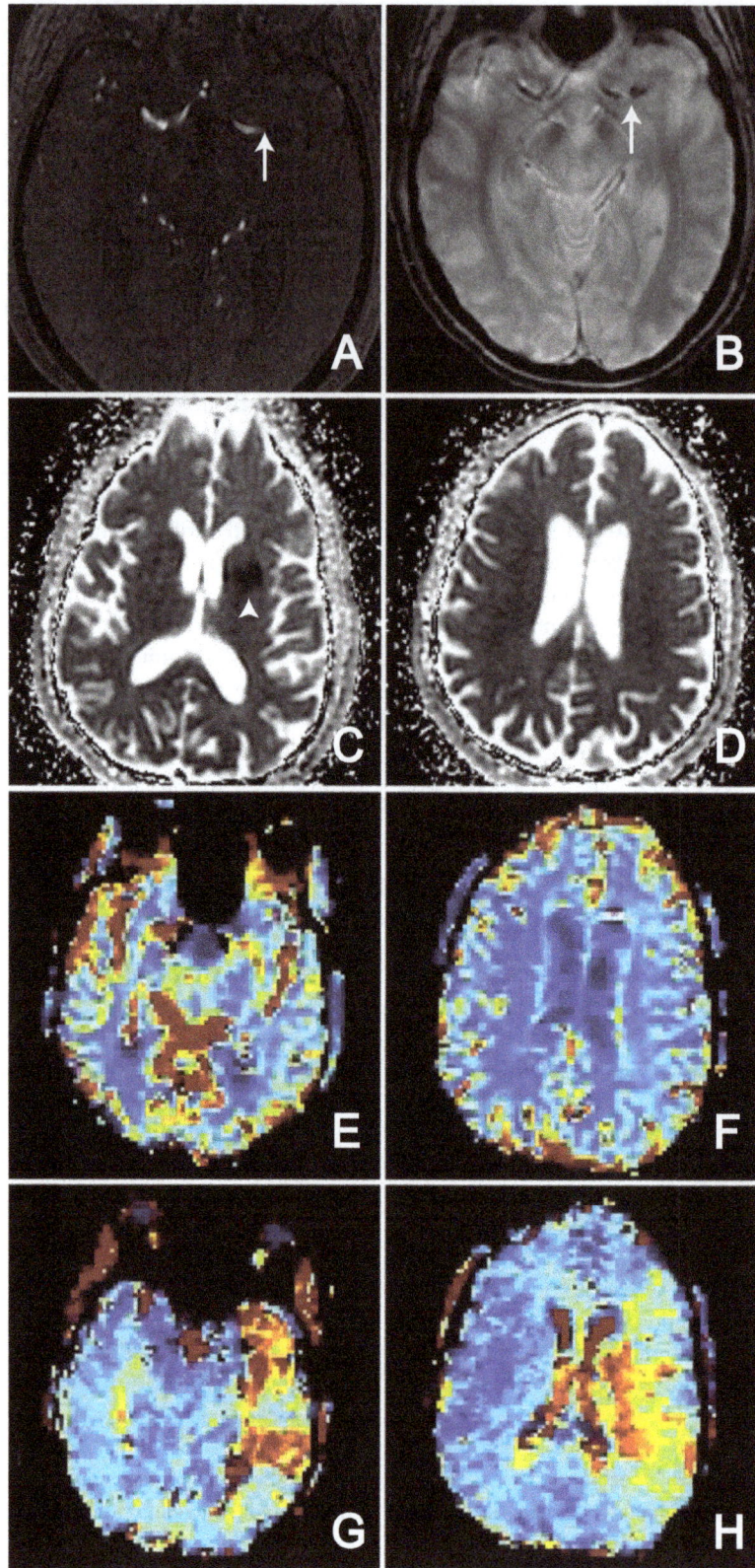

Fig. 4 (See legend on next page.)

(See figure on previous page.)
Fig. 4 Large ischemic penumbra with small core infarct in a 73 year-old with acute stroke. MRA shows acute M1 segment MCA vessel cutoff (arrow, **a**). Blooming artifact localizes to the occlusive thrombus on the GRE image (arrow, **b**). Apparent diffusion coefficient (**a, d, c**) map (**c, d**) demonstrating a small region of core infarct (arrowhead). CBV maps from the PCT show no region of decrease to suggest a large core infarct (**e, f**). Ischemic penumbra comprises the majority of the left MCA territory on the Tmax maps (**g, h**)

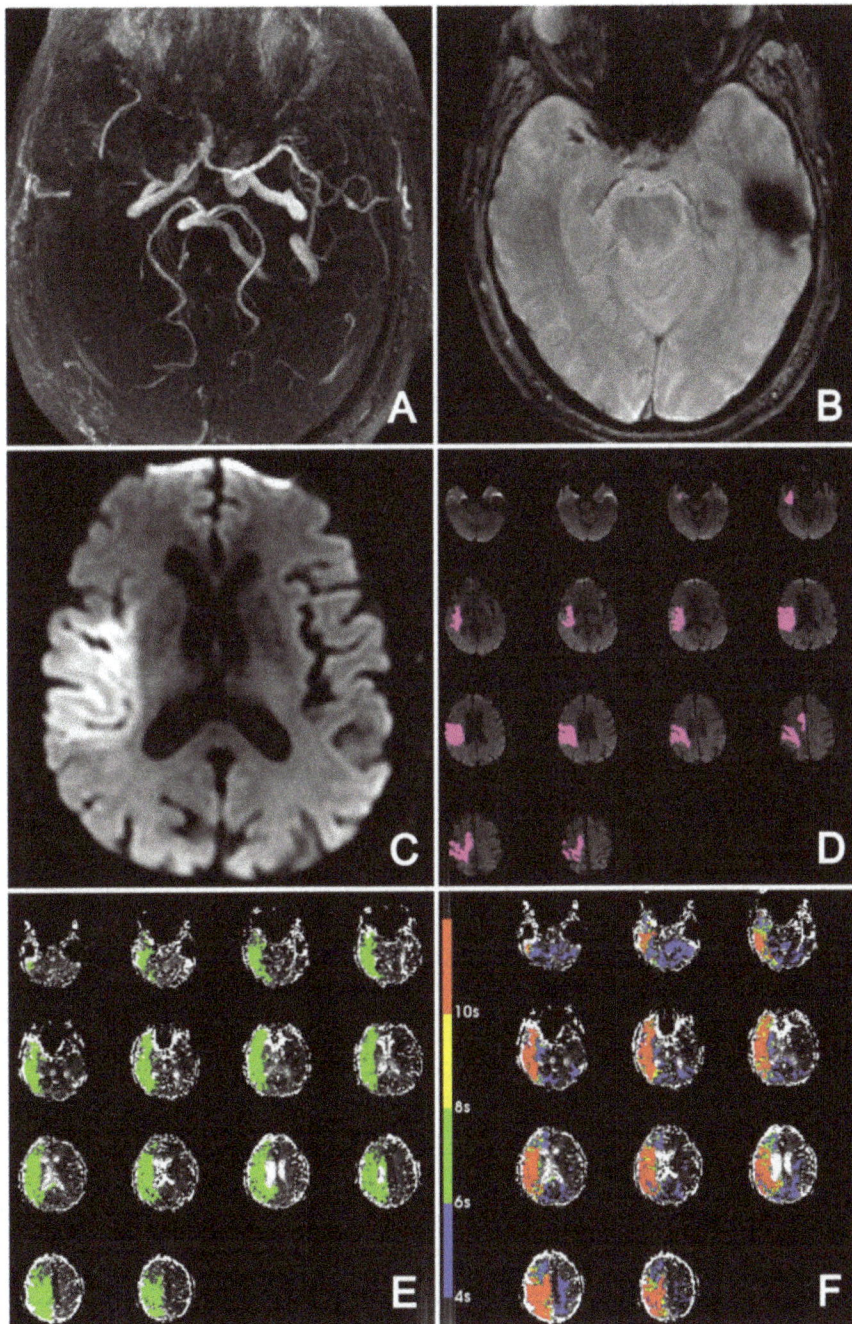

Fig. 5 Malignant perfusion profile in an 82-year-old with a right MCA syndrome. MRA showing a right M1 segment MCA occlusion (**a**). GRE image demonstrates blooming from thrombus at the site of occlusion (**b**, arrow). DWI image demonstrates a moderate-sized ischemic core (**c**), which is colorized on the perfusion map (pink, **d**). The ischemic penumbra is larger than the ischemic core (green, **e**) but in this instance is notable for a large volume of Tmax > 10s consistent with a malignant perfusion profile (**f**)

on FLAIR hours to days after gadolinium administration believed to be caused by accumulation of contrast material in the CSF spaces, and is associated with higher rates of hemorrhagic transformation of stroke [56]. Unfortunately since HARM is seen hours to days after an initial MRI, this is not useful for triage of interventional therapies. Blood brain barrier permeability increases with increasing neuronal injury as a result of ischemia-induced break down of tight junctions, and can be measured with perfusion imaging as expressed by a permeability surface area product (PS). This tool can prospectively stratify patients into those who will or will not go on to develop hemorrhagic conversion using a PS threshold of 0.23 mL/min/100 g [57]. Another study observed an odds ratio of 28 for hemorrhagic transformation discriminating with a PS of >0.84 mL/100 g/min [58]. While not in widespread use, this information is in theory readily available in centers that triage stroke with perfusion imaging.

Conclusion

Level I evidence showing a powerful benefit for endovascular stroke therapy makes this an exciting time for endovascular stroke therapy. On the other hand this evidence has created a need for consistent, effective and rapid triage of stroke patients to properly select those who will most benefit from endovascular stroke therapy. Recent trials have highlighted the need to select patients for endovascular stroke therapy based on the presence of a proximal arterial occlusive lesion, a small-to-moderate sized core infarct, and evidence of ischemic penumbra. While this is simple and quick to perform, it is not nuanced and many other useful imaging predictors of stroke outcome are not taken into consideration in such a simple model. This review has highlighted specific anatomical factors, imaging signs, and stroke physiology that have predictive value in the setting of the triage of a patient presenting with acute stroke. Looking forward, these imaging-specific factors could be included along with demographic factors such as patient age and baseline functional status in a more comprehensive prognostic model to assist in the triage of stroke patients.

Competing interests
The authors declare that they have no competing interests.

Authors' contributions
MW and NT each contributed to text. All authors read and approved the final manuscript.

References

1. Go AS, Mozaffarian D, Roger VL, Benjamin EJ, Berry JD, Blaha MJ, et al. Heart disease and stroke statistics–2014 update: a report from the American Heart Association. Circulation. 2014;129:e28–292.
2. Berkhemer OA, Fransen PS, Beumer D, van den Berg LA, Lingsma HF, Yoo AJ, et al. A randomized trial of intraarterial treatment for acute ischemic stroke. The New England journal of medicine. 2015;372:11–20.
3. Campbell BC, Mitchell PJ, Kleinig TJ, Dewey HM, Churilov L, Yassi N, et al. Endovascular therapy for ischemic stroke with perfusion-imaging selection. The New England journal of medicine. 2015;372:1009–18.
4. Jovin TG, Chamorro A, Cobo E, de Miquel MA, Molina CA, Rovira A, et al. Thrombectomy within 8 Hours after Symptom Onset in Ischemic Stroke. New Engl J Med. 2015;372:2296–2306.
5. Goyal M, Demchuk AM, Menon BK, Eesa M, Rempel JL, Thornton J, et al. Randomized assessment of rapid endovascular treatment of ischemic stroke. New Engl J Med. 2015;372:1019–30.
6. Furlan A, Higashida R, Wechsler L, Gent M, Rowley H, Kase C, et al. Intra-arterial Prourokinase for Acute Ischemic Stroke. Jama. 1999;282:2003.
7. U.S. Dept. of Health and Human Services. [http://www.fda.gov/drugs/developmentapprovalprocess/howdrugsaredevelopedandapproved/approvalapplications/therapeuticbiologicapplications/ucm113568.htm]
8. Broderick JP, Palesch YY, Demchuk AM, Yeatts SD, Khatri P, Hill MD, et al. Endovascular therapy after intravenous t-PA versus t-PA alone for stroke. New Engl J Med. 2013;368:893–903.
9. Ciccone A, Valvassori L, Nichelatti M, Sgoifo A, Ponzio M, Sterzi R, et al. Endovascular treatment for acute ischemic stroke. New Engl J Med. 2013;368:904–13.
10. Kidwell CS, Jahan R, Gornbein J, Alger JR, Nenov V, Ajani Z, et al. A trial of imaging selection and endovascular treatment for ischemic stroke. New Engl J Med. 2013;368:914–23.
11. Heit JJ, Wintermark M. Imaging selection for reperfusion therapy in acute ischemic stroke. Current treatment options in neurology. 2015;17:332.
12. Saver JL, Goyal M, Bonafe A, Diener HC, Levy EI, Pereira VM, et al. Solitaire with the Intention for Thrombectomy as Primary Endovascular Treatment for Acute Ischemic Stroke (SWIFT PRIME) trial: protocol for a randomized, controlled, multicenter study comparing the Solitaire revascularization device with IV tPA with IV tPA alone in acute ischemic stroke. Int J Stroke. 2015;10:439–48.
13. Rankin J. Cerebral vascular accidents in patients over the age of 60. II. Prognosis. Scot Med J. 1957;2:200–15.
14. Farrell B, Godwin J, Richards S, Warlow C. The United Kingdom transient ischaemic attack (UK-TIA) aspirin trial: final results. J Neurol Neurosurg Psychiatr. 1991;54:1044–54.
15. Gerber JC, Miaux YJ, von Kummer R. Scoring flow restoration in cerebral angiograms after endovascular revascularization in acute ischemic stroke patients. Neuroradiology. 2015;57:227–40.
16. Schaefer PW, Pulli B, Copen WA, Hirsch JA, Leslie-Mazwi T, Schwamm LH, et al. Combining MRI with NIHSS thresholds to predict outcome in acute ischemic stroke: value for patient selection. AJNR Am J Neuroradiol. 2015;36:259–64.
17. Zaidi SF, Aghaebrahim A, Urra X, Jumaa MA, Jankowitz B, Hammer M, et al. Final infarct volume is a stronger predictor of outcome than recanalization in patients with proximal middle cerebral artery occlusion treated with endovascular therapy. Stroke; a journal of cerebral circulation.2012;43:3238–44.
18. Thijs VN, Lansberg MG, Beaulieu C, Marks MP, Moseley ME, Albers GW. Is early ischemic lesion volume on diffusion-weighted imaging an independent predictor of stroke outcome? A multivariable analysis. Stroke; a journal of cerebral circulation. 2000;31:2597–602.
19. Saver JL, Johnston KC, Homer D, Wityk R, Koroshetz W, Truskowski LL, et al. Infarct volume as a surrogate or auxiliary outcome measure in ischemic stroke clinical trials. The RANTTAS Investigators. Stroke; a journal of cerebral circulation. 1999;30:293–8.
20. Vogt G, Laage R, Shuaib A, Schneider A, Collaboration V. Initial lesion volume is an independent predictor of clinical stroke outcome at day 90: an analysis of the Virtual International Stroke Trials Archive (VISTA) database. Stroke; a journal of cerebral circulation. 2012;43:1266–72.
21. Parsons MW, Christensen S, McElduff P, Levi CR, Butcher KS, De Silva DA, et al. Pretreatment diffusion- and perfusion-MR lesion volumes have a crucial influence on clinical response to stroke thrombolysis. J Cerebr Blood Flow Metab. 2010;30:1214–25.

22. Campbell BC, Purushotham A, Christensen S, Desmond PM, Nagakane Y, Parsons MW, et al. The infarct core is well represented by the acute diffusion lesion: sustained reversal is infrequent. J Cerebr Blood Flow Metabol. 2012;32:50–6.

23. Barber PA, Demchuk AM, Zhang J, Buchan AM. Validity and reliability of a quantitative computed tomography score in predicting outcome of hyperacute stroke before thrombolytic therapy. The Lancet. 2000;355:1670–4.

24. Puetz V, Dzialowski I, Hill MD, Demchuk AM. The Alberta Stroke Program Early CT Score in clinical practice: what have we learned? Int J Stroke. 2009;4:354–64.

25. Sun CH, Connelly K, Nogueira RG, Glenn BA, Zimmermann S, Anda K, et al. ASPECTS decay during inter-facility transfer predicts patient outcomes in endovascular reperfusion for ischemic stroke: a unique assessment of dynamic physiologic change over time. Journal of Neurointerventional Surgery. 2015;7:22–6.

26. Wintermark M. Brain perfusion-CT in acute stroke patients. Eur Radiol Suppl. 2005;15:d28–31.

27. Wintermark M, Flanders AE, Velthuis B, Meuli R, van Leeuwen M, Goldsher D, et al. Perfusion-CT assessment of infarct core and penumbra: receiver operating characteristic curve analysis in 130 patients suspected of acute hemispheric stroke. Stroke; a journal of cerebral circulation. 2006;37:979–85.

28. Computed Tomography Perfusion (CTP) to Predict Response to Recanalization in Ischemic Stroke Project (CRISP). [https://clinicaltrials.gov/ct2/show/NCT01622517]

29. Smith WS, Lev MH, English JD, Camargo EC, Chou M, Johnston SC, et al. Significance of large vessel intracranial occlusion causing acute ischemic stroke and TIA. Stroke; a journal of cerebral circulation. 2009;40:3834–40.

30. Mendonca N, Rodriguez-Luna D, Rubiera M, Boned-Riera S, Ribo M, Pagola J, et al. Predictors of tissue-type plasminogen activator nonresponders according to location of vessel occlusion. Stroke; a journal of cerebral circulation. 2012;43:417–21.

31. Saver JL, Jahan R, Levy EI, Jovin TG, Baxter B, Nogueira RG, et al. Solitaire flow restoration device versus the Merci Retriever in patients with acute ischaemic stroke (SWIFT): a randomised, parallel-group, non-inferiority trial. The Lancet. 2012;380:1241–9.

32. Nogueira RG, Lutsep HL, Gupta R, Jovin TG, Albers GW, Walker GA, et al. Trevo versus Merci retrievers for thrombectomy revascularisation of large vessel occlusions in acute ischaemic stroke (TREVO 2): a randomised trial. The Lancet. 2012;380:1231–40.

33. Lemmens R, Mlynash M, Straka M, Kemp S, Bammer R, Marks MP, et al. Comparison of the response to endovascular reperfusion in relation to site of arterial occlusion. Neurology. 2013;81:614–8.

34. Behme D, Kowoll A, Weber W, Mpotsaris A. M1 is not M1 in ischemic stroke: the disability-free survival after mechanical thrombectomy differs significantly between proximal and distal occlusions of the middle cerebral artery M1 segment. Journal of Neurointerventional Surgery. 2014;7:559–563.

35. Man S, Hussain MS, Wisco D, Katzan IL, Aoki J, Tateishi Y, et al. The location of pretreatment hyperdense middle cerebral artery sign predicts the outcome of intraarterial thrombectomy for acute stroke. J Neuroimaging. 2015;25:263–8.

36. Moftakhar P, English JD, Cooke DL, Kim WT, Stout C, Smith WS, et al. Density of thrombus on admission CT predicts revascularization efficacy in large vessel occlusion acute ischemic stroke. Stroke; a journal of cerebral circulation. 2013;44:243–5.

37. Liebeskind DS, Sanossian N, Yong WH, Starkman S, Tsang MP, Moya AL, et al. CT and MRI early vessel signs reflect clot composition in acute stroke. Stroke; a journal of cerebral circulation. 2011;42:1237–43.

38. Riedel CH, Zimmermann P, Jensen-Kondering U, Stingele R, Deuschl G, Jansen O. The importance of size: successful recanalization by intravenous thrombolysis in acute anterior stroke depends on thrombus length. Stroke; a journal of cerebral circulation. 2011;42:1775–7.

39. Shobha N, Bal S, Boyko M, Kroshus E, Menon BK, Bhatia R, et al. Measurement of length of hyperdense MCA sign in acute ischemic stroke predicts disappearance after IV tPA. J Neuroimaging. 2014;24:7–10.

40. Puetz V, Dzialowski I, Hill MD, Subramaniam S, Sylaja PN, Krol A, et al. Intracranial thrombus extent predicts clinical outcome, final infarct size and hemorrhagic transformation in ischemic stroke: the clot burden score. Int J Stroke. 2008;3:230–6.

41. Saver JL. Time is brain–quantified. Stroke; a journal of cerebral circulation. 2006;37:263–6.

42. Higashida RT, Furlan AJ, Roberts H, Tomsick T, Connors B, Barr J, et al. Trial design and reporting standards for intra-arterial cerebral thrombolysis for acute ischemic stroke. Stroke; a journal of cerebral circulation. 2003;34:e109–37.

43. Kucinski T, Koch C, Eckert B, Becker V, Kromer H, Heesen C, et al. Collateral circulation is an independent radiological predictor of outcome after thrombolysis in acute ischaemic stroke. Neuroradiology. 2003;45:11–8.

44. Bang OY, Saver JL, Kim SJ, Kim GM, Chung CS, Ovbiagele B, et al. Collateral flow predicts response to endovascular therapy for acute ischemic stroke. Stroke; a journal of cerebral circulation. 2011;42:693–9.

45. Maas MB, Lev MH, Ay H, Singhal AB, Greer DM, Smith WS, et al. Collateral vessels on CT angiography predict outcome in acute ischemic stroke. Stroke; a journal of cerebral circulation. 2009;40:3001–5.

46. McVerry F, Liebeskind DS, Muir KW. Systematic review of methods for assessing leptomeningeal collateral flow. AJNR Am J Neuroradiol. 2012;33:576–82.

47. Souza LC, Yoo AJ, Chaudhry ZA, Payabvash S, Kemmling A, Schaefer PW, et al. Malignant CTA collateral profile is highly specific for large admission DWI infarct core and poor outcome in acute stroke. AJNR Am J Neuroradiol. 2012;33:1331–6.

48. Liebeskind DS, Tomsick TA, Foster LD, Yeatts SD, Carrozzella J, Demchuk AM, et al. Collaterals at angiography and outcomes in the Interventional Management of Stroke (IMS) III trial. Stroke; a journal of cerebral circulation. 2014;45:759–64.

49. Liebeskind DS, Jahan R, Nogueira RG, Zaidat OO, Saver JL, Investigators S. Impact of collaterals on successful revascularization in Solitaire FR with the intention for thrombectomy. Stroke; a journal of cerebral circulation. 2014;45:2036–40.

50. Singer OC, Berkefeld J, Nolte CH, Bohner G, Reich A, Wiesmann M, et al. Collateral vessels in proximal middle cerebral artery occlusion: the ENDOSTROKE study. Radiology. 2015;274:851–8.

51. Nambiar V, Sohn SI, Almekhlafi MA, Chang HW, Mishra S, Qazi E, et al. CTA collateral status and response to recanalization in patients with acute ischemic stroke. AJNR Am J Neuroradiol. 2014;35:884–90.

52. Albers GW, Thijs VN, Wechsler L, Kemp S, Schlaug G, Skalabrin E, et al. Magnetic resonance imaging profiles predict clinical response to early reperfusion: the diffusion and perfusion imaging evaluation for understanding stroke evolution (DEFUSE) study. Ann Neurol. 2006;60:508–17.

53. Cho SH, Kim DG, Kim DS, Kim YH, Lee CH, Jang SH. Motor outcome according to the integrity of the corticospinal tract determined by diffusion tensor tractography in the early stage of corona radiata infarct. Neurosci Lett. 2007;426:123–7.

54. Lindenberg R, Zhu LL, Ruber T, Schlaug G. Predicting functional motor potential in chronic stroke patients using diffusion tensor imaging. Hum Brain Mapp. 2012;33:1040–51.

55. Puig J, Pedraza S, Blasco G, Daunis IEJ, Prados F, Remollo S, et al. Acute damage to the posterior limb of the internal capsule on diffusion tensor tractography as an early imaging predictor of motor outcome after stroke. AJNR Am J Neuroradiol. 2011;32:857–63.

56. Warach S, Latour LL. Evidence of reperfusion injury, exacerbated by thrombolytic therapy, in human focal brain ischemia using a novel imaging marker of early blood-brain barrier disruption. Stroke; a journal of cerebral circulation. 2004;35:2659–61.

57. Aviv RI, d'Esterre CD, Murphy BD, Hopyan JJ, Buck B, Mallia G, et al. Hemorrhagic transformation of ischemic stroke: prediction with CT perfusion. Radiology. 2009;250:867–77.

58. Ozkul-Wermester O, Guegan-Massardier E, Triquenot A, Borden A, Perot G, Gerardin E. Increased blood-brain barrier permeability on perfusion computed tomography predicts hemorrhagic transformation in acute ischemic stroke. Eur Neurol. 2014;72:45–53.

7

Accidental microembolic signals: prevalence and clinical relevance

Jie Chen[1,2], Ying-Huan Hu[1], Shan Gao[1] and Wei-Hai Xu[1*]

Abstract

Background: The purpose of this study was to examine the occurrence of accidental microembolic signals (MES) and its clinical relevance in patients receiving routine transcranial Doppler (TCD) examinations.

Methods: We retrospectively reviewed our institutional TCD database (from January 2007–November 2012). The arteries with positive MES, the presumed sources of emboli and the clinical backgrounds were analyzed.

Results: A total of 10,067 patients received routine TCD examinations in our laboratory during the research period. MES were detected in 98 arteries of 78 patients, with a frequency of 0.77 % of all the recruited patients. A high percentage of MES (64.3 %) were detected in MCAs. Sixty five (83.33 %) accidental emboli were from arterial sources, including atherosclerotic cerebral or carotid artery stenosis ($n = 45$), moyamoya disease ($n = 11$), intracranial arteries ($n = 3$) and Takayasu arteritis ($n = 3$). Thirteen (16.67 %) emboli were from cardiac sources, including atrial fibrillation ($n = 3$), artificial valves ($n = 8$), infective endocarditis ($n = 2$), patent foramen ovale ($n = 2$), and systemic lupus erythematosus ($n = 1$). In artificial valves disease, all patients with MES were asymptomatic, while in atherosclerotic cerebral or carotid artery stenosis, 66.67 % ($n = 30$) patients with MES were symptomatic. In different diseases with accidental MES, the proportion of symptomatic patients and asymptomatic patients were different ($p < 0.001$).

Conclusions: MES are not uncommon during routine TCD examinations, the clinical value of which varied in different diseases.

Keywords: Emboli, Microembolic signal, Stroke, Transcranial Doppler

Background

Microembolic signals (MES) - the high-intensity transient signals detected by transcranial Doppler (TCD) - have been shown to correspond to microembolic materials within the cerebral arteries [1]. MES can be detected in various clinical settings, such as carotid or intracranial stenosis, atrial fibrillation, and mechanical heart valves etc. Although most of these microemboli are clinically silent, many studies found that MES indicate increased risk of ischemic stroke, transient ischemic attack (TIA) or cognitive decline [2, 3].

According to the consensus on microembolus detection by TCD, the preferred recording time for patients with carotid stenosis or atrial fibrillation is at least 1 h

[4]. However, it is difficult to monitor the arteries for such a long time for each patient. During routine TCD examinations, MES can be detected occasionally. The occurrence and its clinical relevance have remained unknown. The goal of this study was to investigate accidental MES in a large TCD database.

Patients and methods

We retrospectively reviewed our institutional TCD database for hospitalized patients from January 2007–November 2012. During this period, the presence of accidental MES in routine TCD examinations was regularly recorded. All the patients in the database were unselectively recruited, including the patients from neurology, endocrine, cardiology and surgery departments. The reasons for TCD examinations varied, depending on the clinicians' intention. According to the practice standards for TCD, the clinical indications included cerebral ischemia, intracranial arterial

* Correspondence: xuwh@pumch.cn
[1]Department of Neurology, Peking Union Medical College Hospital, Chinese Academy of Medical Sciences and Peking Union Medical College, Shuaifuyuan 1, Dongcheng District, Beijing 100730, China
Full list of author information is available at the end of the article

disease, detection of right-to-left shunts, sub-arachnoid hemorrhage, brain death, and periprocedural or surgical monitoring [5]. All the recruited patients underwent a careful review of previous ischemic stroke and TIA history. Thorough evaluations were performed to determine the cause of stroke or TIA, including magnetic resonance image, carotid duplex, TCD, and electrocardiogram.

Ethics, consent and permissions

The study was approved by the Peking Union Medical College Hospital Research Ethics Committee. All the patients signed a consent form.

Transcranial doppler examination

Cerebral arteries were examined with 2-MHz Doppler instrument (Pioneer TC-8080 and Companion III, Nicolet-EME) according to standard protocol, including middle cerebral arteries (MCA), anterior cerebral arteries (ACA), posterior cerebral arteries (PCA), and C1 segment of the internal carotid arteries (ICA) through cranial temporal bone windows; ophthalmic arteries (OA) and ICA siphon through orbital windows; terminal vertebral arteries (VA) and basilar arteries (BA) through foraminal window [4]. And carotid arteries were also insonated by using 4-MHz probe, including extracranial ICA, external carotid arteries (ECA) [6]. All TCD examinations were performed by an experienced sonographer.

Microembolic signals detection

MES data were recorded and analyzed by an experienced observer, who was blinded to the clinical information. The following definitions for MES were used: typical visible and audible (click, chirp, whistle), short-duration, unidirectional, high-intensity signal (≥ 5 dB) within the Doppler flow spectrum with its occurrence at random in the cardiac cycle [7].

Statistical analysis

Student's t-test was performed to compare continuous variables; Pearson $\chi 2$ and Fisher's exact test were used to compare categorical variables between groups. A p value less than 0.05 was considered statistically significant. All statistical analyses were done with SPSS 16.0 (SPSS Inc).

Results

During the study period, a total of 10,067 patients (5162 male, mean age 56.7 ± 17.4) received routine TCD examinations in our laboratory. Among them, 2305 (22.90 %) patients had previous ischemic events or TIA.

MES was detected in 98 arteries of 78 patients, with a frequency of 0.77 % of all the recruited patients. The MES positive arteries including MCA ($n = 63$), ACA ($n = 8$), SCA ($n = 8$), extracranial ICA ($n = 8$), PCA ($n = 5$),

BA ($n = 2$), VA ($n = 2$), ECA ($n = 1$) and OA ($n = 1$, Table 1).

Sixty five (83.33 %) accidental emboli were presumed to come from arterial sources, including atherosclerotic cerebral or carotid artery stenosis ($n = 45$), moyamoya disease ($n = 11$, Fig. 1), intracranial arteries ($n = 3$) and Takayasu arteries ($n = 3$). Thirteen (16.67 %) emboli were presumed to come from cardiac sources, including atrial fibrillation ($n = 3$), artificial valves ($n = 8$), infective endocarditis ($n = 2$), patent foramen ovale ($n = 2$), and systemic Lupus Erythematosus ($n = 1$, Table 2).

In different diseases with accidental MES, the proportion of symptomatic patients and asymptomatic patients were different (Fisher exact test, $p < 0.001$). In artificial valves disease, all patients with MES were asymptomatic, while in atherosclerotic cerebral or carotid artery stenosis, 66.67 % ($n = 30$) patients with MES were symptomatic (Table 2).

Discussion

In this study, accidental MES during routine TCD examinations were investigated in hospitalized patients with a large sample size. Overall, MES can be detected in 3 of 400 unselected hospitalized patients. A high percentage of MES (64.3 %) were detected in MCAs. It was not only because MCA is the common site of intracranial atherosclerosis and the largest artery that distributes blood to the cerebrum, but also the testing time of MCA was the longest, as the whole M1 segment could be detected by TCD.

The clinical significance of MES varied, as MES span a broad spectrum, ranging from harmless air bubbles to the large solid emboli [8]. In patients with artificial valves, none of the 8 patients with MES had the symptoms of cerebral ischemia, probably because the air bubbles produced by artificial valves are harmless. In atherosclerotic cerebral or carotid artery stenosis, however, 66.67 %

Table 1 Arteries with microembolic signals

Arteries MES(+)	n (%)
MCA	63 (64.3)
SCA	8 (8.2)
ACA	8 (8.2)
ICAex	8 (8.2)
PCA	5 (5.1)
BA	2 (2.0)
VA	2 (2.0)
ECA	1 (1.0)
OA	1 (1.0)

MCA middle cerebral artery, *SCA* internal carotid artery siphon segment, *ACA* anterior cerebral artery, *ICAex* extracranial internal carotid artery, *PCA* posterior cerebral artery, *BA* basilar artery, *VA* vertebral artery, *ECA* external carotid artery, *OA* ophthalmic artery

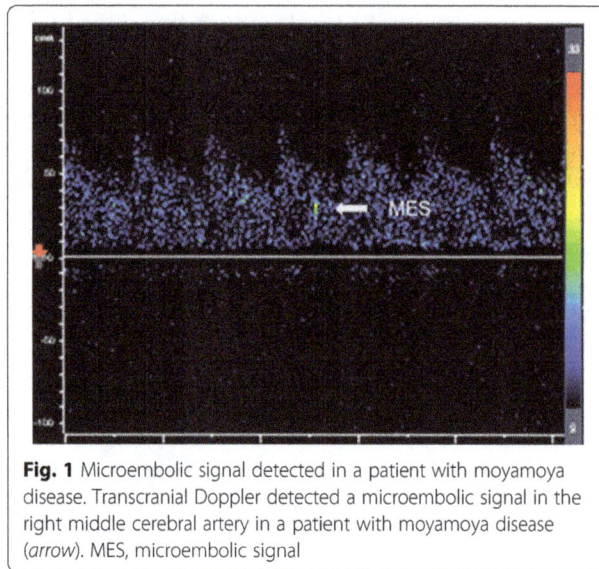

Fig. 1 Microembolic signal detected in a patient with moyamoya disease. Transcranial Doppler detected a microembolic signal in the right middle cerebral artery in a patient with moyamoya disease (*arrow*). MES, microembolic signal

patients with MES were symptomatic. It has been confirmed that the presence of MES was an independent predictor of future stroke in atherosclerotic occlusive cerebrovascular diseases [2, 7]. According to the practice standards for TCD, in patients with symptomatic and asymptomatic extracranial or intracranial large artery disease, the MES information could be used to detect, localize, and quantify cerebral embolization, which may be helpful to establish the diagnosis and change management strategy [5]. For example, one study demonstrated that in patients with MCA stenosis, the presence of an MES was associate with cerebral ischemia on diffusion weighted magnetic resonance imaging [9]. Thus the diffusion weighted imaging procedure might be helpful for these patients to detect cerebral ischemia. As to the therapy strategy, two randomized clinical trials demonstrated that in patients with symptomatic carotid stenosis (≥50 %) and

symptomatic cerebral or carotid artery stenosis, combination therapy with clopidogrel and aspirin was more effective than aspirin alone in reducing MES [10, 11]. Accidental MES in routine TCD examinations may also be an indicator for robust antiplatelet therapy.

It is interesting that MES were also observed in non-atherosclerotic artery stenosis including moyamoya disease, Takayasu's arteritis, and intracranial arteries. It provide evidence that artery-to-artery embolism may also play an important role in the underlying mechanism of ischemic stroke in these patients [12].

This study was a single-center retrospective investigation. There was a possibility of selection bias and information bias.

Conclusions

In conclusion, our study suggests that MES are not uncommon during routine TCD examinations, the clinical value of which varied in different diseases. MES detection during routine TCD examinations may be of potential clinical value in the management of patients.

Abbreviations
ACA: anterior cerebral arteries; BA: basilar arteries; ECA: external carotid arteries; ICA: internal carotid arteries; MCA: middle cerebral arteries; MES: accidental microembolic signals; OA: ophthalmic arteries; PCA: posterior cerebral arteries; TCD: transcranial doppler; TIA: transient ischemic attack; VA: vertebral arteries.

Competing interests
The authors declare no financial or other conflict of interests.

Authors' contributions
This study was designed by WHX and SG. JC, YQH conducted experiments and performed data analysis. The manuscript was written by JC and revision form WHX. All authors read and approved the final manuscript.

Author details
[1]Department of Neurology, Peking Union Medical College Hospital, Chinese Academy of Medical Sciences and Peking Union Medical College, Shuaifuyuan 1, Dongcheng District, Beijing 100730, China. [2]Department of Neurology, Beijing Tiantan Hospital, Capital Medical University, Beijing 10050, China.

Table 2 Sources of accidental emboli

	Symptomatic	Asymptomatic
Arterial Sources		
Atherosclerotic cerebral or carotid artery stenosis	30	15
Moyamoya disease	9	2
Intracranial arteries	3	0
Takayasu arteries	0	3
Cardiac Sources		
Atrial fibrillation	2	1
Artificial valves	0	8
Infective endocarditis	1	1
Patent foramen ovale	1	1
Systemic Lupus Erythematosus	1	0

References
1. Spencer MP, Thomas GI, Nicholls SC, Sauvage LR. Detection of middle cerebral artery emboli during carotid endarterectomy using transcranial Doppler ultrasonography. Stroke. 1990;21:415–23.
2. Ritter MA. Prevalence and prognostic impact of microembolic signals in arterial sources of embolism. J Neurol. 2008;255:953–61.
3. Purandare N, Voshaar RC, Morris J, Byrne JE, Wren J, Heller RF, et al. Asymptomatic spontaneous cerebral emboli predict cognitive and functional decline in dementia. Biol Psychiatry. 2007;62:339–44.
4. Ringelstein EB, Droste DW, Babikian VL, Evans DH, Grosset DG, Kaps M, et al. Consensus on microembolus detection by TCD. International Consensus Group on Microembolus Detection. Stroke. 1998;29:725–9.
5. Alexandrov AV, Sloan MA, Tegeler CH, Newell DN, Lumsden A, Garami Z, et al. Practice standards for transcranial Doppler (TCD) ultrasound. Part II. Clinical indications and expected outcomes. J Neuroimaging. 2012;22:215–24.
6. Sloan MA, Alexandrov AV, Tegeler CH, Spencer MP, Caplan LR, Feldmann E, et al. Assessment: transcranial Doppler ultrasonography: report of the

Therapeutics and Technology Assessment Subcommittee of the American Academy of Neurology. Neurology. 2004;62:468–81.

7. Gao S, Wong KS, Hansberg T, Lam WW, Droste DW, Ringelstein EB. Microembolic signal predicts recurrent cerebral ischemic events in acute stroke patients with middle cerebral artery stenosis. Stroke. 2004;35:2832–6.

8. Choi Y, Saqqur M, Stewart E, Stephenson C, Roy J, Boulanger JM, et al. Relative energy index of microembolic signal can predict malignant microemboli. Stroke. 2010;41:700–6.

9. Wong KS, Gao S, Chan YL, Hansberg T, Lam WW, Droste DW, et al. Mechanisms of acute cerebral infarctions in patients with middle cerebral artery stenosis: a diffusion-weighted imaging and microemboli monitoring study. Ann Neurol. 2002;52:74–81.

10. Markus HS, Droste DW, Kaps M, Larrue V, Lees KR, Siebler M, et al. Dual antiplatelet therapy with clopidogrel and aspirin in symptomatic carotid stenosis evaluated using doppler embolic signal detection: the Clopidogrel and Aspirin for Reduction of Emboli in Symptomatic Carotid Stenosis (CARESS) trial. Circulation. 2005;111:2233–40.

11. Wong KS, Chen C, Fu J, Chang HM, Suwanwela NC, Huang YN, et al. Clopidogrel plus aspirin versus aspirin alone for reducing embolisation in patients with acute symptomatic cerebral or carotid artery stenosis (CLAIR study): a randomised, open-label, blinded-endpoint trial. Lancet Neurol. 2010;9:489–97.

12. Chen J, Duan L, Xu WH, Han YQ, Cui LY, Gao S. Microembolic signals predict cerebral ischaemic events in patients with moyamoya disease. Eur J Neurol. 2014;21:785–90.

8

The predictive value of a targeted posterior fossa multimodal stroke protocol for the diagnosis of acute posterior ischemic stroke

Michal Sharon[1], Karl Boyle[2], Robert Yeung[1], Liying zhang[1], Sean P. Symons[1], Mark I. Boulos[2] and Richard I. Aviv[1*]

Abstract

Background: There is limited but growing research regarding the accuracy of CTP in diagnosing acute posterior ischemia stroke. We sought to evaluate the diagnostic accuracy of an incremental multimodal CT protocol in acute posterior ischemic stroke.

Methods: Retrospective review of incremental NCCT, CTA-source images and CTP use in 82 consecutive patients with acute posterior ischemic stroke. Readers were blinded to infarct status on follow-up imaging (MRI or CT). Predictive effects of observed diagnostic accuracy and confidence score were quantified with the entropy r^2 value. Sensitivity, specificity, and CI were calculated accounting for multiple reader assessments. Receiver Operating Characteristic analyses, including Area Under the Curve, were conducted for the three modalities. Inter-reader agreement was established with Intraclass Correlation Coefficient.

Results: Follow-up imaging confirmed infarct in 69/82 (84 %) patients. Multimodal protocol with CTP, outperforms CTA-source images and NCCT for correct acute posterior ischemia stroke diagnosis. The Area Under the Curve was 0.741 (95 % CI 0.708–0.773); 0.70 (95 % CI 0.663–0.731, $P = 0.03$) and 0.62 (95 % CI 0.588–0.659, $P < 0.0001$), respectively. Incrementally improved correlation between observed and actual diagnosis ($r^2 = 0.09$, 0.26 and 0.32) and a higher rate of certainty (51.4, 69.3 and 81.7 %) was demonstrated for NCCT, CTA-source images and CTP respectively. Inter-reader agreement for the actual diagnosis was good and improved from 0.68 to 0.83 with incremental multimodal CT use.

Conclusions: CTP enhances confident and correct infarct diagnosis over NCCT and CTA-source images in acute posterior ischemia stroke.

Keywords: Posterior fossa stroke, Ischemia, Infarct, CTP, Acute ischemic stroke, Multimodal CT, Posterior circulation

Background

Acute posterior ischemia stroke accounts for 20 % of ischemic stroke [1] and is most commonly cardioembolic followed by large-artery atherosclerosis [2]. Non contrast CT (NCCT) performs poorly at detecting acute posterior-fossa stroke even utilizing posterior circulation Alberta stroke program early CT score (ASPECTS) [3], largely due to beam hardening artifacts and insufficient contrast resolution. MRI and particularly DWI remains the mainstay of infarct diagnosis but is not yet widely adopted in acute stroke imaging due to its

reduced availability, increased cost and scan time. Although the reference standard, DWI demonstrates reduced sensitivity in the context of small and posterior fossa infarction [4]. Both CT angiography (CTA) and CT perfusion (CTP) are previously evaluated in the posterior fossa. CTA-source image (CTA-SI) hypoattenuation is shown to improve detection of posterior fossa infarction and is predictive of clinical outcome [5]. CTP is fast and effective in the emergency evaluation of acute anterior-circulation infarction [6–8] and increases diagnostic certainty for clinical stroke by expert and nonexpert readers over CTA-SI [7] and correlates with MRI DWI [9]. Drawbacks of CT include radiation dose and limited spatial coverage with many centres omitting the posterior-fossa by necessity in favour of supratentorial

* Correspondence: richard.aviv@sunnybrook.ca
[1]Department of Diagnostic Imaging, Division of Neuroradiology, Room AG 31, Sunnybrook Health Sciences Centre, 2075 Bayview Ave, Toronto, ON M4N 3M5, Canada
Full list of author information is available at the end of the article

coverage. CTP however can be directed to evaluate the posterior fossa according to clinical presentation. Literature regarding the diagnostic performance of posterior-fossa CTP is limited but growing with only three recently published articles [10–12]. Advances in CT such as a table-toggle technique or increase detector number [13], now facilitate more extensive brain coverage with increasing visualization of the posterior fossa. However this extended coverage is not yet widely available. With increasing CTP imaging of the posterior fossa expected, further study of the strengths and limitations of CTP within the context of posterior ischemic stroke is needed. The purpose of this study was therefore to assess the predictive value of each component (NCCT, CTA-SI and CTP) of an incremental CT protocol using targeted posterior fossa CTP for the assessment of posterior ischemic stroke presentation.

Methods

Ethics, consent and permissions

The study was approved by the local institutional research ethics board (Research Ethics Human Research Program, Sunnybrook Health Sciences Centre).

Signed was obtained from each patient or substitute decision maker for study enrollment and publication.

Study design and patients

A retrospective cohort of consecutive acute posterior ischemia stroke patients presenting to a tertiary stroke-center emergency department between 2010 and 2012. Targeted posterior fossa CTP was performed prospectively in patients presenting with signs and symptoms of acute posterior ischemia stroke, diagnosed by an experienced Neurologist (xx, 7 years) within 12 h of symptom onset. Patients were included if their final diagnosis based on clinical and imaging findings was TIA or infarct as arbitrated by the Neurologist. Patients with stroke mimics, fetal posterior cerebral artery on baseline CTA or those with contraindications to iodinated-contrast such as allergy or severe renal impairment (GFR < 20) were excluded. Patients with intracranial stenosis were not excluded from the cohort. Baseline clinical data included gender, age, cardiovascular risk factors, NIHSS (National Institutes of Health Stroke Scale) score, rtPA status and dose.

CT protocol

The CT stroke protocol was performed on a 64-section VCT (GE Healthcare). Aortic-arch to vertex CTA was obtained [7]. CTA source-image (CTA-SI) reformations (4 mm thick, 2-mm gap) were aligned to match the NCCT image. The 40-mm slab biphasic CTP commenced inferior to the frontal horns covering most of the posterior fossa, yet retaining visualization of the bilateral anterior cerebral artery and torcula for ROI placement. First phase was 45 s scan reconstructed at 0.5 s intervals followed by 6 further acquisitions 15 s apart for an additional 90s. CTP parameters are: 80 kVp, 100 mA, 0.5 ml/kg (maximum 50 ml) iodinated contrast agent injected at 4 ml/s with a 3–5 s delay [7]. Effective-doses of individual components are NCCT 1.2mSV, CTA 2.4mSV and CTP 2.5mSV. Lifetime attributable risk of cancer for NCCT at the median age of the studied cohort is 0.01 % [14]. Follow-up was performed at 5–7 days on MRI (57/82; 70 %), unless a readily visible hypodensity involving the affected vascular territory was demonstrated on follow-up NCCT (25/82;30 %). MRI minimally included DWI/ADC maps (TR = 8125 ms/ min TE; 26-cm field of view; 128 × 128 matrix; 5-mm section thickness; no intersection gap) and FLAIR (TR = 8000 ms/ TE = 120 ms/ TI = 200 ms; 22-cm field of view; 320 × 224 matrix; 5-mm section thickness; 1-mm intersection gap).

Image processing

Commercially available software (CTP4; GE Healthcare) was used to calculate CTP maps with color-coding of cerebral blood volume (CBV), cerebral blood flow (CBF) and mean transit time (MTT). Generation of arterial and venous time attenuation curves was based on manual selection of the arterial input function (AIF) within the anterior cerebral artery and the torcula, respectively [7].

Review protocol

Images were reviewed by three readers blinded to imaging outcome; including a neuroradiologist (4 years of experience), a neuroradiology fellow and a neurology fellow (2 years' experience each). The review method simulated the clinical review process, beginning with NCCT, followed by CTA-SI and CTP color maps [7, 15]. Therefore, three DICOM folders were prepared containing NCCT, NCCT + CTA-SI and NCCT + CTA-SI + CTP. In all cases the posterior-circulation ASPECTS [16] regions were specifically reviewed to ensure a systematic approach to scan review and to maximize detection. Images were reviewed independently by the readers in three stages, one for each modality, 2 weeks apart to avoid recall-bias. The readers documented in each step the presence or absence of ischemia/infarction, based on parenchymal hypoattenuation on NCCT (infarct) and CTA-SI (ischemia/infarction) [17] , qualitative MTT prolongation and CTP CBF/CBV reduction. We specifically included qualitative CTP because most centers cannot use thresholded parameters in the acute setting. We justified the inclusion of purely ischemic patterns (MTT prolongation/ CBF reduction in the absence of a visible CBV defect) in addition to overt infarction (CBV reduction) because even in the context of TIA (with clinical

improvement), a perfusion abnormality (signifying ischemia) is associated with an increased probability of DWI/
ADC infarction at presentation or follow-up [18, 19].
This approach has been used before in the supratentor-
ium [7] in a recent study of lacunar infarction [15] and
posterior fossa CTP [12]. For each posterior fossa AS-
PECTS location a positive diagnosis required localization
to right, left or midline and was scored individually for
each modality (total scores 738 for 3 readers). Therefore
a positive diagnosis in an incorrect location was considered a false-positive for that location and a false-negative
observation for the true infarct location. A six-point
level of confidence-score was assigned (1-infarct/ische-
mia definitely present; 2- probably present; 3-equivocal
but suspicious for infarct/ischemia; 4-equivocal but in-
farct/ischemia presumed absent; 5- infarct/ischemia
probably absent; 6- definitely absent). Additionally,
readers indicated the affected vascular territory (basi-
lar/perforator, posterior cerebral artery, PICA, AICA,
superior cerebellar artery) based on standard vascular
anatomy texts. Readers documented their observations
separately for each sequence group, without access to
prior entries. Final infarct status/ clinical diagnosis
was based on DWI/ADC restriction, NCCT hypoattenuation and final clinical diagnosis as assessed by an
experienced Neurologist, XX 4 years.

Statistical analysis

Results were expressed as mean ± standard deviation
or median + interquartile range (IQR) for quantitative
variables and as proportions for categorical findings.
Logistic-regression analysis predicted actual from observed stroke diagnosis for the incremental protocol
adjusting for confidence scores. OR and 95 % CI were
calculated. Actual and observed diagnostic performance was recorded as 0 (absence) and 1 (presence) with
l level of confidence score 1 to 6. Combined predictive
effects of the observed diagnostic performance and
confidence scores in the model were quantified with
the entropy r^2value, where the higher the r^2 value the
better the model. Akaike information criterion (AIC)
was compared among the three incremental review
steps with a lower AIC signifying a better model. Diagnostic accuracy of the incremental protocol was evaluated with Receiver Operating Characteristic (ROC)
curve and Area under the Curve (AUC) comparisons
[20]. Generalized estimating equations calculated real
stroke confirmation from observed diagnosis adjusting for
confidence score. A generalized linear model with a bino-
mial distribution was performed using the generalized
estimating equation method. Quasilikelihood-information
criterion (QIC) was applied to the model fit of the generalized estimating equation with smaller values indicating a
better model fit. Because of the correlation resulting from

multiple reader assessments on the same images and the
various CT protocols applying to the same subject, the individual sensitivity (Se_i) and specificity (Sp_i) were calculated from the cross table of real stroke diagnosis and
observed diagnosis for each sequence [21]. Inter-reader
agreement was established with intraclass-correlation coefficient (ICC) [22] to estimate inter-reader concordance
for the actual diagnosis. ICC of ≤ 0.20, 0.21–0.40, 0.41–
0.60, 0.61–0.80 and 0.81– 1.0 were defined as a poor, fair,
moderate, good and very good concordance. A T-test was
applied to compare ICC generated using the bootstrap
method of 1000 generated and calculated sample sets.
Analyses were performed with statistical software package
(SAS version 9.3; SAS Institute, Cary, NC). Results were
considered significant at $p < 0.05$.

Results

There were 82 patients (43/82; 52 % female) with a mean
age of 70 ± 16 years. Baseline demographic characteristics
are listed in Table 1. Infarct was confirmed on follow up
imaging in 69/82 (84 %) of patients, while the remaining
13 patients were diagnosed with TIA; 35/69 (51 %) were
female. Median posterior-circulation ASPECTS was 10
(IQR range 9–10) with 149/5, 904 (2.5 %) positive regions
(82 patients × 3 readers × 8 regions [16]). Median NIHSS
was 4 (IQR 3–7). No statistically significant difference in
age, gender, NIHSS or cardiovascular risk factors was
present in patients with confirmed infarct versus patients

Table 1 Baseline Demographic Characteristics of 82 patients
with suspected acute posterior ischemic stroke

Female Gender	43 (52)
Cardiovascular risk factors	
Hypertension	28 (34)
Diabetes mellitus	33 (40)
Coronary artery disease	18 (22)
Atrial fibrillation	37 (45)
Smoking	34 (41)
Hypercholesterolemia	15 (18)
Presence of infarct on follow up imaging	69 (84)
Large vessel infarct*	63 (91)
Affected side on follow up imaging	
Right	31 (45)
Left	25 (36)
Midline	5 (7)
Bilateral	8 (12)
Imaging follow up	
MRI	57 (70)
CT	25 (30)

All values represent n (%)
* of 69 patients with confirmed infarct on follow up imaging

without infarct. Median time from symptom-onset to baseline CT was 115 min (IQR 89–215). Median time to follow-up was 1 day (IQR 0–1). IV rtPA was administered in 23/82 (28 %) with mean dose of 56 ± 21 mg and within a median of 144 min (IQR 134–186). No patients received intra-arterial thrombolysis. Twenty (87 %) of the rtPA-treated patients had confirmed infarct on follow-up imaging. The vascular distribution of posterior ischemic stroke using the incremental CT protocol is summarized on Table 2.

NCCT, CTA and CTP abnormality was present in 43/82 (52.4 %), 44 (53.7 %) and 62 (75.6 %) patients and 56 (13.7 %), 93 (22.7 %) and 117 (29 %) of 410 vascular territories (5 vascular territories × 82 patients) on NCCT, CTA and CTP respectively. The AUC was greater for CTP 0.741 (95 % CI 0.708 - 0.773) compared to CTA-SI 0.70 (95 % CI 0.663–0.731, $P = 0.03$) and NCCT 0.62 (95 % CI 0.588–0.659, $P < 0.0001$), respectively (Fig. 1). Similarly, CTA-SI outperformed NCCT ($P = 0.0001$). For confident diagnosis of infarct absence (Table 3) CTP sensitivity trended 12.6 % higher than CTA-SI ($p = 0.072$) and was significantly higher than NCCT. For confident diagnosis of infarct presence, CTP sensitivity was 15.8 and 30.2 % greater than CTA-SI and NCCT respectively ($p = 0.025$ and $p < 0.0001$) (Figs. 2 and 3). No specificity differences were seen for CTP over CTA-SI although both CTA-SI and CTP showed improvement over NCCT. Table 4 depicts the distribution of the readers' confidence scores for each modality. Significant reduction of equivocal diagnoses is demonstrated between NCCT (68; 9.2 %) and CTA-SI/ CTP (30; 4.1 % for each modality). More confident diagnosis or infarct exclusion was seen with multimodal CT use (NCCT 51.4 %, CTA 69.3 % and CTP 81.7 %) with higher entropy r^2 and lower AIC, confirming better correlation between the observed and actual diagnosis.

Progressive entropy r^2 increase occurred from 0.09 (NCCT), to 0.26 (CTA-SI) and 0.32 (CTP; Table 5). Similarly, the QIC declined from NCCT to CTA-SI and CTP indicating increasingly better fit between the readers' observed diagnosis and confirmed infarcts. Inter-reader agreement for actual diagnosis was good and improved incrementally with multimodal CT use from 0.59 to 0.87 (Table 6). CTP inter-reader agreement was significantly improved over both NCCT and CTA-SI.

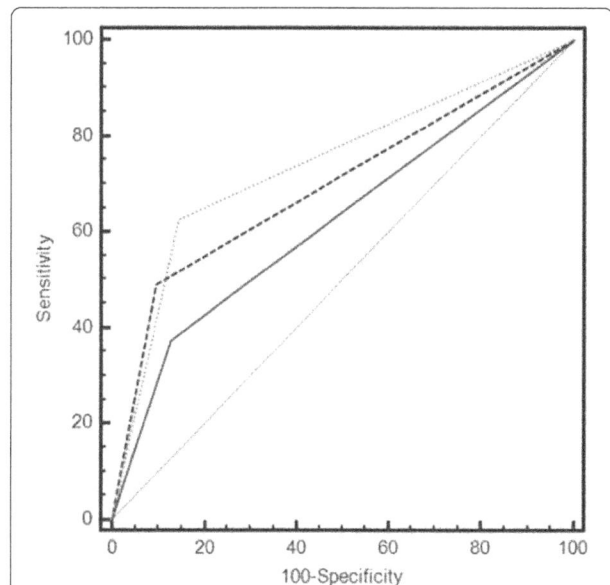

Fig. 1 Receiver Operating Characteristic curves for diagnostic performance of incremental CT protocol for posterior ischemic stroke. The area under the curve of protocol containing targeted posterior fossa CTP (dotted orange line) was greater compared to CTA-SI (dashed brown line, $p = 0.03$) or NCCT (solid blue line $p < 0.0001$)

Discussion

A multimodal CT protocol including targeted posterior-fossa CTP improved acute posterior ischemic stroke diagnosis over NCCT alone or a combination of NCCT/ CTA-SI supporting the addition of CTP to stroke protocols using only NCCT and CTA-SI. This assertion is supported by a recent study showing similar improvement for a multimodal approach in the posterior fossa [11]. Extending on these findings, we demonstrate that multimodal CT demonstrated a greater reader certainty for correct diagnosis, compared to CTA-SI or NCCT with a better inter-reader agreement. Correlation between the observed and actual diagnosis, after adjusting for confidence levels, was 3.75 times greater for CTP than NCCT. Sensitivity of the multimodal protocol for correct diagnosis was increased without significant loss of specificity. The sensitivity for NCCT and CTA-SI is similar to that recently reported in the posterior fossa of 31 % and 33 % but lower on CTP (74 %) while specificity was similar for all modalities (93–98 %). Sensitivity of

Table 2 Vascular distribution of infarct/ischemia at presentation on incremental CT protocol

Vascular territory	Basilar	PCA	PICA	AICA	SCA	Perforator/other
NCCT	0 (0)	10 (0.48)	3 (0.14)	1 (0.05)	3 (0.14)	4 (0.19)
NCCT + CTA-SI	1 (0.17)	2 (0.33)	0 (0)	0 (0)	2 (0.33)	1 (0.17)
NCCT + CTA-SI + CTP	17 (0.18)	39 (0.42)	10 (0.11)	4 (0.04)	12 (0.13)	11 (0.12)

All values represent n (%)
PCA posterior cerebral artery, *SCA* superior cerebellar artery, *CTA-SI* CTA-source images

Table 3 Diagnostic performance for acute posterior stroke absence or presence diagnosed with an incremental stroke protocol

	Sensitivity (Se)		Specificity (Sp)	
	Se % (95 % CI)	p-value*	Sp % (95 % CI)	p-value*
Ischemia/ Infarct absent (Level of confidence score 5 and 6)				
(1) NCCT	41.4 (32.9–50.0)	(1) vs. (2): 0.103	83.7 (80.0–87.4)	(1) vs. (2): < 0.0001
(2) NCCT + CTA-SI	52.3 (43.3–61.2)	(1) vs. (3): 0.0007	95.7 (93.8–97.6)	(1) vs. (3): < 0.0001
(3) NCCT+ CTA-SI + CTP	64.9 (55.7–74.0)	(2) vs. (3): 0.072	92.8 (90.4–95.2)	(2) vs. (3): 0.188
Infarct present (Level of confidence score ≤ 2 vs. > 2)				
(1) NCCT	28.8 (20.6–37.1)	(1) vs. (2): 0.032	91.5 (88.5–94.4)	(1) vs. (2): < 0.0001
(2) NCCT+ CTA-SI	43.2 (33.9–52.6)	(1) vs. (3): < 0.0001	97.7 (96.4–98.9)	(1) vs. (3): 0.002
(3) NCCT+ CTA-SI + CTP	59.0 (49.3–68.7)	(2) vs. (3): 0.025	96.1 (94.2–98.0)	(2) vs. (3): 0.318

NCCT non-contrast CT, CTA-SI CTA Source Images, CTP CT perfusion
*p-value was obtained by linear regression model of natural log(Se) or log(Sp) for each modality

NCCT in posterior ischemic stroke was expectedly lower than that reported in acute anterior ischemic stroke (28 % vs 52 %) with closer approximation of CTA-SI (43 % vs 58 %) and CTP (59 % vs 70 %) sensitivity. There is a small but growing literature discussing the efficacy of CTP in the diagnosis of acute posterior ischemia stroke [10–12]. In part, this is the result of limited CTP spatial coverage, illustrated by a recent sub-analysis of the BASICS study, where complete CTP coverage of all posterior fossa ASPECTS regions was only available in

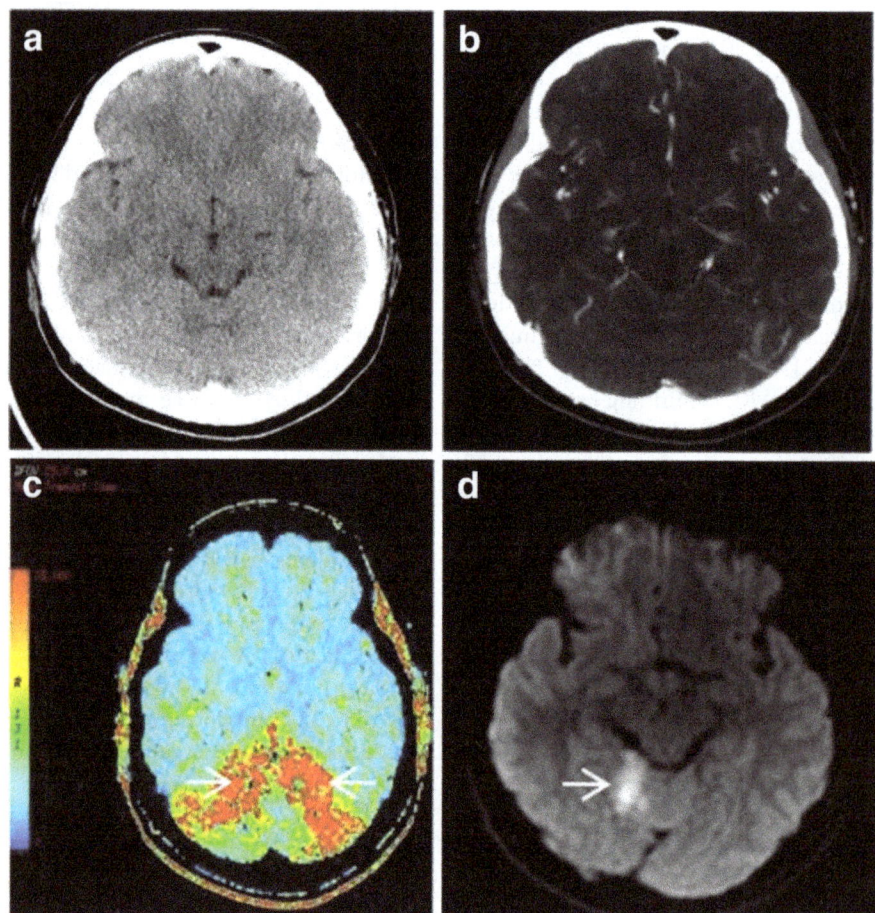

Fig. 2 a NCCT and corresponding (**b**) CTA-SI, (**c**) CTP MTT color maps and (**d**) follow up DWI obtained in 65 year old women presented with posterior ischemic stroke. MTT demonstrates bilateral cerebellar prolongation evolving to right cerebellar hemisphere infarction (arrows). NCCT and CTA-SI are unremarkable

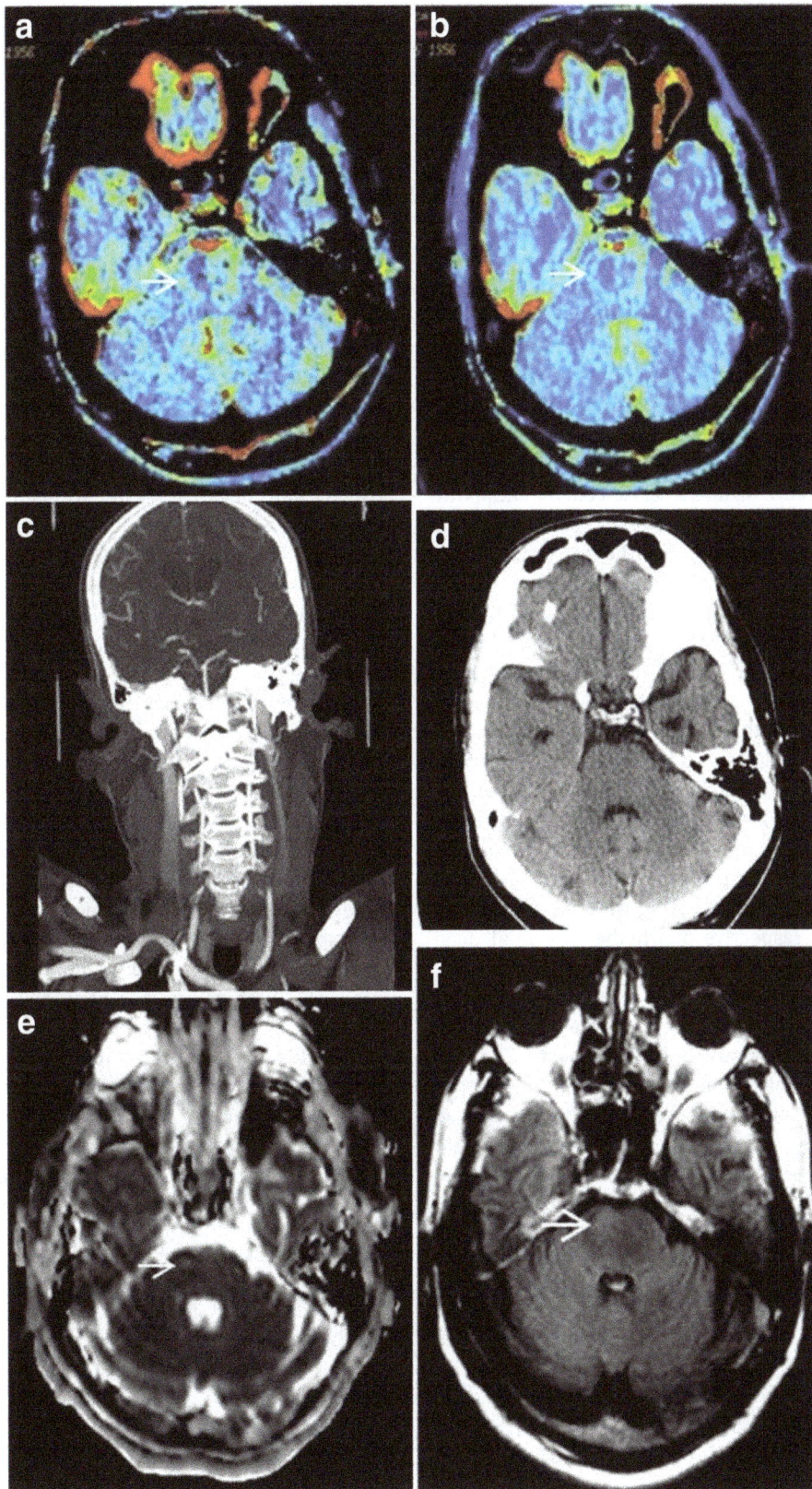

Fig. 3 (See legend on next page.)

(See figure on previous page.)
Fig. 3 Matched areas of decreased CBF (**a**) and CBV (**b**) in the right pons (arrows) indicating an irreversible infraction in a 72 year old man. CTA (**c**) is negative for arterial filling defects, indicating its lacunar nature. NCCT (**d**) is equivocal. A right hemipontine acute infarction was confirmed on MRI that was obtained 4 days later as shown on DWI/ADC (**e**) and corresponding FLAIR (**f**)

15 % of 27 patients. While this limitation is addressed by the table-toggle technique [10, 13, 23] it is associated with reduced sensitivity for detecting small infarcts [23], offset by greater scan coverage contributing to a higher overall detection rate. As 256-multi-detector-CT scanners become increasingly available, whole-brain coverage will become routine [24, 25]. A prior study, utilizing table-toggle CTP concluded that the performance of infratentorial CTP is comparable to that of supratentorial CTP [10]. In our study we adopted a pragmatic solution to scanning for centres that do not have a table-toggle option or large array detector scanners. Close collaboration with the stroke team enabled us to alter our traditional supratentorial CTP coverage to the posterior fossa. While stroke triage reflects a typical management pathway in major stroke-centres, targeted posterior fossa CTP is unique and allows simultaneous visualization of lower basal ganglia and posterior fossa assisting in diagnosis of posterior ischemic stroke. This imaging approach represents the application of anatomically and clinically directed scanning, maximizing diagnostic benefit over the risk of radiation exposure. Other important differences between the prior study and this should be noted. Previously, only patients with confirmed infarct on follow-up were investigated whereas we included all patients presenting with acute posterior ischemia stroke irrespective of whether the final diagnosis was TIA or infarction. This approach is supported by the importance of DWI abnormality in the context of clinical TIA [26, 27] and studies demonstrating higher recurrent stroke and TIA risk in TIA patients with initial perfusion abnormality [18]. Further, up to 30 % of patients not receiving rtPA because of mild or rapidly improving ischemic stroke have poor functional outcome [28, 29]. These findings are supported by the high number (87 %) of patients included

in the present series that demonstrated infarction. The high proportion of patients with posterior ischemic stroke in the current study is attributable to careful clinical screening and is similar to the 86 % prevalence recently reported in a post hoc analysis of posterior fossa infarcts reported by the DUST investigators [11]. To mitigate against a potential performance bias associated with high infarct presence we required precise lateralization for positive infarct designation. Indeed, only 29 % of the vascular territories assessed were affected. This requirement increases the number of false positive and negative designations if overcalling occurred for a particular modality. Prevalence of CTP and CTA-SI abnormality in the context of known posterior fossa infarct in the BASICS sub-study demonstrated MTT, CBF, CBV and CTA-SI changes in 93, 78, 46 and 78 % of patients respectively [12]. These values are higher than 76 and 54 % for any CTP and CTA-SI abnormality reported in this study. The higher prevalence in BASICS is consistent with recruitment of patients with known basilar occlusion rather than any posterior circulatory vessel occlusion included in the present study.

The present cohort size is approximately double that of the prior single center study and included a 12-h compared to 24-h time to presentation. The CT approach therefore reflects the performance of each modality within a screened cohort, assessed within a clinically meaningful time period with greater potential for successful outcome [30].

CTP adds 30 % to the total effective dose of 6.1 mSv for the CTP protocol. Incremental dose, although small, must confer benefit towards diagnosis because even small radiation doses are important in terms of overall population burden. Conscientious effort should therefore be made to conform to the as low as reasonably

Table 4 Distribution of confidence scores for side-specific presence of infarct/ischemia for each modality (levels 1 and 2 indicate definite and probable presence of ischemia/infarction, levels 5 and 6 indicate definite and probable absence of ischemia/infarction)

Modality	Distribution of each score, n (%)					
Confidence Score	1	2	3	4	5	6
NCCT (n = 738)	61 (8.3)	47 (6.4)	40 (5.4)	28 (3.8)	244 (33.1)	318 (43.1)
CTA-SI (n = 738)	74 (10.0)	34 (4.6)	14 (1.9)	16 (2.2)	162 (22.0)	438 (59.3)
CTP (n = 738)	133 (18.0)	18 (2.4)	10 (1.4)	20 (2.7)	87 (11.8)	470 (63.7)

NCCT non-contrast CT, *CTA-SI* CTA Source Images, *CTP* CT perfusion

Table 5 Logistic regression analysis and generalized estimating equations were used to model the real infarct diagnosis on different observed confidence scores for the corresponding modality

	Logistic regression model			GEEs method		
	r^2	AIC	p-value	OR (95 % CI)	QIC	p-value
NCCT						
Model fit statistics	0.0856	840.6			840.6	
Observed Confidence Score			< 0.0001	0.67 (0.61–0.74)		< 0.0001
NCCT + CTA-SI						
Model fit statistics	0.2578	686.7			686.7	
Observed Confidence Score			< 0.0001	0.45 (0.39–0.51)		< 0.0001
NCCT + CTA-SI + CTP						
Model fit statistics	0.321	621			620.9	
Observed Confidence Score			< 0.0001	0.47 (0.41–0.52)		< 0.0001

AIC Akaike information criterion, *QIC* quasilikelihood information criterion, *NCCT* non-contrast CT, *CTA-SI* CTA Source Images, *CTP* CT perfusion

achievable (ALARA) principle. A recent study shows that no quantitative CTP parameter differences were demonstrated when CTP dose was reduced by 50 % from 100 mA to 50 mA, however it remains unclear whether performance for infarct detection will remain the same at this reduced dose [31]. Scan obliquity ensures that no significant lens dose exposure occurs unlike CTA which remains the largest single dose contributor. MRI DWI remains the reference standard in acute infarct and provides superior infarct delineation but acute MRI access is limited in many institutions [32]. Therefore, although a recent consensus recommends MRI triage, the decision to treat with IV rtPA is still usually based on NCCT findings [32]. We suggest that CTA and CTP use may improve initial infarct detection over NCCT with the possibility of progressing to MRI where available.

Limitations include the relatively small sample size in comparison to anterior-circulation series. However the present study represents the largest single-center series evaluating pure acute posterior ischemia stroke. In comparison to the DUST study recruiting 88 patients from 14 centers over 4 years we recruited 82 patients in 3 years reflective of a high-volume tertiary institute and arguing against any selection bias. We purposefully utilized multidisciplinary readers of different levels of expertise, reflecting the diversity of everyday practice, where radiology trainees and non-radiologists may be the first to interpret emergency scans before a Neuroradiology staff opinion is sought. The majority of patients received MRI follow-up, with NCCT follow up used only where a radiologically-obvious acute infarct was present. DWI demonstrates high accuracy for stroke detection, but false-negative studies are documented in small and posterior infarcts [4, 33, 34]. It is plausible that a small number of patients may have been misclassified by MRI as negative in the context of a true clinical stroke. Similarly, because any CTP abnormality was considered positive, TIA associated with perfusion deficit, fully recanalized ischemia with residual perfusion defect and intracranial stenosis could all be potentially result in false positive abnormality in the absence of DWI abnormality. The impact of a systematic misclassification error is likely to affect each modality similarly and the effect on modality comparison is presumed negligible.

Conclusions

In conclusion, in centers with limited CTP coverage, targeted posterior fossa CTP in clinically selected patients enhances confident and correct infarct diagnosis and inter-reader reliability.

Table 6 Inter-reader agreement for three readers as reflected by ICC. ICC of 0.61–0.80 and 0.81– 1.0 were defined as good and very good concordance, respectively

Modality	ICC	95 % CI	Interpretation	p-value
NCCT	0.6796	0.6034–0.7432	Good	reference
NCCT + CTA-SI	0.7829	0.7312–0.8260	Good	120.4 (< 0.0001)
NCCT + CTA-SI + CTP	0.8337	0.7941–0.8667	Very Good	145.9 (< 0.0001)

ICC intraclass-correlation coefficient, *NCCT* Non-contrast CT, *CTA-SI* CTA Source Images, *CTP* CT perfusion

Competing interests
The authors declare that they have no competing interests.

Authors' contributions
MS - data acquisition, CT interpretation, literature research, data analysis and interpretation, manuscript writing. KB - data acquisition, CT interpretation, manuscript revising. RY - CT interpretation, manuscript revising. LZ - performed the statistical analysis and tables, manuscript revising. SS - participated in the design of the study, manuscript revising. MB - data acquisition, manuscript revising. RA - data acquisition, study design, literature research, data analysis and interpretation, manuscript writing. All authors read and approved the final manuscript.

Author details
[1]Department of Diagnostic Imaging, Division of Neuroradiology, Room AG 31, Sunnybrook Health Sciences Centre, 2075 Bayview Ave, Toronto, ON M4N 3M5, Canada. [2]Department of Medicine, Division of Neurology, Sunnybrook Health Sciences Centre, 2075 Bayview Ave, Toronto, ON M4N 3M5, Canada.

References
1. Savitz SI, Caplan LR. Vertebrobasilar disease. N Engl J Med. 2005;352:2618–26.
2. Caplan L. Posterior circulation ischemia: then, now, and tomorrow. The Thomas Willis Lecture. Stroke. 2000;31:2011–23.
3. Hwang DY, Silva GS, Furie KL, Greer DM. Comparative sensitivity of computed tomography vs. magnetic resonance imaging for detecting acute posterior fossa infarct. J Emerg Med. 2012;42:559–65.
4. Oppenheim C, Stanescu R, Dormont D, Crozier S, Marro B, Samson Y, et al. False-negative diffusion-weighted MR findings in acute ischemic stroke. AJNR Am J Neuroradiol. 2000;21:1434–40.
5. Schaefer PW, Yoo AJ, Bell D, Barak ER, Romero JM, Nogueira RG, et al. CT angiography-source image hypoattenuation predicts clinical outcome in posterior circulation strokes treated with intra-arterial therapy. Stroke. 2008; 39:3107–9.
6. Koenig M, Klotz E, Luka B, Venderink DJ, Spittler JF, Heuser L, Perfusion CT of the brain: diagnostic approach for early detection of ischemic stroke. Radiology. 1998;209:85–93.
7. Hopyan J, Ciarallo A, Dowlatshahi D, Howard P, John V, Yeung R, et al. Certainty of stroke diagnosis: incremental benefit with CT perfusion over noncontrast CT and CT angiography. Radiology. 2010;255:142–53.
8. Ledezma CJ, Wintermark M. Multimodal CT in stroke imaging: new concepts. Radiol Clin North Am. 2009;47:109–16.
9. Wintermark M, Reichhart M, Cuisenaire O, Maeder P, Thiran JP, Schnyder P, et al. Comparison of admission perfusion computed tomography and qualitative diffusion- and perfusion-weighted magnetic resonance imaging in acute stroke patients. Stroke. 2002;33:2025–31.
10. Lee IH, You JH, Lee JY, Whang K, Kim MS, Kim YJ, et al. Accuracy of the detection of infratentorial stroke lesions using perfusion CT: an experimenter-blinded study. Neuroradiology. 2010;52:1095–100.
11. van der Hoeven EJ, Dankbaar JW, Algra A, Vos JA, Niesten JM, van Seeters T, et al. Additional diagnostic value of computed tomography perfusion for detection of acute ischemic stroke in the posterior circulation. Stroke. 2015; 46:1113–5.
12. Pallesen LP, Gerber J, Dzialowski I, van der Hoeven EJ, Michel P, Pfefferkorn T, et al. Diagnostic and Prognostic Impact of pc-ASPECTS Applied to Perfusion CT in the Basilar Artery International Cooperation Study. J Neuroimaging. 2014;25:384–9.
13. Roberts HC, Roberts TP, Smith WS, Lee TJ, Fischbein NJ, Dillon WP, Multisection dynamic CT perfusion for acute cerebral ischemia: the "toggling-table" technique. AJNR Am J Neuroradiol. 2001;22:1077–80.
14. Brenner DJ, Hall EJ. Computed tomography-an increasing source of radiation exposure. N Engl J Med. 2007;357:2277–84.
15. Das T, Settecase F, Boulos M, Huynh T, d'Esterre CD, Symons SP, et al. Multimodal CT provides improved. performance for lacunar infarct detection. AJNR Am J Neuroradiol. 2015;36:1069–75.
16. Puetz V, Sylaja PN, Coutts SB, Hill MD, Dzialowski I, Mueller P, et al. Extent of hypoattenuation on CT angiography source images predicts functional outcome in patients with basilar artery occlusion. Stroke. 2008;39:2485–90.
17. Sharma M, Fox AJ, Symons S, Jairath A, Aviv RI. CT angiographic source images: flow- or volume-weighted? AJNR Am J Neuroradiol. 2011;32:359–64.
18. Coutts SB, Eliasziw M, Hill MD, Scott JN, Subramaniam S, Buchan AM, et al. An improved scoring system for identifying patients at high early risk of stroke and functional impairment after an acute transient ischemic attack or minor stroke. Int J Stroke. 2008;3:3–10.
19. Asdaghi N, Coutts SB. Imaging predictors of outcome in patients with transient ischemic attacks and minor stroke: review of published data from the VISION study. Eur J Cardiovasc Med. 2011;1:22–5.
20. DeLong ER, DeLong DM, Clarke-Pearson DL. Comparing the areas under two or more correlated receiveroperating characteristic curves: a nonparametric approach. Biometrics. 1988;44:837–45.
21. Zhou XH, Obuchowski NA, McClish DK. The sensitivity and specificity of clustered binary data. In: BaldingDJ, Bloomfield P, Cressie NAC, editors. Statistical methods in diagnostic medicine. New York: Wiley; 2002. p. 104–6.
22. Shrout PE, Fleiss JL. Intraclass correlations: uses in assessing rater reliability. Psychol Bull. 1979;86:420–8.
23. Youn SW, Kim JH, Weon YC, Kim SH, Han MK, Bae HJ. Perfusion CT of the brain using 40–mm-wide detector and toggling table technique for initial imaging of acute stroke. AJR Am J Roentgenol. 2008;191:120–6.
24. Mori S, Obata T, Nakajima N, Ichihara N, Endo M. Volumetric perfusion CT using prototype 256-detector row CT scanner: preliminary study with healthy porcine model. AJNR Am J Neuroradiol. 2005;26:2536–41.
25. Murayama K, Katada K, Nakane M, Toyama H, Anno H, Hayakawa M, et al. Whole-brain perfusion CTperformed with a prototype 256-detector row CT system: initial experience. Radiology. 2009;250:202–11.
26. Coutts SB, Hill MD, Simon JE, Sohn CH, Scott JN, Demchuk AM. Silent ischemia in minor stroke and TIApatients identified on mr imaging. Neurology. 2005;65:513–7.
27. Rovira A, Rovira-Gols A, Pedraza S, Grivé E, Molina C, Alvarez-Sabín J. Diffusion-weighted mr imaging inthe acute phase of transient ischemic attacks. AJNR Am J Neuroradiol. 2002;23:77–83.
28. Rajajee V, Kidwell C, Starkman S, Ovbiagele B, Alger JR, Villablanca P. Early MRI and outcomes of untreated patients with mild or improving ischemic stroke. Neurology. 2006;67:980–4.
29. Barber PA, Zhang J, Demchuk AM, Hill MD, Buchan AM. Why are stroke patients excluded from TPA therapy? An analysis of patient eligibility. Neurology. 2001;56:1015–20.
30. Versnick EJ, Do HM, Albers GW, Tong DC, Marks MP. Mechanical thrombectomy for acute stroke. AJNR Am J Neuroradiol. 2005;26:875–9.
31. Murphy A, So A, Lee TY, Symons S, Jakubovic R, Zhang L, et al. Low dose CT perfusion in acute ischemic stroke. Neuroradiology. 2014;56:1055–62.
32. Wintermark M, Sanelli PC, Albers GW, Bello J, Derdeyn C, Hetts SW, et al. Imaging recommendations for acute stroke and transient ischemic attack patients: A joint statement by the American Society of Neuroradiology, the American College of Radiology, and the Society of NeuroInterventional Surgery. AJNR. 2013;34:117–27.
33. Linfante I, Llinas RH, Schlaug G, Chaves C, Warach S, Caplan LR. Diffusion-weighted imaging and National Institutes of Health Stroke Scale in the acute phase of posterior-circulation stroke. Arch Neurol. 2001;58:621–8.
34. Lövblad KO, Laubach HJ, Baird AE, Curtin F, Schlaug G, Edelman RR, et al. Clinical experience with diffusion-weighted MR in patients with acute stroke. AJNR Am J Neuroradiol. 1998;19:1061–6.

9

Can CT perfusion accurately assess infarct core?

Dan C. Huynh[1], Mark W. Parsons[2], Max Wintermark[3], Achala Vagal[4], Christopher D. d'Esterre[5], Rita Vitorino[1], Daniel Efkehari[1], Jesse Knight[1], Thien J. Huynh[1], Andrew Bivard[6], Rick Swartz[7], Sean Symons[1] and Richard I. Aviv[1]*

Abstract

Background: We sought to quantify CTP-derived infarct core applying previously published perfusion thresholds to multi-institutional CTP data to assess the margin of error for 25 mL and 70 mL critical volume thresholds using early DWI as a reference standard.

Methods: 60 patients with acute ischemic stroke undergoing CTP and DWI within 6 and 24 h of symptom onset, respectively, were retrospectively analyzed from 3 tertiary care centers. CTP-derived infarct core was calculated using published thresholds for absolute and relative CBF and CBV in addition to manual CBV tracing. Using DWI as the reference standard, performance of CTP-derived measures of infarct core was assessed using co-registered voxel-by-voxel analysis and total infarct volume comparison. Volumes of each CTP infarct core estimate were compared against DWI to determine the degree of infarct core over or underestimation at the critical volumes of 25 mL and 70 mL.

Results: Median core infarct volume was 10.8 mL. Mean CTP-derived infarct core volumes were similar to DWI for all CTP threshold methods to within ± 1 mL. CBV tracing demonstrated an overall significant core overestimation compared to DWI ($p = 0.017$). All CTP core volume estimations showed robust correlation with DWI (Pearson p-value < 0.001). As core volume increased, CTP demonstrated increased deviation from DWI. At the critical cut-offs of 25 mL and 70 mL, relative CBF demonstrated the best agreement with DWI for infarct core compared to the other CTP-derived measures of infarct core.

Conclusion: Our study demonstrates close approximation between multiple CTP-derived measures of infarct core and DWI infarct volume, Especially relative CBF.

Background

There is a continued interest in physiological imaging to select patients for reperfusion therapies in acute ischemic stroke (AIS) [1]. DWI is considered the reference standard for identifying permanently infarcted brain tissue while CTP is an alternative, although hotly debated surrogate [2–6]. Identification of potentially salvageable brain tissue facilitates a more personalized approach to thrombolytic therapy administration [1] and could improve outcomes beyond the traditional 4.5 h time window [7].

Infarct core volume is an increasingly important determinant in success of reperfusion therapy. A planimetrically measured core infarct volume of 70 mL is considered a critical upper limit above which poor outcome is experienced, despite high recanalization rates [8–11]. Additionally, a core infarct volume of ≤25 mL recently demonstrates very high rates of good outcomes with recanalization [12]. Accuracy of acute infarct core volume estimation is clinically important especially given recent studies demonstrating a degree infarct core volume overestimation using CTP compared to MR perfusion (MRP) and DWI within 1 h of CTP [1, 13]. There is ongoing debate over the validity of CTP to identify infarct core and while no clear consensus exists on the optimal parameter most predictive of tissue viability and outcome, CBF thresholds appear most promising [4, 5, 14–16]. Acknowledging that CTP processing methods

* Correspondence: richard.aviv@sunnybrook.ca
[1]Division of Neuroradiology, Department of Medical Imaging, University of Toronto and Sunnybrook Health Sciences Centre, 2075 Bayview Avenue, Room AG 31, Toronto, ON M4N 3M5, Canada
Full list of author information is available at the end of the article

are affected by many technical challenges such as threshold value used, type of CTP processing software and post-processing protocols [4, 5, 15, 17] a pragmatic argument could be made that the correlation between CTP and DWI core infarct determination need only be accurate enough to distinguish critical lesion volume thresholds such as 25 and 70 mL [15]. CTP utilization remains attractive because of widespread CT availability in the acute clinical setting especially in non-tertiary hospitals. We sought to quantify CTP-derived infarct core applying previously published perfusion thresholds to multi-institutional CTP data [18] to assess the margin of error for 25 mL and 70 mL critical volume thresholds using early DWI as a reference standard.

Methods

Study design and patient cohort

This retrospective study was approved by the local institutional research ethics board. Stroke patients were collected from the databases of three separate institutions between 2008 and 2010. Patients presenting with AIS who underwent NCCT and CTP within six hours of stroke symptom onset and acute DWI <24 h of presentation were included in the study. CT angiography was performed at a median of 24 ± 4 h after stroke onset to classify recanalization status.63 patients were identified. Three (3/63, 5 %) were excluded as the infarct core on DWI was beyond CTP coverage. Baseline characteristics including age, gender, NIHSS and 90-day mRS were recorded.

Scan protocol

Multicenter stroke imaging was obtained with a 64-slice CT scanner (8*5 mm), 16-slice and 64-slice scanners (single 4*5 mm acquisition or 2 contiguous acquisitions of 4*5 mm). Follow-up DWI was obtained with 1.5 T at all institutions (7000 ms/min [repetition time (TR)/echo time (TE)], field of view [FOV] of 24 cm, matrix 128*128, section thickness (ST) of 5 mm, no gap; 5000 ms/min [TR/TE], FOV of 13 cm, matrix 128*128, ST of 5 mm, 1.5 mm gap; 6000 ms/107 min [TR/TE], FOV of 40 cm, matrix 128*128/256*256, 1 mm gap). CTA angiogram was performed at baseline with parameters: aortic arch to the vertex, 0.7-mL/kg iodinated contrast agent up to a maximum of 90 mL (iohexol, Omnipaque 300 mg iodine/mL; GE Healthcare, Piscataway, New Jersey), 5- to 10- second delay, 120 kVp, 270 mA, 1 s/rotation, 1.25-mm-thick sections, and table speed of 3.7 mm/rotation. CTP was performed locally as a biphasic examination [45 s acquisition, 0.5 s intervals, 8 slices followed by 120 s acquisition, 15 s intervals, 8 slices] [19]. Other CTP acquisition were performed as 45-75 s acquisition, 1.3 s intervals, 2*2 slices and 50-70s

acquisition, 1-2 s intervals [4, 20]. In all cases 40-50 mL of iodinated contrast was injected at 4–5 mL/s.

Imaging processing

Analysis of all CTP studies was performed using CT Perfusion 4 software (GE Healthcare). Gaussian smoothing using a kernel width of 4 pixels was applied to the processed maps (Fig. 1) [1, 4]. Using Statistical Parametric Mapping (SPM8, Wellcome Trust Centre, United Kingdom), CTP and DWI maps were coregistered using tri-linear interpolation to baseline NCCT. Grey and white matter NCCT segmentation was additionally performed using SPM8.

Imaging analysis

To identify infarct core on CTP, previously validated gray and white matter specific absolute and relative voxel-intensity thresholds (relative CBF threshold (relCBF), relative CBV threshold (relCBV), absolute CBF threshold (AbsCBF), absolute CBV threshold (AbsCBV); Table 1) were applied to CBF and CBV maps respectively with upper thresholds of <100 mL/100 g/min and <8 mL/100 g respectively to eliminate vasculature [18]. To compare visual CBV abnormality tracing compared to thresholded measures to identify infarct core an experienced neuroradiologist (XX, 10 years), blinded to DWI, manually traced areas of CBV abnormality (designated CBV tracing) using Medical Image Processing, Analysis, and Visualization (MIPAV; version: 7.0.2, National Institutes of Health, Bethesda, MD). Voxel-by-voxel comparison of the 5 generated CTP measures of infarct core was made to determine performance of each measure against the DWI reference standard utilizing MATLAB (version: 2012b, The MathWorks, Inc., Natick, MA). Finally, the volume of each CTP core estimate was compared against DWI to determine the degree of infarct core over or underestimation.

Statistical analysis

All analyses were performed using SPSS (Version 17.0. SPSS Inc., Chicago, IL). Descriptive results and quantitative baseline patient characteristics were reported as mean ± SD or median (IQR). Sensitivity and specificity were calculated for each patient for all CTP techniques and compared to DWI. Paired Student's t-test or Wilcoxon signed-rank test compared parametric and nonparametric data respectively. Mean differences between CTP predicted infarct core and DWI infarct core volumes were compared. A correlation matrix using Pearson's R test was performed for volumetric measures of infarct core between predicted and DWI infarct core volumes. A volumetric agreement comparison (Bland-Altman) between CTP parameters and DWI for infarct core was performed for each patient. To account for the

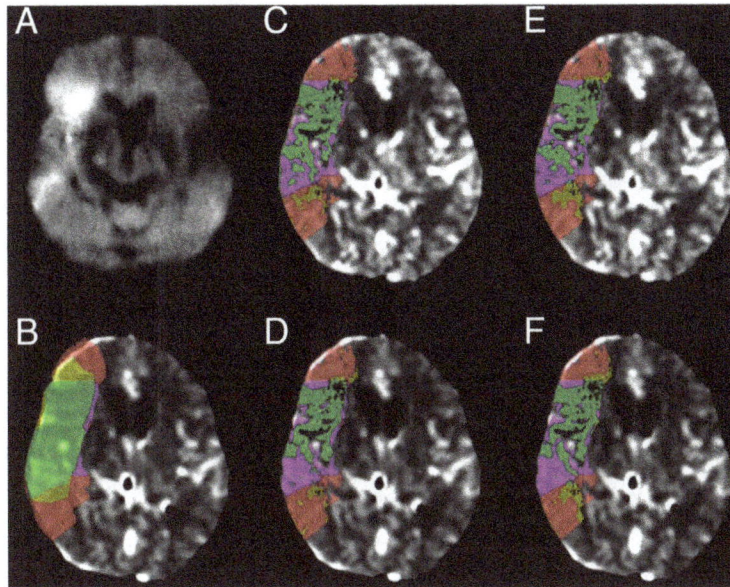

Fig. 1 A comparison of computed tomography perfusion (CTP) parameters. **a** Diffusion-weighted imaging (DWI) in identifying a right-sided infarct core. **b** CBV tracing, (**c**) absolute CBF threshold, (**d**) absolute CBV threshold, (**e**) relative CBF threshold, (**f**) relative CBV threshold vs. Shaded areas correspond to true-positive (*green*), false-positive (*yellow*), false-negative (*purple*), and true-negative (*red*) voxels

potential of recanalization between onset and DWI, DWI/CTP differences were initially compared after dichotomizing by recanalization status. Patients were subdivided by time interval between CTP and DWI into acute (≤4 h) and subacute (>4 h) groups. A 4-h mark was chosen because this represents the upper time limit in our institution within the clinically significant therapeutic window for assessing an AIS patient while retaining sufficient time to still administer reperfusion therapy. Mean sensitivity and specificity were compared between acute and delayed group patients. Within each CTP technique, a volumetric comparison of infarct core between the acute and delayed patients was performed. Differences between predicted and actual infarct core volumes were calculated. Furthermore, patients were partitioned according to CTP scan acquisition time (<60s or ≥60s) to study the artificial reduction of CBV due to venous time density curve (TDC) truncation [15]. Lastly, cases with CTP infarct core estimation >70 mL, but DWI <70 mL (overestimation), and cases with CTP <70 mL, but DWI >70 mL (underestimation) were noted and used as a critical value for Cohen's kappa inter-

modality agreement [8, 9]. The same inter-modality agreement was also assessed using a critical infarct volume of 25 mL [12]. Kappa statistics of 0.21 to 0.4, 0.41 to 0.6, 0.61 to 0.8, and 0.81 to 1 were considered fair, moderate, substantial, and nearly perfect, respectively [21]. A value of $p < 0.05$ was considered statistically significant.

Results

Mean patient age was 67.6 ± 13.3 and 33 % (20/60) were male. Median time from stroke symptom onset to CTP was 2.5 (IQR 1.6-3.8) hours while median time to DWI was 3.9 (IQR 1.12-15.3) hours. Recanalization occurred in 38 (63 %) of patients. Median baseline NIHSS and 90-day mRS was 16 (IQR 9–19), and 3.5 (IQR 2–5) respectively. Median core infarct volume was 10.8 mL (IQR 6.8-41.5). Figure 1 illustrates an example of the calculation of CTP performance for DWI infarct core. Mean sensitivity, specificity, and accuracy for each CTP parameter are demonstrated in Table 2. A comparison of DWI- and CTP-derived infarct core volume estimations and volumetric differences is presented in Table 3. CBV tracing demonstrated a significant core overestimation of 6.8 mL compared to DWI ($p = 0.017$), while CTP threshold parameters demonstrated insignificant differences (<1 mL) in comparison to DWI. All CTP core volume estimations showed robust correlation with DWI ($p < 0.001$). Bland-Altman plots demonstrating CTP-DWI volume difference for each CTP parameter are shown in Fig. 2. Mean volumetric 95 % confidence interval differences were: −48.7 - 48.5 mL (absCBF), −45.9 – 46.9 mL

Table 1 Threshold values used to determine infarct core in grey matter (GM) and white matter (WM) for each CTP technique [18]

Threshold technique	Core volume definition			
	AbsCBF	AbsCBV	rCBF	rCBV
Gray Matter (GM)	≤13.80	≤1.31	≤0.42	≤0.89
White Matter (WM)	≤9.80	≤0.85	≤0.56	≤0.81

Table 2 Overall, acute (CTP-DWI ≤ 4 h) and delayed (CTP-DWI > 4 h) mean sensitivities (SE), specificities (SP), and accuracies (ACC) for each CTP parameter (left to right) when compared spatially with DWI on a voxel by voxel basis

Parameter	Overall (n = 60)			≤4 h (n = 31)			>4 h (n = 29)		
	SE	SP	ACC	SE	SP	ACC	SE	SP	ACC
AbsCBF	50 %	68 %	54 %	49 %	69 %	47 %	51 %	66 %	62 %
AbsCBV	56 %	64 %	53 %¥	54 %	68 %	45 %	58 %ε	61 %	61 %
rCBF	48 %*§	71 %	57 %	52 %	68 %	49 %	44 %ε	73 %	67 %
rCBV	54 %*	67 %	57 %	57 %	67 %	49 %	50 %	67 %	66 %
CBV Tracing	61 %§	70 %	60 %¥	65 %	67 %	48 %	56 %	74 %	72 %

Values with the same superscript symbol demonstrate a significant difference between parameters (p < 0.05)

(absCBV), −44.7 – 43.2 mL (relCBF), −42.5 – 41.6 mL (relCBV), −34.5 – 48.2 mL (CBV tracing). For small (<25 mL) core volumes all CTP measures showed minimal differences in comparison to DWI. However as DWI volume increased, CTP threshold parameters tended to underestimate infarct core volume. There were no significant differences in baseline infarct core volume estimation between patients with and without recanalization.

Thirty one patients underwent DWI within 4 h of CTP (acute DWI) whereas 29 received delayed DWI (>4 h). Median time to DWI after CTP for acute and delayed groups was 1.2 (IQR 0.6-2.7) hours and 15.4 (IQR 8.0-24.9) hours, respectively. There was no significant difference in time from stroke onset to initial CTP between the two groups. Mean core infarct volumes and CTP/DWI differences for the two groups are displayed in Table 4. No significant sensitivity and specificity differences when comparing early versus late DWI within each CTP technique (Table 2). Compared to early DWI only CBV tracing significantly overestimated infarct core (p = 0.039). Compared to delayed DWI no significant differences for any CTP parameter and DWI was observed. When dichotomizing patients by CTP acquisition time (<60s, n = 19 vs. ≥60s, n = 41), CBV tracing on shorter acquisition time data, trended to DWI overestimation compared to the ≥60s group (13.0 mL vs. 3.6 mL; p = 0.07).

The inter-modality agreement for 25 mL and 70 mL is presented in Table 5. rCBF threshold demonstrated the best agreement for 25 mL (κ = 0.610) while rCBV and CBV tracing showed moderate agreement. AbsCBF and

Table 3 Volumetric mean for predicted infarct core in all CTP parameters and their difference to DWI

Parameter	Mean (mL)	CTP-DWI difference (mL)	p-value
AbsCBF	24.6 ± 20.6	0.11	0.970
AbsCBV	24.9 ± 20.5	0.46	0.879
rCBF	23.7 ± 20.9	−0.76	0.789
rCBV	24.0 ± 21.6	−0.44	0.873
CBV Tracing	31.3 ± 33.6	6.81	0.017

AbsCBV thresholds demonstrated fair agreement. Discordance was due to a CTP overestimation of core infarct compared to DWI. Similarly for 70 mL rCBF threshold demonstrated a substantial agreement while all other CTP parameters demonstrated moderate agreement (Table 5). While CTP threshold parameters had minimal overestimation (1 case), there were 4 (7 %) cases where CTP CBV tracing overestimated infarct core at the critical volume.

Discussion

The strength of the present study is the application of previously determined thresholds from a large stroke population to data from three different stroke institutions utilizing different imaging protocols [18]. This approach undoubtedly diminishes performance for infarct volume determination compared to other studies where thresholds were optimized to study-specific patient cohorts [1, 4, 18]. Nevertheless, our results indicate close agreement with DWI volumes. rCBF demonstrates the highest agreement whereas traced CBV overestimates infarct volume particularly where scan duration is <60 s.

CBV tracing demonstrated the highest volumetric correlation to DWI, but significantly overestimate infarct core. To understand this overestimation, patients were dichotomized by length of CTP acquisition to assess the influence of truncation [15, 22]. Our results show that CTP acquisitions with acquisition times <60s overestimate infarct core due to underestimation of true CBV values. CBV underestimation due to TDC truncation is important and the need for longer CTP acquisitions that capture more of the venous phase is recently highlighted [15]. Sanelli et al. demonstrated that premature TDC cut off resulted in higher CBF and lower CBV values within the infarct core [23]. This artifact remains a significant cause of infarct volume overestimation and TDC should routinely be reviewed for adequate TDC coverage prior to CTP CBV analysis or interpretation.

An underestimation of infarct core at higher DWI volumes is attributed to the limited coverage of CTP compared to DWI with extension of infarcted tissue beyond the imaged CTP slices. This could be an important

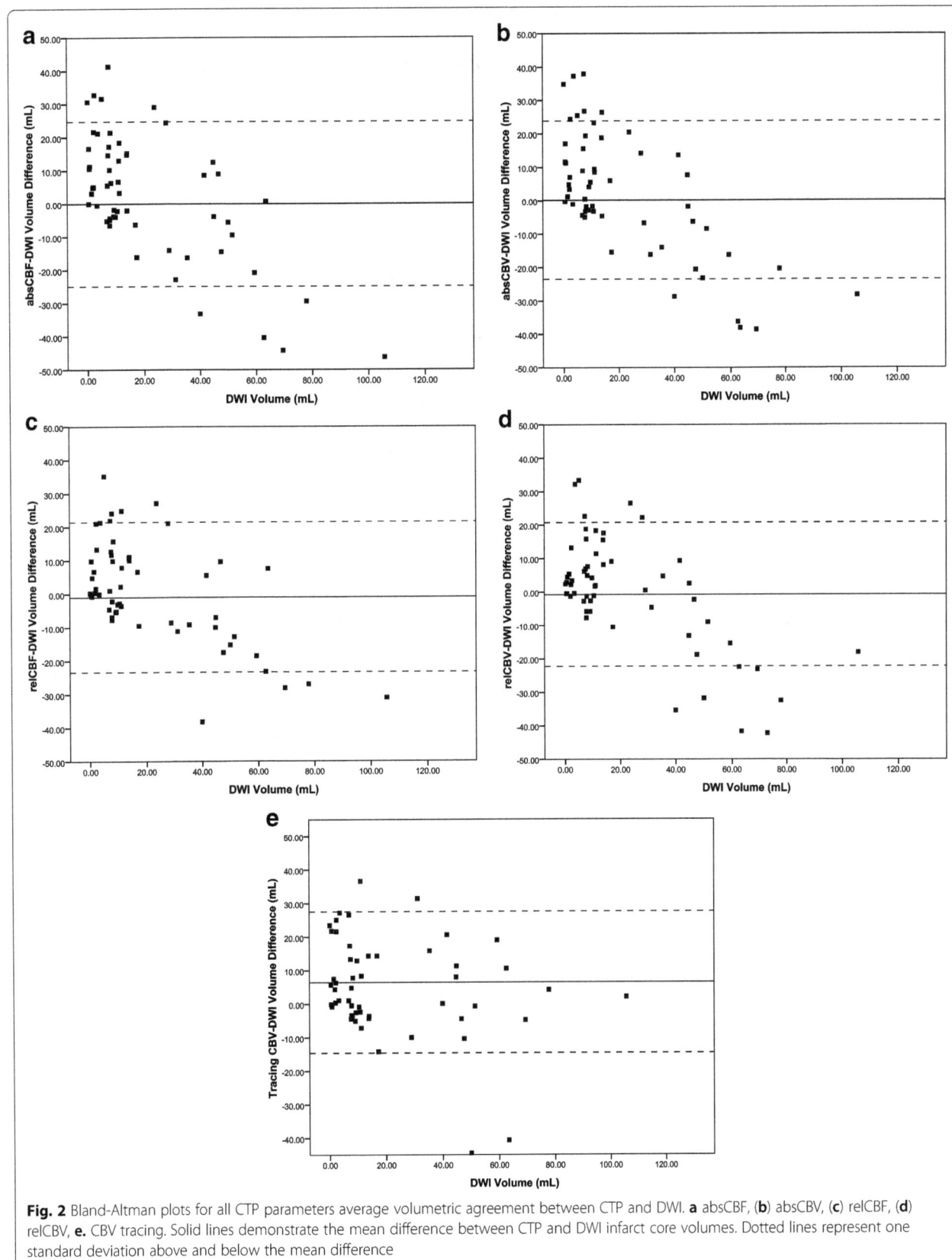

Fig. 2 Bland-Altman plots for all CTP parameters average volumetric agreement between CTP and DWI. **a** absCBF, (**b**) absCBV, (**c**) relCBF, (**d**) relCBV, **e.** CBV tracing. Solid lines demonstrate the mean difference between CTP and DWI infarct core volumes. Dotted lines represent one standard deviation above and below the mean difference

Table 4 Predicted mean core infarct volumes and the mean difference between CTP and DWI for acute and delayed MRI follow up

Parameter	≤4 h			>4 h		
	Mean (mL)	CTP-DWI difference (mL)	Correlation to DWI	Mean (mL)	CTP-DWI difference (mL)	Correlation to DWI
AbsCBF	26.5	0.76 ± 47.9	0.516	22.6	−0.55 ± 50.2	0.765
AbsCBV	25.6	−0.10 ± 44.1	0.603	24.1	1.03 ± 49.7	0.770
rCBF	27.5	1.73 ± 39.2	0.705	19.8	−3.33 ± 48.8	0.794
rCBV	26.8	1.05 ± 37.4	0.738	21.2	−1.97 ± 47.1	0.800
CBV Tracing	35.9	10.2 ± 48.6	0.634	26.4	3.31 ± 30.3	0.918

limitation of CTP if the volume approximates an upper threshold where treatment may be of no benefit, but is easily addressed by extended coverage techniques such as table toggle, tandem CTP techniques or full brain coverage with 320 slice scanners [24, 25]. Increased dose concerns may be addressed by imaging at 50 mA rather than 100mAs, nulling any increased radiation dose by halving MA and doubling spatial coverage [26]. CTP (2.5 mSV) contributes approximately 30 % of total CT Stroke protocol dose (6.1 mSv) with CTA an equal contributor (2.4 mSV). Differences between CTP and early or late DWI demonstrated significant differences only for CBV tracing. Differences reduced over time reflecting infarct evolution on later DWI offsetting the effect of baseline CBV overestimation.

Clinical importance of volume disagreement using critical thresholds demonstrated moderate to substantial intermodality agreement. Threshold selection was based on data from EXTEND, DEFUSE, and Yoo et al. [8–12]. At the critical volume of 25 mL, all CTP parameters demonstrated similar false-negative underestimation of core infarct compared to DWI. However, AbsCBF, AbsCBV, and rCBV demonstrated higher false-positive overestimation for true core infarct compared to rCBF and CBV tracing. rCBF demonstrated relatively low over- and under-estimation and the best inter-modality agreement. Using 70 mL, CBV tracing demonstrated a higher false-positive overestimation of infarct core

compared to DWI than other CTP parameters. Highest agreement was demonstrated for rCBF. At both critical volumes, rCBF displayed the best agreement, reinforcing the utility of this measure for infarct core determination [4]. It is notable that this parameter has been identified as the best predictor of infarct core by a number of studies irrespective of post-processing technique or particular threshold used [4, 16, 18]. rCBF is also recently used to defined core in EXTEND-IA [11] Our results vary from a recent publication that showed larger confidence intervals for DWI versus CBF and CBV differences [27]. That study employed a non-traditional approach to CTP map by applying a threshold relative to the thalamus and not accounting for threshold differences between gray and white matter - likely contributed to their wider confidence intervals.

Limitations of this study include small sample size, due to the restrictive entry criteria, limiting the power to detect potential small differences in infarct volumes between modalities. A small percentage of our patient cohort demonstrated infarct core volumes exceeding 70 mL highlighting a limitation for this threshold, however new data suggests that a 25 mL core volume may be a better threshold. Retrospective analysis limited this study due to variation in DWI time, however the median time to DWI was approximately 1 h. CBV and DWI volumes were manually traced without testing the intra-observer agreement of this measurement. This could

Table 5 Patient misclassification using 25 mL and 70 mL (EXTEND criteria) as the critical infarct volume

		DWI				DWI		
		≤25 mL	>25 mL	Kappa		≤70 mL	>70 mL	Kappa
AbsCBF	≤25 mL	29	6	0.439	≤70 mL	57	2	0.487
	>25 mL	10	15		>70 mL	0	1	
AbsCBV	≤25 mL	27	5	0.422	≤70 mL	57	2	
	>25 mL	12	15		>70 mL	0	1	0.487
rCBF	≤25 mL	32	4	0.610	≤70 mL	56	1	
	>25 mL	7	17		>70 mL	1	2	0.649
rCBV	≤25 mL	29	3	0.558	≤70 mL	57	2	
	>25 mL	10	18		>70 mL	0	1	0.487
CBV Tracing	≤25 mL	31	4	0.579	≤70 mL	53	1	
	>25 mL	8	17		>70 mL	4	2	0.405

potentially introduce a margin of error into the measurements and their correlation with perfusion parameters. Finally, thresholds used in the current paper represent validated thresholds utilizing the image processing techniques described. We eliminated variability due to different post processing techniques by using the same pipeline for all studies. Similar results may not be obtained with other vendors' post processing techniques.

Conclusion

In conclusion, our study demonstrates close approximation of DWI-derived infarct volume assessment with multiple CTP parameters, especially rCBF. Infarct overestimation is greatest for CBV tracing likely attributable to CBV underestimation from technical factors relating to short CTP acquisition times.

Ethical standards and patient consent

We declare that all human and animal studies have been approved by the Sunnybrook Research Institute Ethics Board and have therefore been performed in accordance with the ethical standards laid down in the 1964 Declaration of Helsinki and its later amendments. We declare that all patients gave informed consent prior to inclusion in this study.

Competing interests
The authors declare that they have no competing interests.

Authors' contributions
DCH: Literature review, Project development, Data collection, Image processing, Data analysis, Manuscript writing. MWP: Literature review, Project development, Data collection, Manuscript review. MW: Literature review, Project development, Data collection, Manuscript review. AV: Data collection, Manuscript review. CDd'E: Project development, Manuscript review. RV: Data collection, Data analysis, Manuscript review. DE: Image processing, Data analysis, Manuscript review. JK: Image processing, Data analysis, Manuscript review. TJH: Data analysis, Manuscript review. AB: Data collection, Manuscript review. SS: Project development, Manuscript review. RIA: Literature review, Project development, Data collection, Manuscript writing, Manuscript review. All authors read and approved the final manuscript.

Disclosures/grant support
AV received funding support from Imaging Core Lab, PRISMS Trial, Genentech, Inc.

Author details
[1]Division of Neuroradiology, Department of Medical Imaging, University of Toronto and Sunnybrook Health Sciences Centre, 2075 Bayview Avenue, Room AG 31, Toronto, ON M4N 3M5, Canada. [2]Department of Neurology, John Hunter Hospital, The University of Newcastle, Newcastle, NSW, Australia. [3]Department of Radiology, Neuroradiology Division, Stanford University, California, USA. [4]Department of Radiology, Section of Neuroradiology, University of Cincinnati College of Medicine, Cincinnati, OH, USA. [5]Calgary Stroke Program, Department of Radiology, University of Calgary, Alberta, Canada. [6]Melbourne Brain Centre, University of Melbourne, Melbourne, VIC, Australia. [7]Department of Medicine (Neurology), Sunnybrook Health Sciences Centre, University of Toronto, Toronto, ON, Canada.

References

1. Campbell BCV et al. Comparison of computed tomography perfusion and magnetic resonance imaging perfusion-diffusion mismatch in ischemic stroke. Stroke. 2012;43(10):2648–53.
2. Fiebach JB et al. CT and diffusion-weighted MR Imaging in randomized order: diffusion-weighted imaging results in higher accuracy and lower interrater variability in the diagnosis of hyperacute ischemic stroke. Stroke. 2002;33(9):2206–10.
3. Campbell BCV et al. The infarct core is well represented by the acute diffusion lesion: sustained reversal is infrequent. J Cereb Blood Flow Metab. 2012;32(1):50–6.
4. Campbell BCV et al. Cerebral blood flow is the optimal CT perfusion parameter for assessing infarct core. Stroke. 2011;42(12):3435–40.
5. Kamalian S et al. CT cerebral blood flow maps optimally correlate with admission diffusion-weighted imaging in acute stroke but thresholds vary by postprocessing platform. Stroke. 2011;42(7):1923–8.
6. Young KC, Benesch CG, Jahromi BS. Cost-effectiveness of multimodal CT for evaluating acute stroke. Neurology. 2010;75(19):1678–85.
7. Picanço MR et al. Reperfusion after 4·5 hours reduces infarct growth and improves clinical outcomes. Int J Stroke. 2014;9(3):266–9.
8. Campbell BCV et al. A multicenter, randomized, controlled study to investigate EXtending the time for Thrombolysis in Emergency Neurological Deficits with Intra-Arterial therapy (EXTEND-IA). Int J Stroke. 2014;9(1):126–32.
9. Lansberg MG et al. MRI profile and response to endovascular reperfusion after stroke (DEFUSE 2): a prospective cohort study. Lancet Neurol. 2012;11(10):860–7.
10. Yoo AJ et al. MRI-based selection for intra-arterial stroke therapy: value of pretreatment diffusion-weighted imaging lesion volume in selecting patients with acute stroke who will benefit from early recanalization. Stroke. 2009;40(6):2046–54.
11. Campbell BC et al. Endovascular therapy for ischemic stroke with perfusion-imaging selection. N Engl J Med. 2015;372(11):1009–18.
12. Parsons MW et al. Pretreatment diffusion- and perfusion-MR lesion volumes have a crucial influence on clinical response to stroke thrombolysis. J Cereb Blood Flow Metab. 2010;30(6):1214–25.
13. Lin L et al. Comparison of computed tomographic and magnetic resonance perfusion measurements in acute ischemic stroke: back-to-back quantitative analysis. Stroke. 2014;45(6):1727–32.
14. Bivard A et al. Defining the extent of irreversible brain ischemia using perfusion computed tomography. Cerebrovasc Dis. 2011;31(3):238–45.
15. Lev MH. Acute stroke imaging: what is sufficient for triage to endovascular therapies? Am J Neuroradiol. 2012;33(5):790–2.
16. Wintermark M et al. Imaging recommendations for acute stroke and transient ischemic attack patients: a joint statement by the American Society of Neuroradiology, the American College of Radiology, and the Society of Neurointerventional Surgery. Am J Neuroradiol. 2013;34(11):E117–27.
17. Fahmi F et al. Differences in CT perfusion summary maps for patients with acute ischemic stroke generated by 2 software packages. Am J Neuroradiol. 2012;33(11):2074–80.
18. Eilaghi A et al. Toward patient-tailored perfusion thresholds for prediction of stroke outcome. Am J Neuroradiol. 2014;35(3):472–7.
19. Aviv RI et al. Hemorrhagic transformation of ischemic stroke: prediction with CT perfusion. Radiology. 2009;250(3):867–77.
20. Zhu G et al. Computed tomography workup of patients suspected of acute ischemic stroke: perfusion computed tomography adds value compared with clinical evaluation, noncontrast computed tomography, and computed tomography angiogram in terms of predicting outcome. Stroke. 2013;44(4):1049–55.
21. Landis JR, Koch GG. The measurement of observer agreement for categorical data. Biometrics. 1977;33(1):159–74.
22. Lev MH. Perfusion imaging of acute stroke: its role in current and future clinical practice. Radiology. 2013;266(1):22–7.
23. Sanelli PC et al. The effect of varying user-selected input parameters on quantitative values in CT perfusion maps1. Acad Radiol. 2004;11(10):1085–92.
24. Roberts HC et al. Multisection dynamic CT perfusion for acute cerebral ischemia: the "toggling-table" technique. Am J Neuroradiol. 2001;22(6):1077–80.
25. Wintermark M et al. Dynamic perfusion CT: optimizing the temporal resolution and contrast volume for calculation of perfusion ct parameters in stroke patients. Am J Neuroradiol. 2004;25(5):720–9.
26. Murphy A et al. Low dose CT perfusion in acute ischemic stroke. Neuroradiology. 2014;56(12):1055–62.
27. Schaefer PW et al. Limited reliability of computed tomographic perfusion acute infarct volume measurements compared with diffusion-weighted imaging in anterior circulation stroke. Stroke. 2015;46(2):419–24.

10

Swirls and spots: relationship between qualitative and quantitative hematoma heterogeneity, hematoma expansion, and the spot sign

Dale Connor[1], Thien J. Huynh[1], Andrew M. Demchuk[2], Dar Dowlatshahi[3], David J. Gladstone[4], Sivaniya Subramaniapillai[1], Sean P. Symons[1] and Richard I. Aviv[1*]

Abstract

Background: Acute intracerebral hemorrhage (ICH) heterogeneity on NCCT, characterized by qualitative and quantitative methods, is predictive of hematoma expansion and mortality however association with the spot sign is not well-described. We sought to validate and determine the association between qualitative and quantitative hematoma heterogeneity with expansion and the spot sign, respectively.

Methods: We retrospectively studied 71 ICH patients presenting <24 h post-ictus with baseline NCCT, CTA and 24-hour follow-up CT available. Baseline NCCT was assessed qualitatively for presence of swirl sign or hematoma heterogeneity by two independent readers blinded to CTA findings and quantitatively using CT densitometry (CTD). Associations with 24-hour hematoma expansion ≥6 ml or ≥33 % and spot sign were assessed using logistic regression and diagnostic performance was assessed. Association between qualitative and quantitative densitometry parameters was also examined.

Results: Swirl sign and quantitative CTD standard deviation were independently associated with expansion on multivariable analysis (p = 0.037 and p = 0.032, respectively). Swirl sign and hematoma heterogeneity were predictive of CTA spot sign (p = 0.020 and p = 0.035, respectively) while CTD standard deviation demonstrated only trend univariate association. CTD parameters were not significantly associated with swirl sign while only CTD skewness was associated with hematoma heterogeneity. Agreement for swirl sign and hematoma heterogeneity identification was nearly perfect (κ = 0.81) and substantial (κ = 0.79) respectively.

Conclusion: NCCT qualitative parameters predict hematoma expansion and CTA spot sign presence. Quantitative markers independently predict hematoma expansion but not CTA spot sign presence.

Background

Hematoma expansion occurs in up to 73 % of patients with primary intracerebral hemorrhage (ICH) and is independently associated with early neurological deterioration, death, and disability [1, 2]. Prevention of expansion is an attractive therapeutic target however improved means for expansion prediction are needed to guide potential acute interventions [3, 4]. Previous studies have identified heterogeneity or low-attenuation within a hematoma on hyperacute NCCT, coined the 'swirl sign,' to be predictive of expansion and poor outcome [5–11]. Hematoma heterogeneity may partially reflect the presence of active extravasation within the hematoma in which uncoagulated blood appears iso- or hypodense relative to the brain parenchyma on CT [11]. Quantitative hematoma heterogeneity analysis using CT densitometry (CTD) is theoretically more robust, reproducible, and less prone to interpretation bias compared to qualitative techniques [5, 6]. CTD may also facilitate rapid and reliable expansion prediction in the acute setting using semi-automated techniques [12].

* Correspondence: richard.aviv@sunnybrook.ca
[1]Division of Neuroradiology and Department of Medical Imaging, Sunnybrook Health Sciences Centre, University of Toronto, 2075 Bayview Avenue, Room AG 31, Toronto, ON M4N 3M5, Canada
Full list of author information is available at the end of the article

Recently CTD parameters, including the coefficient of variation (CV) and standard deviation (SD), were found be predictive of hematoma expansion independent of initial ICH volume and time from symptom onset [6]. These promising results however have yet to be validated. The association between qualitative and quantitative parameters of hematoma heterogeneity and the CTA spot sign, a potent marker of active hemorrhage expansion [13, 14], has also not been well-studied. NCCT predictors of hematoma expansion and the CTA spot sign could theoretically mitigate the need for CTA in patients at low risk of harboring vascular lesions or alert the clinician to the suspicion of underlying CTA spot sign and potentially facilitate earlier prothrombotic or hypotensive management thereby reducing the magnitude of expansion [15]. Importantly, many centers especially in the community do not or cannot perform emergent CTA in the setting of acute ICH. We therefore attempted to validate the association between quantitative and qualitative hematoma heterogeneity, hematoma expansion and the CTA spot sign in an acute ICH population. We further sought to determine the association between quantitative CTD parameters and qualitatively assessed hematoma heterogeneity.

Methods
Study cohort
Sunnybrook Hospital Research ethics board approved study retrospectively reviewed all ICH patients entered into a departmental stroke database between September 2010 and December 2012. Study inclusion criteria were all patients presenting to our tertiary care hospital emergency department with stroke symptoms attributable to primary ICH demonstrated on non-contrast CT with follow-up 24-hour CT available. Patients with evidence of secondary ICH such as ICH from trauma, aneurysm, vascular malformation, hemorrhagic transformation of ischemic stroke, venous sinus thrombosis and tumor were excluded. Patients with isolated intraventricular hemorrhage (IVH) were also excluded. Of 106 eligible cases, 35 were excluded due to lack of 24-hour follow-up ($n = 6$), surgical intervention before follow-up ($n = 12$), administration of recombinant factor VIIa ($n = 2$), isolated IVH ($n = 4$), unknown time of onset ($n = 4$), and poor scan quality/motion artifact ($n = 7$). Seventy-one (67 %) patients were therefore included in final analysis.

Clinical data
Baseline variables were recorded in an ICH database at time of presentation and any missing data retrieved by chart review. Clinical variables included were: patient age, gender, history of anticoagulation or hypertension, baseline neurological status (NIHSS), mean arterial blood pressure (MABP), time from symptom onset to baseline CT and follow-up. Hemoglobin, platelet and white blood cell count, serum glucose, International Normalized Ratio (INR) and partial thromboplastin time (PTT) were also recorded.

Image acquisition
All patients underwent standard institutional acute ICH CT protocol, performed on a 64-slice CT scanner (LightSpeed Plus and VCT; GE Healthcare), including baseline head NCCT, CTA of the neck and intracranial circulation, and follow-up 24-hour NCCT. All NCCT was performed from the skull base to the vertex with the following parameters: 120 kVp, 340 mA, 4 × 5 mm collimation, 1 s/rotation, and table speed of 15 mm/rotation. CTA studies were acquired from the aortic arch to the vertex in helical half-scan mode with the following parameters: 0.7 mL/kg of iodinated contrast (maximum 90 mL via antecubital fossa through 18- or 20-G angiocatheter), 120 kVp, 280 mA, 1 s/rotation, 1.25-mm section thickness at 0.625-mm intervals, and table speed of 3.75 mm/rotation. CTA contrast bolus timing was performed using SmartPrep (GE Healthcare) semi-automated attenuation-triggered technique.

Imaging analysis
Individual patient hematoma volumes and quantitative CTD parameters were measured from three-dimensional ROIs on baseline and follow-up NCCT studies. Measured CTD parameters included mean hematoma density in HU, SD, CV, skewness, and kurtosis [6]. ROIs were generated using a semi-automated seeding algorithm coded in MATLAB (Version R2012b; MathWorks, Natick, Massachusetts). The ROI generation algorithm started with an operator selected seed ROI created within the confines of the hematoma and then was coded to expand into adjacent voxels meeting a minimum attenuation threshold set to 44 HU. A secondary ROI growth phase was used to expand up to 3 voxels further with minimum attenuation threshold of 38 HU in order to adequately capture the hematoma periphery and lower density details within the hematoma. Low-density voxels inside the hematoma not meeting minimum threshold attenuation, potentially representing swirl signs, were included in the ROI by a reverse growing algorithm which included all voxels not connected with the exterior of the hematoma on each axial slice. Manually defined ROI margin constraints were applied where the hematoma margins were contiguous with adjacent bone, dura, or intraventricular hemorrhage. Accuracy of all ROIs was validated by a staff neuroradiologist (XX) with 10 years of experience. Hematoma volumes were compared against the validated Quantomo technique [12, 14] for a subset of 28 cases to further ensure accuracy. Hematoma appearance on NCCT was qualitatively assessed and dichotomized into homogeneous

and heterogeneous appearance. All hematomas demonstrating enclosed regions that were iso- or hypodense to brain parenchyma were classified as heterogeneous. Heterogeneous hematomas were further subdivided into swirl sign positive or negative according to Selariu [9]. Specifically, the swirl sign was defined as an intrahematoma region of hypo or isoattenuation compared to the attenuation of brain parenchyma and may be rounded, streak-like, or irregular. If the heterogeneity was inconsistent with the swirl sign definition the hematoma was considered heterogeneous but swirl negative. To facilitate classification, standard windowing settings were used (width 30, level 30). CTA was assessed by the staff neuroradiologist for presence and number of spot signs by identifying intrahematoma contrast density on CTA, having either a serpiginous and/or spot-like appearance, without connection to an outside vessel [14, 16]. ICH location (ie. deep, lobar, and infratentorial) and IVH presence was also recorded. Baseline CT review was performed 8 weeks prior to assessment of 24-hour follow-up imaging results to avoid bias.

Statistical analysis

Outcomes for the study were 1) hematoma expansion, 2) presence of the spot sign, and 3) swirl sign and hematoma heterogeneity presence. Hematoma expansion was defined as ICH growth of >6 ml or >33 % from baseline to 24-hour CT [14, 17, 18]. Univariate associations between clinical and NCCT radiographic variables with hematoma expansion were assessed using bivariate logistic regression. Variables demonstrating significant or trend association ($p < 0.10$) were included in a multivariable logistic regression model using backwards stepwise selection. Predictors of the CTA spot sign and heterogeneity were also examined using the same approach. Prior to multivariable modelling, multicollinearity was assessed with the variance inflation factor statistic. Diagnostic performance of the swirl sign was assessed for hematoma expansion prediction with and without spot sign presence. Diagnostic performance of the swirl sign for spot sign prediction was also examined. Interobserver agreement of the swirl sign and heterogeneity was assessed using the Cohen's κ statistic. Values of κ from 0.21 to 0.4, 0.41 to 0.6, 0.61 to 0.8, and 0.81 to 1 were considered fair, moderate, substantial, and nearly perfect, respectively [19]. Pearson's correlation coefficient and intraclass correlation coefficient (ICC) compared baseline volumes obtained by the semiautomated ROI generation algorithm and the validated Quantomo technique [12]. ICC values of <0.4, 0.4 to 0.75, and >0.75 were considered to demonstrate poor, fair to good, and excellent agreement. Differences between included and excluded patients were examined with the Wilcoxon rank sum and x^2 tests for continuous and categorical/dichotomous variables respectively.

Statistical significance was defined as $p < 0.05$ for all tests. Statistical analysis was performed using SAS 9.2 (SAS Institute Inc, Cary, NC) and R, version 2.13.2 (http://www.r-project.org).

Results

Patient characteristics are summarized in Table 1. In brief, mean (SD) patient age was 68.2 ± 15.6 years and 46 (65 %) patients were male respectively. Median (interquartile range [IQR]) time from onset to baseline CT was 1.9 (1.3–4.6) hours and median (IQR) NIHSS at presentation was 10 (6–16). Hypertension and anticoagulation history was present in 57 (80 %) and 9 (13 %) patients respectively. Median (IQR) baseline ICH volume was 18.1 (5.3–37.6). Thirty-six (51 %) patients had a deep ICH location and 36 (51 %) had IVH.

There were no significant differences in patient age, gender, time from symptom onset to baseline CT, anticoagulation history, or baseline ICH volume between included and excluded patients (all $p > 0.05$). Excluded patients however had a greater IVH frequency (71 % vs. 51 %; x^2 $p = 0.042$) and higher baseline NIHSS (median [IQR] 18 [8–23] vs. 10 [6–16]; $p = 0.020$). Semiautomated hematoma volume measurements demonstrated near perfect correlation and high agreement with the previously validated Quantomo technique [12] for baseline hematoma volume measurements ($\rho = 0.90$, 95 % CI 0.80–0.95; ICC 0.84, 95 % CI 0.68–0.92 respectively). Thirty-three (46 %) and 35 (49 %) patients demonstrated a swirl sign and heterogeneous hematoma respectively. Interobserver agreement for the swirl sign and qualitatively assessed hematoma heterogeneity was nearly perfect (κ = 0.81, 95 % CI 0.67–0.96) and substantial respectively (κ = 0.79, 95 % CI 0.63–0.93).

Prediction of hematoma expansion

Hematoma expansion of >6 ml or >33 % occurred in 21 (30 %) patients. Univariate associations between clinical and radiographic predictors of hematoma expansion are summarized in Table 1.

Significant NCCT predictors of hematoma expansion included swirl sign (OR 3.3, 95 % CI 1.2–10; $p = 0.031$) and CTD SD (OR 0.65, 95 % CI 0.43–0.94; $p = 0.029$). Additionally CTD CV ($p = 0.059$), CTD mean density ($p = 0.052$), and hematoma heterogeneity ($p = 0.062$) trended to significance. No significant clinical predictors of expansion were detected, although time from onset to baseline CT of <3 h ($p = 0.059$), and baseline INR >1.5 ($p = 0.057$) trended towards significance. Collinearity was noted between the swirl sign and hematoma heterogeneity in addition to CTD SD and CTD CV and accordingly these variables were assessed in separate multivariable models. Multivariable analysis including swirl sign and CTD SD in addition to other NCCT and clinical

Table 1 Patient characteristics and univariate associations with hematoma expansion

Variable	All patients (n = 71)	Hematoma expansion* (n = 21)	No hematoma expansion (n = 50)	p-value**
Clinical Variables				
Age, years (mean ± SD)	68.2 ± 15.6	71.1 ± 14.0	66.9 ± 16.2	0.295
Gender, male (%)	46 (65)	13 (62)	33 (66)	0.742
Hypertension (%)	57 (80)	16 (76)	41 (82)	0.574
Anticoagulation (%)	9 (13)	2 (10)	7 (14)	0.605
Time to Baseline CT, hours	1.9 (1.3–4.6)	1.4 (1.2–1.9)	2.1 (1.4–6.4)	0.361
<3 h n (%)	49 (69)	18 (86)	31 (62)	0.059
NIHSS	10 (6–16)	11 (8–15)	10 (5–16)	0.751
MABP, mmHg	146 (130–172)	150 (137–172)	144 (129–169)	0.773
Laboratory Values				
Hemoglobin, g/L	142 (131–150)	142 (117–150)	142 (135–149)	0.317
Platelets, x10^9/L	228 (180–286)	239 (181–297)	227 (175–268)	0.173
WBC, x10^9/L	8.1 (6.8–10.8)	7.5 (6.7–9.1)	8.6 (6.8–10.9)	0.257
INR	1.03 (0.99–1.12)	1.06 (0.99–1.20)	1.02 (0.99–1.11)	0.243
INR >1.5 (%)	6 (8)	4 (19)	2 (4)	0.057
PTT (sec)	31 (28–34)	32 (28–36)	30 (28–33)	0.455
Glucose (mmol/L)	7.1 (6.0–8.3)	7.0 (6.1–7.8)	7.1 (6.0–8.4)	0.529
Radiological Characteristics				
NCCT characteristics				
Baseline Hematoma Volume (cm^3)	18.1 (5.3–37.6)	8.0 (4.3–42.9)	18.5 (6.2–36.3)	0.633
ICH Location				0.211
Deep (%)	36 (51)	13 (62)	23 (46)	–
Lobar (%)	29 (41)	7 (33)	22 (44)	–
Infratentorial (%)	6 (8)	1 (5)	5 (10)	–
IVH presence (%)	36 (51)	10 (48)	26 (52)	0.736
Swirl Sign (%)	33 (46)	14 (67)	19 (38)	**0.031**
Heterogeneous Hematoma (%)	35 (49)	14 (67)	21 (42)	0.062
Quantitative NCCT Densitometry Values				
Mean HU (mean ± SD)	55.1 ± 3.9	53.7 ± 3.7	55.7 ± 3.9	0.052
SD (mean ± SD)	10.1 ± 1.5	9.4 ± 1.7	10.4 ± 1.4	**0.029**
CV (mean ± SD)	0.182 ± 0.021	0.174 ± 0.024	0.185 ± 0.019	0.059
Skewness (mean ± SD)	−0.23 ± 0.26	−0.18 ± 0.18	−0.24 ± 0.29	0.383
Kurtosis (mean ± SD)	2.31 ± 0.37	2.30 ± 0.24	2.31 ± 0.41	0.952
CTA variables				
CTA spot sign presence (%)	26 (37)	12 (57)	14 (28)	**0.023**
CTA spot sign number	0 (0–1)	1 (0–3)	0 (0–1)	**0.009**

All values represent median (IQR) or n (%) unless specified
*Hematoma expansion defined as >6 mL or >33 %
**p-value calculated from bivariate logistic regression
Bold font indicates statistical significance

predictors of expansion with trend association yielded a final model including swirl sign (OR 3.3, 95 % CI 1.1–10.6; p = 0.037) and CTD SD (OR 0.66, 95 % CI 0.43–0.94; p = 0.032). Substitution of CTD CV for CTD SD yielded a final model including swirl sign (OR 3.8, 95 % CI 1.3–12.8; p = 0.020) and CTD mean density (OR 0.8, 95 % CI 0.70–0.97; p = 0.033). Substitution of swirl sign with hematoma heterogeneity in the multivariable regression with CTD SD or CTD CV yielded final models that included CTD SD alone or hematoma heterogeneity (OR

3.4, 95 % CI 1.1–11.2; $p = 0.040$) and CTD mean density (OR 0.84, 95 % CI 0.70–0.97; $p = 0.032$), respectively.

Multivariable model area under the curve ranged from 0.64 for the model with swirl sign alone to 0.73 for a model with swirl sign and CTD SD. There was no statistically significant difference in expansion discrimination between multivariable models.

Diagnostic performance of swirl sign and hematoma heterogeneity for hematoma expansion prediction with and without the presence of a spot sign are listed in Table 2.

Predictors of CTA spot sign

A CTA spot sign was present in 26 (37 %) patients. Significant NCCT predictors of the spot sign on univariate analysis included the swirl sign (OR 4.5, 95 % CI 1.6–12.7; $p = 0.005$) and heterogeneous hematomas (OR 4.9, 95 % CI 1.7–15; $p = 0.003$). Trend associations were noted for CTD SD (OR 0.73, 95 % CI 0.51–1.0; $p = 0.067$) and CTD CV (OR 0.01, 95 % CI 0.00–10.7; $p = 0.076$). Significant clinical predictors of spot sign presence included time from onset to baseline CT <3 h (OR = 9.6; 95 % CI = 2.0–46; $p = 0.004$) and NIHSS (OR 1.1; 95 % CI 1.0–1.2; $p = 0.009$). Collinearity was noted between the swirl sign and hematoma heterogeneity in addition to CTD SD and CV. Multivariable analysis including swirl sign and CTD SD in addition to other NCCT and clinical predictors of the spot sign with trend association demonstrated a final model including swirl sign (OR 3.2; 95 % CI 1.1–10; $p = 0.020$) and time from symptom onset to baseline CT <3 h (OR 7.1; 95 % CI 1.7–48; $p = 0.035$). Substitution of CTD CV for CTD SD yielded the same final model. Substitution of swirl sign with hematoma heterogeneity in multivariable regression with CTD SD or CTD CV yielded final models that included hematoma heterogeneity (OR 3.4, 95 % CI 1.1–11; $p = 0.035$) and time from symptom onset to baseline CT <3 h (OR 6.7, 95 % CI 1.6–46; $p = 0.020$). Both multivariable models demonstrated a model area under the curve of 0.75. Diagnostic performance of the swirl sign and hematoma heterogeneity for spot sign presence is demonstrated in Table 3.

Association between CTD parameters and qualitative hematoma heterogeneity

Univariate analysis between CTD predictors and the swirl sign and hematoma heterogeneity separately demonstrated trend association between CTD skewness and swirl sign ($p = 0.079$) and significant association CTD skewness and hematoma heterogeneity (OR 0.1, 95 % CI 0.01–0.63; $p = 0.021$). The remaining CTD parameters, including CTD SD, CV, mean, and kurtosis were not significantly associated with either outcome (all $p > 0.10$).

Discussion

Previous studies of the swirl sign and hematoma heterogeneity in acute ICH, assessed both qualitatively and quantitatively on NCCT, demonstrated significant statistical associations with hematoma expansion [5, 6]. Our study findings are concordant with these findings demonstrating that both qualitative (swirl sign) and quantitative (CTD SD) measures independently predict hematoma expansion. Other quantitative predictors of expansion included CTD mean density and qualitative hematoma heterogeneity. For both CTD SD and CTD mean density, an inverse relationship with expansion was noted such that the risk of expansion was increased when either CTD SD or CTD mean density decreased as demonstrated in densitometry histograms from Fig. 1. The inverse relationship between CTD SD and greater hematoma expansion was also noted by Barras et al. in their previous CTD study of 81 acute ICH patients in the placebo arm of the Phase 2 recombinant Factor VIIa trial [6]. The same study identified CTD CV as the greatest individual predictor of expansion although this only demonstrated trend association in the present study ($p = 0.059$). The differences between the two studies remains unclear, but both studies confirm the potential for quantitative prediction of hematoma expansion.

To our knowledge, the association between the swirl sign, hematoma heterogeneity and the CTA spot sign is not previously studied. A significant association between the swirl sign and qualitative hematoma heterogeneity and the spot sign independent of time from symptom onset was demonstrated. These findings further support the importance of recognizing the swirl sign and hematoma heterogeneity for predicting spot sign

Table 2 Diagnostic performance of qualitative hematoma heterogeneity for hematoma expansion

	Sensitivity	Specificity	Positive predictive value	Negative predictive value
Spot Sign	57 (34–78)	72 (58–84)	46 (27–67)	80 (65–90)
Swirl Sign	67 (43–85)	62 (47–75)	42 (25–61)	82 (66–92)
Either	76 (53–92)	50 (36–64)	39 (24–55)	83 (65–94)
Both	48 (26–70)	84 (71–93)	56 (31–78)	79 (66–89)

All values listed in percentage with 95 % confidence intervals listed in parentheses

Table 3 Diagnostic performance of qualitative hematoma heterogeneity for spot sign presence

	Sensitivity	Specificity	Positive predictive value	Negative predictive value
Swirl Sign	69 (48–86)	67 (51–80)	55 (36–72)	79 (63–90)
Hematoma Heterogeneity	73 (52–88)	64 (49–78)	54 (37–71)	80 (37–71)

All values listed in percentage with 95 % confidence intervals listed in parentheses

presence. The inability of quantitative measures to predict the spot sign or the swirl sign but independent association with hematoma expansion suggests that qualitative and quantitative measures may be capturing different imaging features of potential for hematoma expansion. Therefore, optimal NCCT ICH expansion prediction, in the absence of CTA, may benefit from both qualitative and quantitative measures of hematoma heterogeneity. An important limitation of swirl sign recognition is that platelet-fibrin thrombi may mimic a swirl sign in vitro by reducing attenuation relative to retracted blood clot [20]. CTA may therefore be preferable, by facilitating direct contrast extravasation visualization. In the absence of CTA availability, the swirl sign and hematoma heterogeneity may however aide in hematoma expansion prediction.

Interobserver agreement of the swirl sign and hematoma heterogeneity was nearly perfect ($\kappa = 0.81$) and substantial ($\kappa = 0.79$), respectively, similar to results demonstrated by Selariu for the swirl sign ($\kappa = 0.80$). To facilitate high interobserver agreement, a pre-specified viewing window width and level of 30 and 30 respectively is recommended similar to strategies employed in NCCT evaluation for ischemic stroke and for CTA spot sign identification [17, 21]. Utilization of thin slice CT may further improve agreement or alter performance

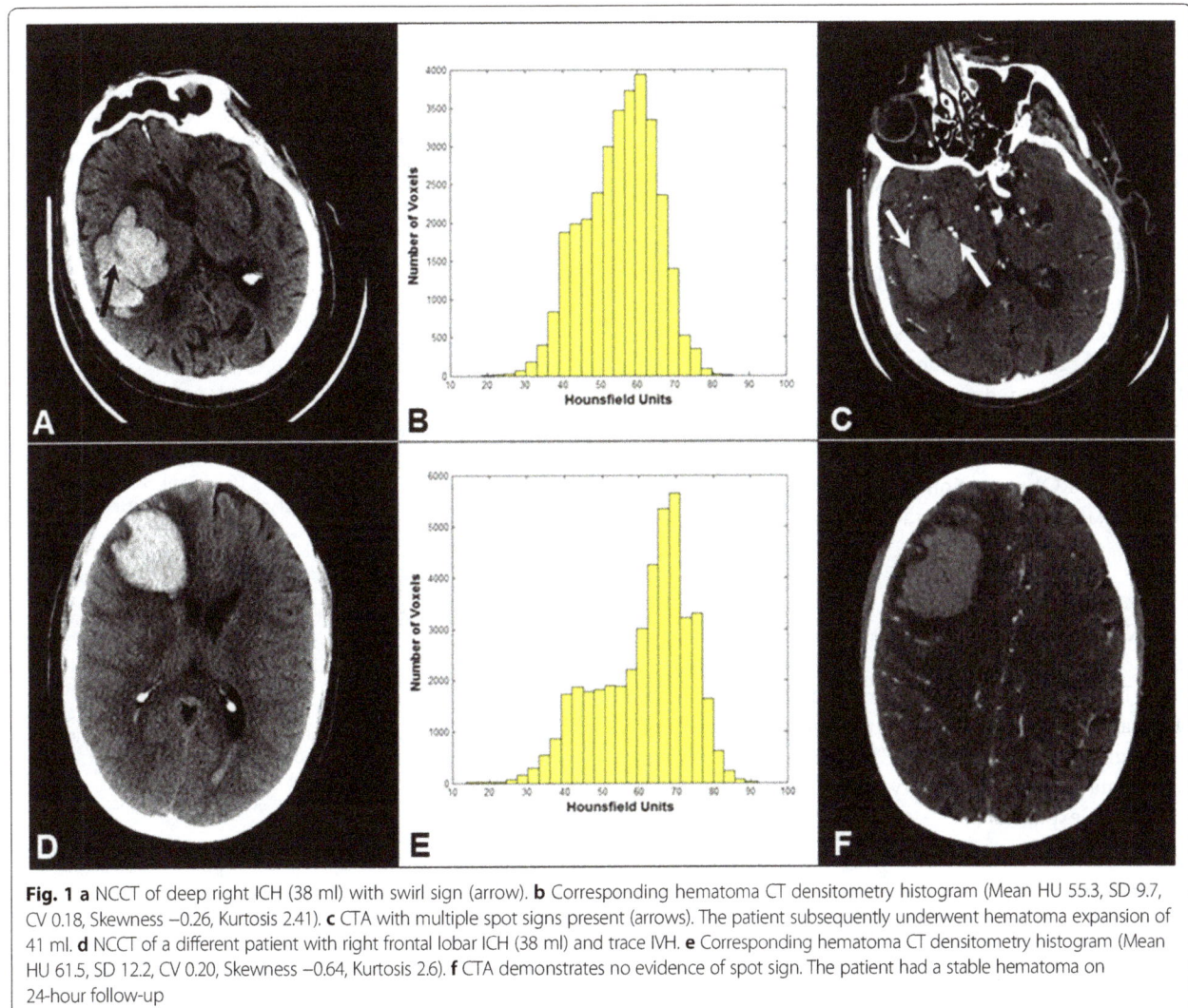

Fig. 1 a NCCT of deep right ICH (38 ml) with swirl sign (arrow). **b** Corresponding hematoma CT densitometry histogram (Mean HU 55.3, SD 9.7, CV 0.18, Skewness −0.26, Kurtosis 2.41). **c** CTA with multiple spot signs present (arrows). The patient subsequently underwent hematoma expansion of 41 ml. **d** NCCT of a different patient with right frontal lobar ICH (38 ml) and trace IVH. **e** Corresponding hematoma CT densitometry histogram (Mean HU 61.5, SD 12.2, CV 0.20, Skewness −0.64, Kurtosis 2.6). **f** CTA demonstrates no evidence of spot sign. The patient had a stable hematoma on 24-hour follow-up

but requires further study [22]. Swirl sign prevalence was modestly higher in our study (46 %) compared to Selariu (30 %) and Kim (15 %). Previous radiological-surgical correlation studies in patients with traumatic extra-axial hematomas demonstrate that the swirl sign was associated with evidence of active bleeding at time of surgery evacuation, most commonly arterial hemorrhage [11, 23]. Extravasation of intravenous contrast both on post-contrast CT and conventional angiogram in epidural hematomas has also been shown and further support active bleeding in epidural hematomas [24, 25]. Recently in acute ICH patients, the spot sign was studied using a dynamic 60 s CTA acquisition and demonstrated evolving growth over time consistent with sites of active extravasation [13]. Our finding that swirl signs were associated both hematoma expansion and spot sign is consistent with these previous findings suggesting recent or on-going extravasation and potential risk for further expansion [20].

Our study was limited in sample size with a significant proportion of patients excluded due to surgical intervention, lack of adequate CT follow-up, or severe motion artifact at baseline. This limited our statistical power and number of variables allowable for multivariable analysis. This study was also performed retrospectively and further prospective study is required to determine whether these methods may be employed with high-interobserver agreement real-time in the acute setting. Variations in CT scanners may contribute to heterogeneity in CTD results and further validation in a multicenter setting with CT scanners from different models and manufacturers is needed [6]. The semi-automated ROI generation techniques used in this study demonstrated high correlation with the previously validated Quantomo technique but remains limited by the need for manual seed placement and tracing to prevent ROI extension into areas of IVH and dural or calvarial hematoma contact.

Conclusion

The NCCT swirl sign and hematoma heterogeneity are significantly associated with hematoma expansion and the CTA spot sign. CTD SD is the best CTD predictor of expansion however is not significantly associated with spot sign. In the absence of CTA availability, swirl sign and hematoma heterogeneity recognition may aide in hematoma expansion.

Abbreviations
CTD: CT densitometry; CV: Coefficient of variation; ICC: Intraclass correlation coefficient; ICH: Intracerebral hemorrhage; INR: International Normalized Ratio; MABP: Mean arterial blood pressure; PTT: Partial thromboplastin time; IQR: Interquartile range; IVH: Intraventricular hemorrhage; SD: Standard deviation.

Competing interests
The authors declare that they have no competing interests.

Authors' contributions
Conceived and designed the research RIA, acquired the data DC, AD, TH, SS, DD, DG, SPS. Analyzed and interpreted the data DC, TH, RIA. Performed statistical analysis DC, TH, RIA. Handled funding and supervision DD, AD, RIA. Drafted the manuscript all authors. Made critical revision of the manuscript for important intellectual content all authors. All Authors read and approved the final manuscript.

Acknowledgements
Grant support
Dr. Huynh was supported by a Canadian Institutes of Health Research Masters Award.
Dr. Dowlatshahi was supported by a Canadian Institutes of Health Research Fellowship Award and a University of Ottawa Department of Medicine Research Salary Award.
All remaining authors report no relevant disclosures.

Presentation
Part content of this manuscript was presented at the 2014 American Society of Neuroradiology Annual Meeting.

Author details
[1]Division of Neuroradiology and Department of Medical Imaging, Sunnybrook Health Sciences Centre, University of Toronto, 2075 Bayview Avenue, Room AG 31, Toronto, ON M4N 3M5, Canada. [2]Calgary Stroke Program, Department of Clinical Neurosciences, Department of Radiology, Hotchkiss Brain Institute, University of Calgary, Calgary, Canada. [3]Department of Medicine (Neurology), University of Ottawa, Ottawa Hospital Research Institute, Ottawa, Canada. [4]Division of Neurology, Department of Medicine, and Brain Sciences Program, Sunnybrook Health Sciences Centre, University of Toronto, Toronto, Canada.

References
1. Davis SM, Broderick J, Hennerici M, Brun NC, Diringer MN, Mayer SA, et al. Hematoma growth is a determinant of mortality and poor outcome after intracerebral hemorrhage. Neurology. 2006;66:1175–81.
2. Brott T, Broderick J, Kothari R, Barsan W, Tomsick T, Sauerbeck L, et al. Early hemorrhage growth in patients with intracerebral hemorrhage. Stroke. 1997;28:1–5.
3. Huynh TJ, Symons SP, Aviv RI. Advances in CT for prediction of hematoma expansion in acute intracerebral hemorrhage. Imaging Med. 2013;5:539–51.
4. Mayer SA, Brun NC, Begtrup K, Broderick J, Davis S, Diringer MN, et al. Efficacy and safety of recombinant activated factor VII for acute intracerebral hemorrhage. N Engl J Med. 2008;358:2127–37.
5. Barras CD, Tress BM, Christensen S, MacGregor L, Collins M, Desmond PM, et al. Density and shape as CT predictors of intracerebral hemorrhage growth. Stroke. 2009;40:1325–31.
6. Barras CD, Tress BM, Christensen S, Collins M, Desmond PM, Skolnick BE, et al. Quantitative CT densitometry for predicting intracerebral hemorrhage growth. AJNR Am J Neuroradiol. 2013;34:1139–44.
7. Al-nakshabandi NA. The swirl sign. Radiology. 2001;218:433.
8. Kim J, Smith A, Hemphill JC, Smith WS, Lu Y, Dillon WP, et al. Contrast extravasation on CT predicts mortality in primary intracerebral hemorrhage. AJNR Am J Neuroradiol. 2008;29:520–5.
9. Selariu E, Zia E, Brizzi M, Abul-Kasim K. Swirl sign in intracerebral haemorrhage: definition, prevalence, reliability and prognostic value. BMC Neurol. 2012;12:109.
10. Smith SD, Eskey CJ. Hemorrhagic stroke. Radiol Clin North Am. 2011;49:27–45.
11. Zimmerman RA, Bilaniuk LT. Computed tomographic staging of traumatic epidural bleeding. Radiology. 1982;144:809–12.
12. Kosior JC, Idris S, Dowlatshahi D, Alzawahmah M, Eesa M, Sharma P, et al. Quantomo: validation of a computer-assisted methodology for the volumetric analysis of intracerebral haemorrhage. Int J Stroke. 2011;6:302–5.
13. Dowlatshahi D, Wasserman JK, Momoli F, Petrcich W, Stotts G, Hogan M, et al. Evolution of computed tomography angiography spot sign is consistent with

a site of active hemorrhage in acute intracerebral hemorrhage. Stroke. 2014;45:277–80.

14. Demchuk AM, Dowlatshahi D, Rodriguez-Luna D, Molina CA, Blas YS, Dzialowski I, et al. Prediction of haematoma growth and outcome in patients with intracerebral haemorrhage using the CT-angiography spot sign (PREDICT): a prospective observational study. Lancet Neurol. 2012;11:307–14.

15. Anderson CS, Heeley E, Huang Y, Wang J, Stapf C, Delcourt C, et al. Rapid blood-pressure lowering in patients with acute intracerebral hemorrhage. N Engl J Med. 2013;368:2355–65.

16. Thompson AL, Kosior JC, Gladstone DJ, Hopyan JJ, Symons SP, Romero F, et al. Defining the CT angiography "spot sign" in primary intracerebral hemorrhage. Can J Neurol Sci. 2009;36:456–61.

17. Wada R, Aviv RI, Fox AJ, Sahlas DJ, Gladstone DJ, Tomlinson G, et al. CT angiography "spot sign" predicts hematoma expansion in acute intracerebral hemorrhage. Stroke. 2007;38:1257–62.

18. Dowlatshahi D, Demchuk AM, Flaherty ML, Ali M, Lyden PL, Smith EE. Defining hematoma expansion in intracerebral hemorrhage: Relationship with patient outcomes. Neurology. 2011;76:1238–44.

19. Landis JR, Koch GG. The measurement of observer agreement for categorical data. Biometrics. 1977;33:159–74.

20. New PF, Aronow S. Attenuation measurements of whole blood and blood fractions in computed tomography. Radiology. 1976;121:635–40.

21. Lev MH, Farkas J, Gemmete JJ, Hossain ST, Hunter GJ, Koroshetz WJ, et al. Acute stroke: improved nonenhanced CT detection–benefits of soft-copy interpretation by using variable window width and center level settings. Radiology. 1999;213:150–5.

22. Riedel CH, Zoubie J, Ulmer S, Gierthmuehlen J, Jansen O. Thin-Slice Reconstructions of Nonenhanced CT Images Allow for Detection of Thrombus in Acute Stroke. Stroke. 2012;43:2319–23.

23. Greenberg J, Cohen WA, Cooper PR. The "hyperacute" extraaxial intracranial hematoma: computed tomographic findings and clinical significance. Neurosurgery. 1985;17:48–56.

24. Helmer FA, Sukoff MH, Plaut MR. Angiographic extravasation of contrast medium in an epidural hematoma. Case report. J Neurosurg. 1968;29:652–4.

25. Palmieri A. Extravasation of contrast-enhanced blood in an epidural hematoma. Neuroradiology. 1981;21:163–4.

11

Translational theranostic methodology for diagnostic imaging and the concomitant treatment of malignant solid tumors

Hemant Sarin

Abstract

Pathologic hyperpermeability exists in the spectrum of disease states, including neuro-ischemic, neuro-inflammatory and neuro-oncological. To-date the characterization of disease pathology with T_1-weighted quantitative dynamic contrast-enhanced magnetic resonance imaging has relied on the study of modeled microvascular parameters such as diseased tissue transvascular flow rates of small molecule paramagnetic imaging agents with short plasma half-lives, based on which it is difficult to assess the specific nature of the disease state. Another type of T_1-weighted quantitative dynamic contrast-enhanced magnetic resonance imaging involves the use of paramagnetic heavy metal-chelated dendrimer nanoparticles that possess longer plasma half-lives with pre-determined molar relaxivities to quantitatively image concentration of macromolecular contrast agent accumulation over time in hyperpermeable pathology such as solid tumor tissue with the important advantage of concomitantly treating the pathology, which, in recent years, has been shown to be possible with the use of optimally-sized theranostic dendrimer nanoparticles in the 7 to 10 nanometer size range that are functionalized biocompatibly with a small molecule therapeutic. In this focused review, this translational theranostic methodology for quantitative dynamic contrast-enhanced magnetic resonance imaging and the concomitant treatment of malignant solid tumors with optimally designed theranostic nanoparticles within the 7 to 10 nanometer size range is discussed in context of fine-tuning its suitability for the study and treatment of other disease states with pathologic hyperpermeability and without.

Keywords: Nanoparticle, Functionalized dendrimer, Quantitative magnetic resonance imaging, Bi-compartmental modeling, Intravenous administration, Drug delivery, Blood half-life, Pathologic angiogenesis, Primary brain tumor, Metastases

Introduction

Pathologic angiogenesis is a hallmark of hyperpermeable disease states of chromic hypoxia, particularly solid malignancies, irrespective of type or grade, with there being a physiologic upper limit of pore size greater than that of normal healthy tissue blood capillaries with few exceptions [1-3]. In other disease states of hyperpermeability such as neuro-ischemic disease the character of microvascular barrier dysfunction depends on the time course of hypoxia, whereby acute ischemia results in cytotoxic edema and in secondarily altered diffusion of water molecules within the tissue interstitia [4] followed by varying periods of endothelial cell dysfunction and compromised inter-endothelial junctional complex integrity of varying degrees [5], as may be the case in the hyperpermeability of neuro-inflammatory disease.

Diagnostic imaging with hydrophilic contrast agents enables the detection of pathologic hyperpermeability in the form of abnormal contrast enhancement of the diseased tissue interstitium. This abnormal contrast enhancement of diseased tissue is observable following the intravenous infusion of hydrophilic small molecule contrast agents but requires administration at relatively high doses, of tens of grams of the hydrophilic small molecule contrast agent, and often necessitates the intra-arterial or intra-thecal administration due to the non-selectivity of these contrast agents combined with their relatively short plasma half-lives, which is irrespective of imaging modality, whether

Correspondence: hsmd74@hotmail.com
[1]Charleston, West Virginia (WV), USA

it is computed tomography (CT), positron emission tomography (PET) or magnetic resonance imaging (MRI). Furthermore, due to the sub-optimal pharmacokineticodyamics of small molecule contrast agents and the requirement for the administration of high doses, the issue of systemic toxicity arises and is not uncommon, which can manifests as systemic hypersensitivity, either as immediate or delayed, depending on the biophysical properties of the contrast agent, whereby contrast agents such as Omnipaque 370, an iodinated hexol for CT, can cause immediate-type hypersensitivity reactions, while those such as gadopentetate dimeglumine (Magnevist) or gadodiamide (Omniscan), both being poorly chelated forms of polyvalent heavy metal Gadolinium (Gd3+) cause delayed–type hypersensitivity [6], in contrast to when Gd3+ is introduced into the biological system in its much more stably chelated biocompatible cyclic form of Gd-DOTA (Gd-Gadoteric acid) [7].

Although the mainstay of present day diagnostic neurovascular magnetic resonance imaging in everyday clinical practice remains the acquisition of images in signal space without respect to the quantification of relative contrast enhancement [8], magnetic resonance imaging affords the ability to detect contrast-enhanced signal change in real-time at exquisite resolution as compared to CT or PET imaging, whereby contrast-enhanced signal change can be quantified accurately for MRI contrast agents of appropriate exterior biophysical character [3,9]. Of the select premier academic centers that offer dynamic contrast-enhanced MRI-based quantification, these centers offer bi-compartmental model-based estimates of permeability surface area product parameters such as K$trans$ (forward transvascular flow rate per min; permeability surface area product) [10-12] and Vp (vascular plasma volume) [12], parameters derived on the basis of the bi-compartmental modeling of change in normalized contrast-enhanced plasma signal to that of the change in normalized contrast-enhanced diseased tissue signal over time with contrast agents having short blood half-lives [10,12,13]. Even as model-derived parameters identify areas of hyperpermeability consistent with pathologic hyperpermeability [14] and offer perspective into therapeutic efficacy for pathologies of known etiology [15], these parameters such as K$trans$ are also normally elevated for hyperpermeable healthy tissues [16,17], being non-specific parameters, making it difficult to discriminate solid tumor tissue from normally hyperpermeable tissues such as muscle tissue [18], especially at tumor infiltrating border zones where the permeability surface area product values are marginally elevated [16,18].

The poor diagnostic specificity of dynamic contrast-enhanced MRI-based bi-compartmentally modeled microvascular permeability parameters of small molecule contrast agent pharmacokineticodynamics [19-23] cannot

be overcome by temporarily increasing the blood half-life of a small molecule contrast agent by decreasing its renal filtration fraction [12,24], or alternatively, by increasing the dose, due to the non-selective extravasation of small molecule contrast agents of less than 2 nanometers into healthy tissues with loose macula occludens junctions or fenestrated endothelial cells [1,2]. The poor diagnostic cum therapeutic specificity of small molecule contrast agent pharmacokineticodynamics, however, can be improved by the utilization of biocompatible macromolecular agents of the dendritic sub-class of larger sizes within the optimal size range of 7 to 10 nanometers [3,8,25,26] because even as the per minute forward transvascular flow rate (K$trans$) from blood plasma into the solid tumor interstitium decreases significantly with increasing contrast agent molecular size [27,28], the blood plasma half-life of a contrast agent increases with increasing size, whereby the contrast agent's blood plasma half life becomes the primary determinant of the extensiveness of intratumoral contrast agent accumulation within solid tumor tissue [3,8,28,29], which becomes important for the diagnostic imaging, and importantly, the treatment of solid tumors, in which small molecule chemotherapeutics do not build up to effective concentrations [3,30,31].

The current status of the field of translational theranostics is reviewed herein in context of a methodological discussion of the prototypical quantitative dynamic contrast-enhanced magnetic resonance imaging-based theranostic approach for the concomitant diagnosis and non-invasive treatment of solid tumors, one which has translational potential towards clinical application.

Review
Small molecules and nanoparticles for non- and semi-quantitative diagnostic imaging

Small molecules with biophysical properties of specific character have applications for a variety of diagnostic imaging modalities including dense atom-based for CT imaging, radioisotope-based for PET imaging, photostable luminescent atom- or fluorescent organic biomolecule-based for fluorescent imaging, as well as paramagnetic atom-based such as Gadolinium-based for magnetic resonance imaging [32], however, they possess short blood plasma half-lives and lack polyvalency, in contrast to their commensurate macromolecular nanoparticulate-based forms.

Due to the limitations of small molecule-based diagnostic imaging probes, particularly short blood plasma half-lives and lack polyvalency, over decades, macromolecular and polymeric nanoparticle forms have been developed, including for quantum dot-based fluorescent imaging for *in vivo* applications [33,34], and those of greater probability for biocompatibility investigated for clinical imaging, including for PET imaging, which include radioisotopes conjugated to 150 kDa antibodies that possess longer blood half-lives at a hydrodynamic molecular size of approximately 12 nanometers [35], as well as for diagnostic MRI for the clinical setting, which include: (1) iron oxide core-based ferromagnetic nanoparticles with various types of non-covalent dextran-based coatings, beginning in earlier years with interest in the clinical diagnostic imaging application of individual particles in the 16 to 35 nanometer size range [36-38], and cumulating in most recent years towards the clinical development of very small citrated-dextran coated iron oxide nanoparticles (VSOPs) with an anionic exterior and a molecular size of approximately 8 nanometers for macrophage imaging due to the propensity for de-coating and the uptake of iron oxide cores by cells of the monocycte-macrophage phagocytic system [39]; and (2) a dendritic conjugate of chelated paramagnetic heavy metal Gadolinium, Gadomer-17, a 17 kDa dendrimer-based nanoparticle with anionic exterior polyvalency and an improved blood half-life at a molecular size of approximately 3 nanometers, which has been utilized exclusively as a blood pool contrast agent for perfusion magnetic resonance imaging [40].

In addition to Gadomer-17, other spherical monodisperse nanoparticles of the dendrimer sub-class have been extensively studied in more recent decades, for their applications as blood pool agents for blood and lymphatic perfusion MRI [41-43], as well as for studying microvascular permeability of hyperpermeable pathology [43-45], which include the most biocompatible of the imageable dendrimer sub-class, those employing cyclic tetracarboxylic acid DOTA as the chelate for Gadolinium, and demonstrate biocompatible biophysical character including exterior functionalization, shape and size, happening to fall within the molecular size range of 2 nm to 14 nm: This being the case, however, not much emphasis has been placed on the following two crucial aspects the first being on the applicability of the imageable dendrimer sub-class for therapeutic purposes including those in the optimal size range for selective transvascular drug delivery of chemotherapy into hyperpermeable pathologies such as solid tumors, and the second being, on the applicability of dynamic contrast-enhanced imaging such as dynamic contrast-enhanced MRI to non-invasively quantify therapeutic delivery into hyperpermeable pathologies voxel-by-voxel, until most recently [1,3,8,25,26,28,29].

In the few years from 2006 to 2009, it was determined that imageable dendrimer-based theranostic nanoparticles that possess longer blood plasma half-lives (Figures 1 and 2) achieve effective concentrations in pathologic tissue cells of solid tumors [3,8,28,29], with the optimal size range for nanoparticles with an anionically neutralized exterior being between 7 and 10 nanometers in hydrodynamic diameter [3,8,25], which is due to solid

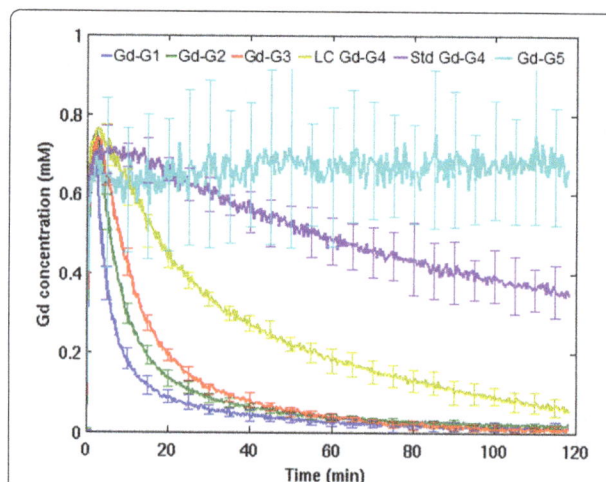

Figure 1 Superior sagittal sinus blood plasma Gd concentration curves over 2 hours following 1 minute bolus intravenous infusion of Gd-DTPA dendrimer generations G1 through G8 infusions at dose of 0.09 mmol Gd/kg body weight (bw). Blood plasma concentrations measured via dynamic contrast-enhanced MRI-based analysis by selection of 5-to-10 voxels in the superior sagittal sinus (SSS) free from partial volume averaging effects. Gd-G1 (n = 5), Gd-G2 (n = 6), Gd-G3 (n = 6), lowly conjugated (LC) Gd-G4 (n = 4), standard (Std) Gd-G4 (n = 6), Gd-G5 (n = 6), Gd-G6 (n = 5), Gd-G7 (n = 5) and Gd-G8 (n = 6). Gd-G5 through Gd-G8 dendrimers rapidly reach and maintain a steady state in blood over 2 hours (G6, G7 and G8 not shown for clarity). Error bars represent standard deviation (s.d.) and are shown once every five minutes for clarity. Adapted from references [3,8,28].

tumor blood capillary microvasculature having a physiologic upper limit of pore size of approximately 12 nanometers [29], it being more defective than the blood capillary microvasculature supplying normal healthy tissues [1]. During the course of this experimental studies, the sensitivity of a prototypical translational theranostic approach for quantifiable dynamic contrast-enhanced imaging-based concomitant imaging and treatment of solid malignancies has been validated in over 150 rodent subjects bearing over 250 orthotopic and ectopic malignant gliomas from volumes beginning at 20 mm^3 (2–3 mm diameter tumors) utilizing 7.5 nanometer diameter-sized Gadolinium-DTPA-dendrimer nanoparticles infused over 1 minute [28,29] (Figures 3, 4, 5, 6, 7; Table 1) and 9 nanometer diameter-sized Gadolinium-DTPA-dendrimer-Doxorubicin nanoparticles infused intravenously over 2 minutes [3,8] (Figure 8; Table 1).

Historical overview on the development of nanoparticles for therapeutic purposes: From liposomes to dendrimers

Beginning in the 1980s, there has been a virtual explosion in the field of polymeric science for biological applications [46-49], which has led to the development of various investigational macromolecular therapeutics as vehicles for the delivery of small molecule chemotherapeutics based

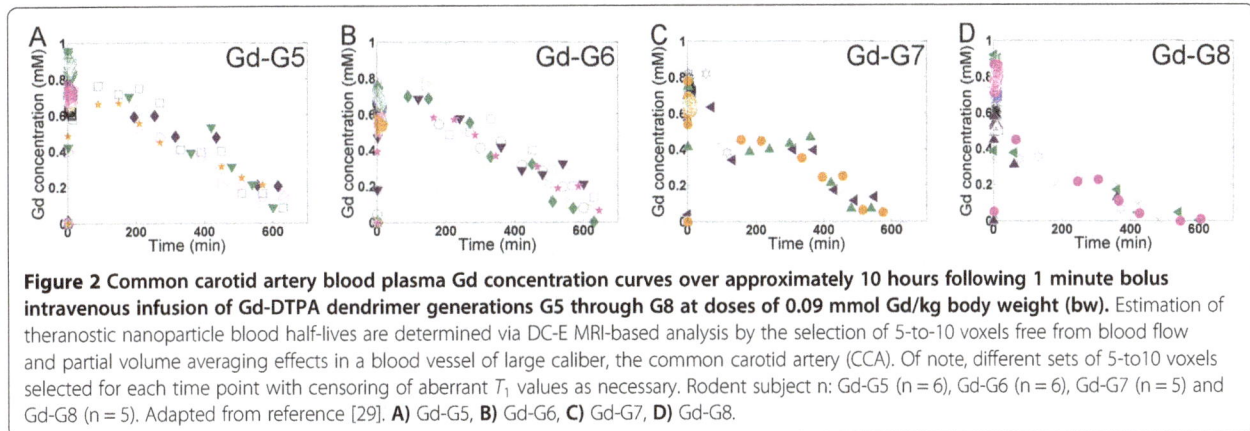

Figure 2 Common carotid artery blood plasma Gd concentration curves over approximately 10 hours following 1 minute bolus intravenous infusion of Gd-DTPA dendrimer generations G5 through G8 at doses of 0.09 mmol Gd/kg body weight (bw). Estimation of theranostic nanoparticle blood half-lives are determined via DC-E MRI-based analysis by the selection of 5-to-10 voxels free from blood flow and partial volume averaging effects in a blood vessel of large caliber, the common carotid artery (CCA). Of note, different sets of 5-to10 voxels selected for each time point with censoring of aberrant T_1 values as necessary. Rodent subject n: Gd-G5 (n = 6), Gd-G6 (n = 6), Gd-G7 (n = 5) and Gd-G8 (n = 5). Adapted from reference [29]. **A)** Gd-G5, **B)** Gd-G6, **C)** Gd-G7, **D)** Gd-G8.

on the enhanced permeation and retention (EPR) phenomenon [47,50] including to overcome multi-drug resistance [51] via local sustained release [52], but without emphasis on the optimal size range or design for biocompatibility in the biological system in the physiologic state, until recently [1-3,7,8,25,26]. However, it has since then been realized that more attention must be paid to the biophysical properties of macromolecular therapeutics such as the purposeful introduction of cationicity to the exterior of sub-optimally sized nanoparticles in order to improve their permeation across the blood-tumor barrier and diffusion through the tumor interstitium [53,54], which results in significant non-selective toxicity to the biological system in the physiologic state [2,3,25,26]. Of the selected subset of these macromolecular drug carriers that have been tested in the clinical setting for therapeutic applications, these include liposomes in the 100 to 200

nanometer size range [55,56]; it is sufficient to re-iterate that for non-pegylated liposomal doxorubicin (Myocet/Doxil), there is the rapid uptake of the non-pegylated forms (Myocet/Doxil) by the monocycte-macrophage phagocytic and reticuloendothelial systems, which results in only micormolar concentrations in blood plasma [57], and that for the pegylated forms (Caelyx) with longer circulatory half lives than that of the non-pegylated form [57], there is a widespread myoinflammatory response manifesting as different grades of palmar-plantar erythro-dysesthesia (hand-foot syndrome) [58], which is likely a form of microvascular inflammatory necrosis (author observation) due to the continuous slow release of low concentrations of doxorubicin, a cationic lipophile anthracycline antibiotic of hydro-lipophilic character, which is directly toxic to cellular membranes, particularly to capillary wall endothelial cell membranes: Importantly, in the cases of

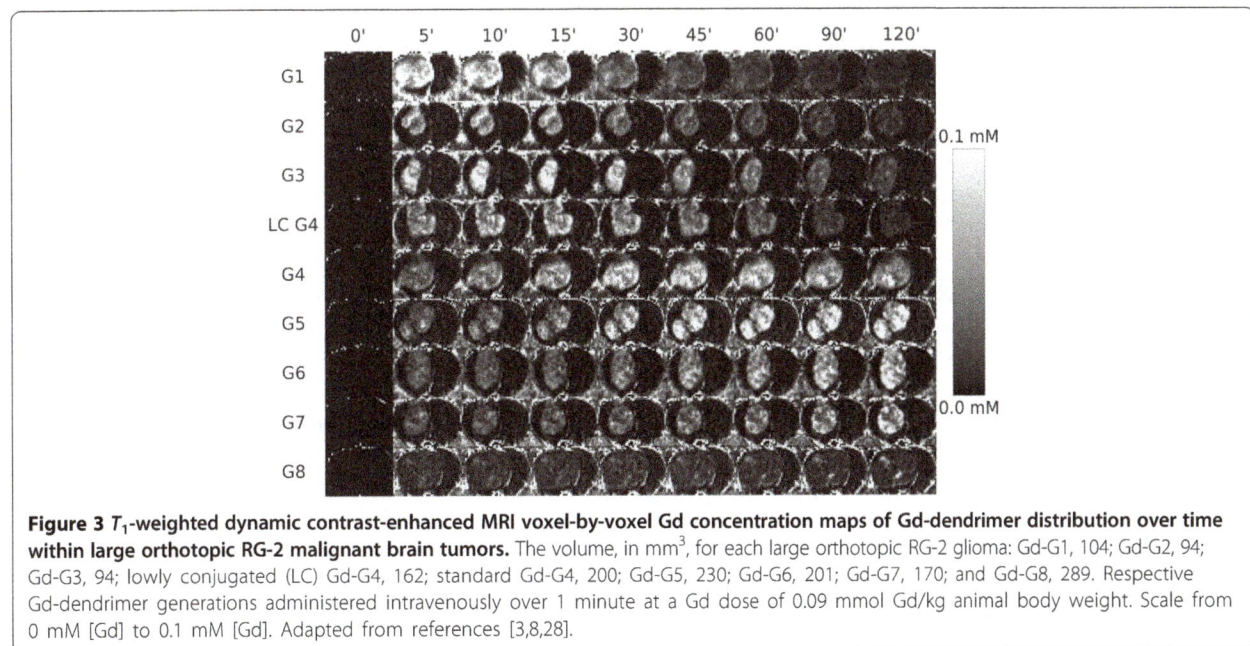

Figure 3 T_1-weighted dynamic contrast-enhanced MRI voxel-by-voxel Gd concentration maps of Gd-dendrimer distribution over time within large orthotopic RG-2 malignant brain tumors. The volume, in mm^3, for each large orthotopic RG-2 glioma: Gd-G1, 104; Gd-G2, 94; Gd-G3, 94; lowly conjugated (LC) Gd-G4, 162; standard Gd-G4, 200; Gd-G5, 230; Gd-G6, 201; Gd-G7, 170; and Gd-G8, 289. Respective Gd-dendrimer generations administered intravenously over 1 minute at a Gd dose of 0.09 mmol Gd/kg animal body weight. Scale from 0 mM [Gd] to 0.1 mM [Gd]. Adapted from references [3,8,28].

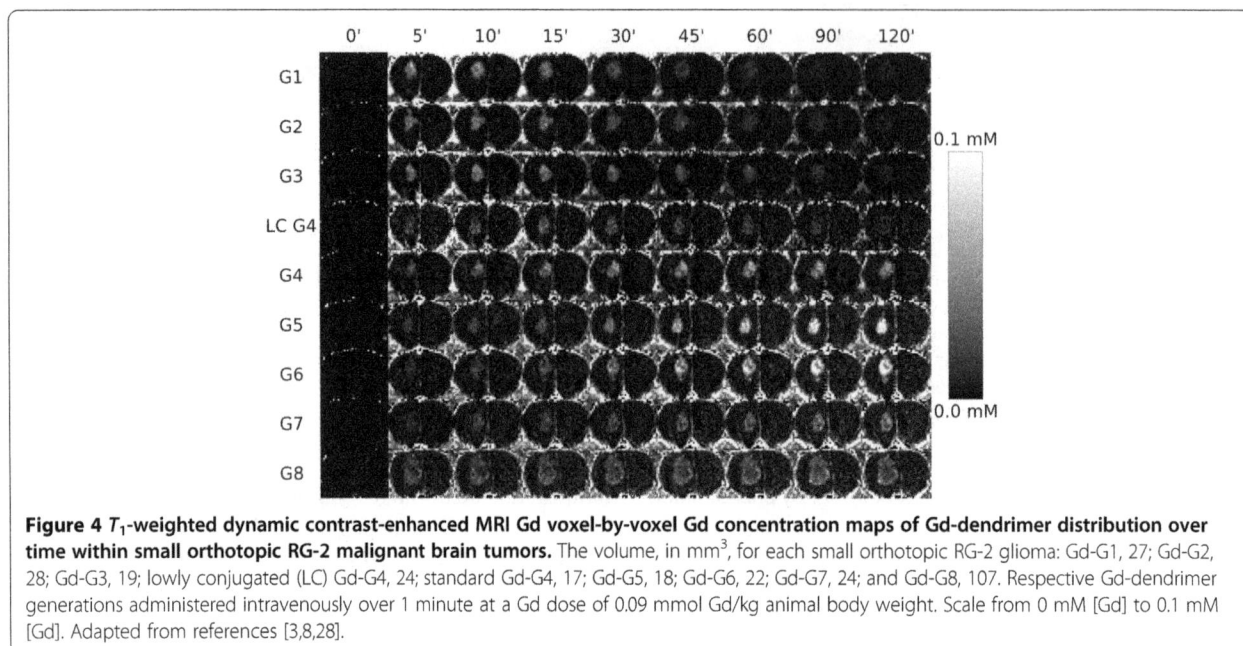

Figure 4 T_1-weighted dynamic contrast-enhanced MRI Gd voxel-by-voxel Gd concentration maps of Gd-dendrimer distribution over time within small orthotopic RG-2 malignant brain tumors. The volume, in mm^3, for each small orthotopic RG-2 glioma: Gd-G1, 27; Gd-G2, 28; Gd-G3, 19; lowly conjugated (LC) Gd-G4, 24; standard Gd-G4, 17; Gd-G5, 18; Gd-G6, 22; Gd-G7, 24; and Gd-G8, 107. Respective Gd-dendrimer generations administered intravenously over 1 minute at a Gd dose of 0.09 mmol Gd/kg animal body weight. Scale from 0 mM [Gd] to 0.1 mM [Gd]. Adapted from references [3,8,28].

both, there is the release of small molecule free drug is into systemic circulation, whereby the free drug itself does not accumulate to effective concentrations within solid tumor tissue itself, due to a upper limit of pore size of approximately 12 nanometers in the hyperpermeable blood capillaries supplying solid tumor tissue [28,29].

In more recent years, there has been exquisite interest in the development of various kinds of biocompatible nanoparticles for therapeutic purposes that remain in the optimal size range of 7 to 10 nanometers upon functionalization, but which has been tempered by the realization that it is difficult to engineer such biocompatibly-sized nanoparticles having covalently-bound stable biocompatible exteriors without toxic metal cores that do not biodegrade. Examples of nanoparticles in the optimal size range that fail to meet this criterion include the 8 nanometer-sized very small Iron Oxide core nanoparticles with a non-covalently-bound dextran organic biomolecule coating (VSOP-C184) [59], as well as the 5 to 10 nanometer-sized Cadmium-Tellurium or Cesium-Selenium core quantum dots, which have non-biocompatible metal cores and require non-covalent capping with Zinc-Sulfur and coated with organic biomolecules that themselves may or may not be biocompatible [33].

In contrast to other nanoparticles within the optimal size range, dendrimers are unique nanoparticles [8,25], as dendrimers are spherical nanoparticles with optimal terminal branch surface area-to-volume ratios and no significant increase in volume upon hydration, with the naked, non-functionalized, dendrimer being a repeating biocompatible monomeric units with terminal branches

increasing exponentially by 2^x units doubling for each successive full-generation, beginning with reference to the dendritic core, the zero generation dendrimer (G0) having 4 terminal branches (x = 2), with the 1st generation dendrimer (G1: 1.4 kDa; 1.9 nm diameter [Dendritic Nanotechnologies, Inc]) having 8 terminal branches (x = 4) and the 5th generation dendrimer (G5: 29 kDa; Diameter est at 5.5 nm [60]) having 128 terminal branches (x = 7) (NH3+), for example, whereas half-generation dendrimers (G1.5, G2.5 etc.) have intermediate numbers of terminal branches (COO-, OH) [61,62]. Even though dendrimer-based nanoparticles have been extensively researched in the past for their potential to be effective at chemotherapeutic drug delivery into solid tumors [63-69], including for folate receptor-targeted chemotherapeutic drug delivery [70-74], these investigations have been without emphasis on the optimal size range of 7 to 10 nanometers, the optimal density or the optimal exterior functionalization for effective, passively selective transvascular delivery, without risk of systemic toxicity, biophysical aspects that have important translational implications [1-3,7,8,25,26] (Table 1).

Optimally sized and designed MRI imageable functionalized dendrimers for theranostic purposes

Nanoparticles of the dendrimer class are monodisperse [60], and functionalized MRI imageable dendrimers with anionically neutralized exteriors maintain their monodispersity within a very narrow size distribution in their respective generation as determined by transmission electron microscopy [28,29,75], whereby the higher generation dendrimers functionalized with paramagnetic heavy metal

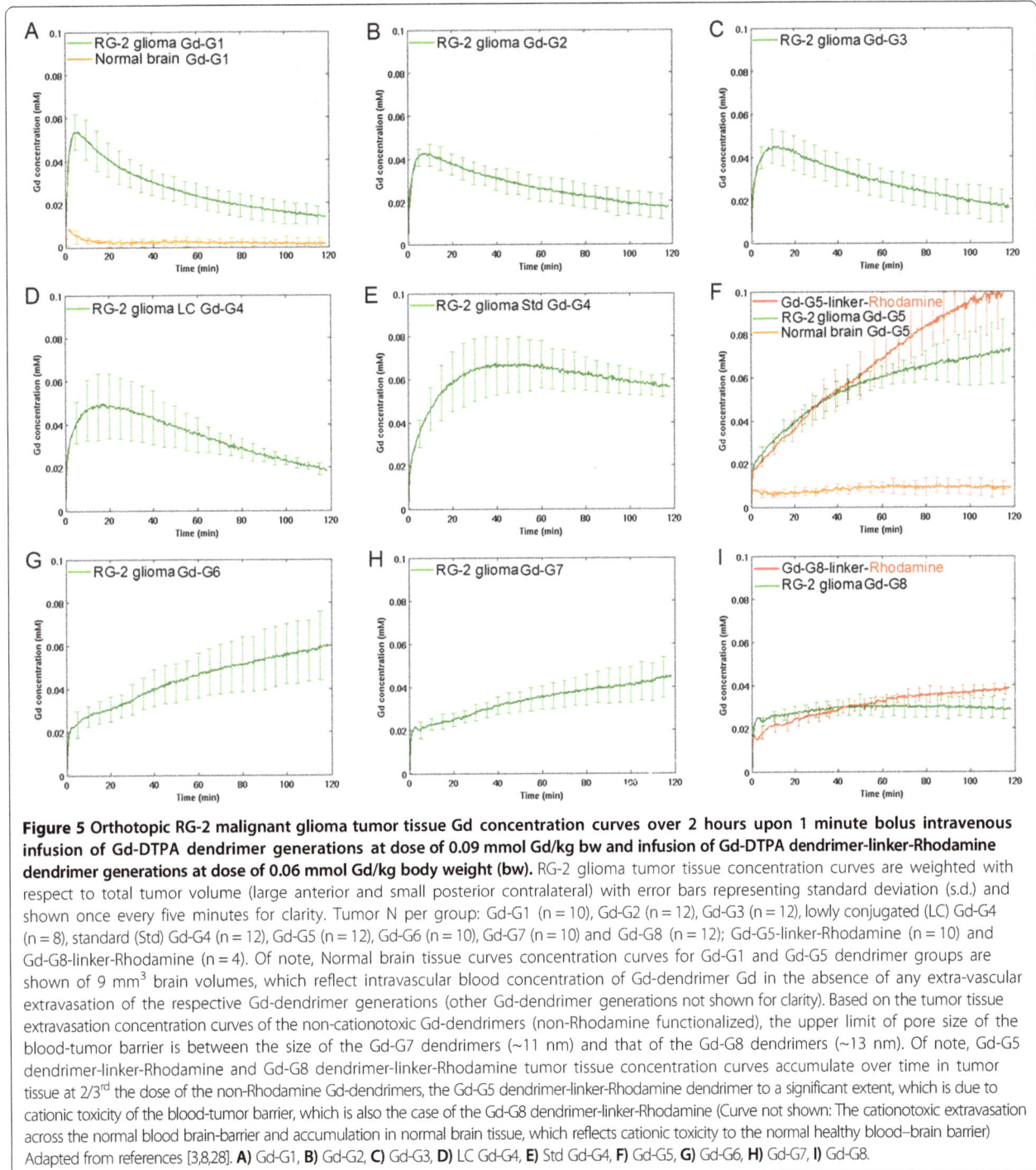

Figure 5 Orthotopic RG-2 malignant glioma tumor tissue Gd concentration curves over 2 hours upon 1 minute bolus intravenous infusion of Gd-DTPA dendrimer generations at dose of 0.09 mmol Gd/kg bw and infusion of Gd-DTPA dendrimer-linker-Rhodamine dendrimer generations at dose of 0.06 mmol Gd/kg body weight (bw). RG-2 glioma tumor tissue concentration curves are weighted with respect to total tumor volume (large anterior and small posterior contralateral) with error bars representing standard deviation (s.d.) and shown once every five minutes for clarity. Tumor N per group: Gd-G1 (n = 10), Gd-G2 (n = 12), Gd-G3 (n = 12), lowly conjugated (LC) Gd-G4 (n = 8), standard (Std) Gd-G4 (n = 12), Gd-G5 (n = 12), Gd-G6 (n = 10), Gd-G7 (n = 10) and Gd-G8 (n = 12); Gd-G5-linker-Rhodamine (n = 10) and Gd-G8-linker-Rhodamine (n = 4). Of note, Normal brain tissue curves concentration curves for Gd-G1 and Gd-G5 dendrimer groups are shown of 9 mm^3 brain volumes, which reflect intravascular blood concentration of Gd-dendrimer Gd in the absence of any extra-vascular extravasation of the respective Gd-dendrimer generations (other Gd-dendrimer generations not shown for clarity). Based on the tumor tissue extravasation concentration curves of the non-cationotoxic Gd-dendrimers (non-Rhodamine functionalized), the upper limit of pore size of the blood-tumor barrier is between the size of the Gd-G7 dendrimers (~11 nm) and that of the Gd-G8 dendrimers (~13 nm). Of note, Gd-G5 dendrimer-linker-Rhodamine and Gd-G8 dendrimer-linker-Rhodamine tumor tissue concentration curves accumulate over time in tumor tissue at 2/3rd the dose of the non-Rhodamine Gd-dendrimers, the Gd-G5 dendrimer-linker-Rhodamine dendrimer to a significant extent, which is due to cationic toxicity of the blood-tumor barrier, which is also the case of the Gd-G8 dendrimer-linker-Rhodamine (Curve not shown: The cationotoxic extravasation across the normal blood brain-barrier and accumulation in normal brain tissue, which reflects cationic toxicity to the normal healthy blood–brain barrier) Adapted from references [3,8,28]. **A)** Gd-G1, **B)** Gd-G2, **C)** Gd-G3, **D)** LC Gd-G4, **E)** Std Gd-G4, **F)** Gd-G5, **G)** Gd-G6, **H)** Gd-G7, **I)** Gd-G8.

chelates on the exterior remain within the 7 to 10 nanometer size range following functionalization, which is the case for the range of Gd-DTPA-G5 dendrimer (80–85 kDa; Diameter est at 7.5 nm) [3,8,28,29,76] (Table 1). In the case of the Gd-DTPA-G5 dendrimer-linker-Doxorubicin (85 kDa), its diameter as measured by dynamic light scattering in serum albumin protein-free solution, is at 9 nanometers [3] (Table 1), due to the linker attachment of

Doxorubicin to the exterior, which protrudes ~1.5 nanometers above the nanoparticles surface.

In the case of MRI imageable functionalized dendrimers, it is notable that there is a significant increase in the density of nanoparticle molecular weight upon the conjugation of chelated paramagnetic heavy metal Gadolinium (0.157 kDa) either by DTPA (0.393 kDa) or by DOTA (0.404 kDa) as when ~50% of the terminal amines of

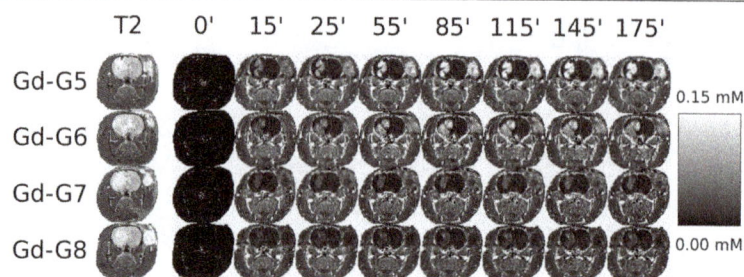

Figure 6 T_2–weighted anatomical MRI images and T_1-weighted dynamic contrast-enhanced MRI voxel-by-voxel Gd concentration maps of higher generation Gd-dendrimer distribution over approximately 3 hours within orthotopic and ectopic RG-2 malignant solid tumors. The volume, in mm^3, for each orthotopic and ectopic RG-2 glioma: First row, Gd-G5; 45 mm^3 (brain), 113 mm^3 (peripheral); Second row, Gd-G6; 97 mm^3 (brain), 184 mm^3 (peripheral); Third row, Gd-G7; 53 mm^3 (brain), 135 mm^3 (peripheral); Fourth row, Gd-G8; 50 mm^3 (brain); 163 mm^3 (peripheral). Respective Gd-dendrimer generations administered intravenously over 1 minute at a Gd dose of 0.09 mmol Gd/kg animal body weight. Scale from 0.00 mM [Gd] to 0.15 mM [Gd]. Adapted from references [8,29].

naked polyamidoamine dendrimer generation 5 (G5) are conjugated the cationic exterior of the naked polyamidoamine dendrimer (Table 1), it is anionically neutralized due to the presence of 2- charges of the Gd-DTPA/DOTA chelates protruding on the exterior of the MRI imageable functionalized dendrimer. Furthermore, the Gd-DTPA functionalized molecular weight is ~2.6-fold that of the naked dendrimer weight (Table 1), and importantly, the functionalized dendrimer size is only ~1.5 nanometers larger than that of the naked dendrimer (Table 1), which is superior to method of exterior pegylation to increase molecular weight in which case the overall size of the molecule increases disproportionately to greater than that of the 7 to 10 nanometer size range. Therefore, imageable

heavy metal chelate-based functionalization helps maintain a compact configuration that becomes important for optimally prolonged blood plasma half life as the densely chelated compact nanoparticle does not proteolytically degrade as rapidly in systemic circulation, which has an anionically neutralized exterior.

The other important consideration with regards to the optimal overall design of MRI imageable functionalized theranostic dendrimer nanoparticles within the 7 to 10 nanometer size range towards clinical application is the biophysical character of the functionalized nanoparticle exterior upon outermost exterior covalent functionalization of small molecule probes with inherent lipophilic cationicity such as fluorescent dye, linker-Rhodamine or

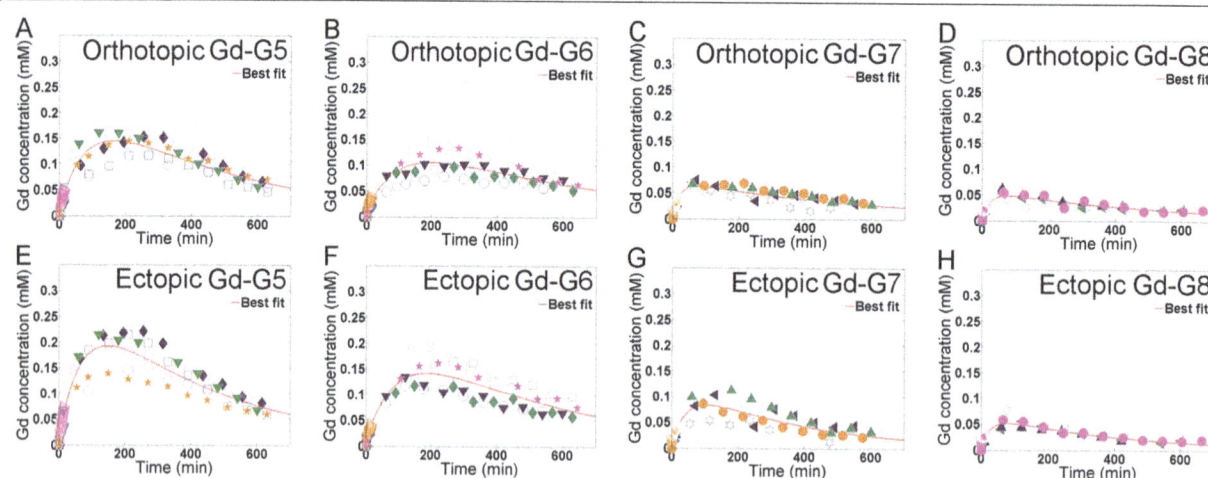

Figure 7 Orthotopic and ectopic RG-2 malignant glioma tumor tissue Gd concentration cures over 10 hours following 1 minute bolus intravenous infusion of Gd-DTPA dendrimer generations G5 through G8 at doses of 0.09 mmol Gd/kg body weight (bw). Orthotopic and ectopic RG-2 malignant solid tumor tissue concentration curves of intra-cranial caudate nucleus tumors (average volume ~100 mm^3) and contralateral extra-cranial temporalis muscle tumors (average volume ~150 mm^3) grown in the same rodent subjects. The Gd concentration values of free moving rodent subjects in-between scans represent whole tumor average Gd concentrations determined on the basis of co-registered tumor slice volume region-of-interest values for entire tumor volumes and not voxel-by-voxel. Shown is the best fit curve by least squares minimization. Orthotopic n: Gd-G5 (n = 6), Gd-G6 (n = 6), Gd-G7 (n = 5) and Gd-G8 (n = 5); Ectopic n: Gd-G5 (n = 6), Gd-G6 (n = 6), Gd-G7 (n = 5) and Gd-G8 (n = 5). Adapted from reference [8,29]. A) Gd-G5 Orthotopic RG-2 tumor, B) Gd-G6 Orthotopic RG-2 tumor, C) Gd-G7 Orthotopic RG-2 tumor, D) Gd-G8 Orthotopic RG-2 tumor, E) Gd-G5 Ectopic RG-2 tumor, F) Gd-G6 Ectopic RG-2 tumor, G) Gd-G7 Ectopic RG-2 tumor, H) Gd-G8 Ectopic RG-2 tumor.

Table 1 Biophysical properties of naked dendrimers and functionalized dendrimer-based theranostic nanoparticles

Polyamidoamine dendrimer (G)	Terminal groups (#)	Naked dendrimer weight (kDa)	Naked dendrimer size (nm) &	Gd-DTPA conjugation (%)~1	Small molecule drug conjugation (%)~2	Funtionalized dendrimer weight (kDa)^	Gd-DTPA dendrimer size (nm)	Theranostic dendrimer size (nm)*	Molar relaxivity (r:ms-1/mM)
Gt-dtpa-G1	8	1.43	1.9	67.1		5.63			9.8
Gt-dtpa-G2	16	3.26	2.6	65.9		11.2			10.1
Gt-dtpa-G3	32	6.91	3.6	47.7		18.6			10.4
Low Gd-dtpa-G4	64	14.2	4.4	29.8		24.4			7.8
Std Gd-dtpa-G4	64	14.2	5.7	47.5		39.8			12.2
Gd-dtpa-G5	128	28.8	est 5.5	47.2		79.8	est 7.5		109
Theranostic G5	128	28.8	est 5.5	48.1	7.8	85.0	n/a	9	10.1
Gd-dtpa-G6	256	58.0	6.9	39.9		133	est 10		10.6
Gd-dtpa-G7	512	116	8.0	50		330^	11		10.3
Gd-dtpa-G8	1024	233	10.3	37.8		597^	13		9.4

Blank = not available.

G = Dendrimer Genaration.

& = Combination of outside data from Dynamic light scattering and TEM findings of Ref 60 and Dendritic Nanotechnologies,Inc.

~1 = Based on (MALDI TOF Functionalized Dendrimer Weight - Naked Dendrimer Weight) / 725; Gd-DTPA unit Weight = 725 Daltons.

Doxorubicin (544 Da) + Linker Weight (278 Da) = 822 Daltons (8 Doxorubicin per Funtionalized Dendrimer).

* = Dynamic light scattering measurement for Gd-DTPA-dendrimer-Hydrazone LINKER-Doxorubicin; Otherwise estimated or measured per ADF TEM.

^ = Measured by ADF TEM; Otherwise measured by MADLI TOF spectroscopy.

chemotherapeutic antibiotic, linker-Doxorubicin, which is a form of hydro-lipophilicity [7]: Nanoparticles with cationic exteriors are particularly toxic to cellular membranes, due to the presence of multivalent exterior cationicity protruding outwards from the nanoparticle (Figure 5, Panels F and I; Figure 8), which, when present on the exterior of circulating nanoparticles cause systemic blood-endothelial cell capillary barrier damage as evidenced by non-selective contrast enhancement of the normal blood–brain barrier on dynamic contrast-enhanced MRI [3,8]; this is the case for the prototype of a MRI imageable theranostic dendrimer, whose biophysical character is altered due to the introduction of cationic lipophilicity onto its surface that protrudes above the biocompatible anionicity of its pre-existing chelated exterior [2,3,7,8], which results in non-selective systemic toxicity to normal healthy microvascular barriers including to the normal blood–brain barrier [3,8] (Figure 8) and is the likely reason for the observed

dose-limiting systemic toxicities in experimental studies with dendrimer-based therapeutics with targeting or therapeutic moieties of cationic lipophilic character on the exterior [72,77-79].

It can therefore be surmised that dendrimers are truly unique nanoparticles in that they possess the inherent inner architecture to proteolytically biodegrade along with the potential to be functionalized on the exterior via covalent modifications whereby their biophysical properties can be fine-tuned for: (1) Optimizing size to within the 7 to 10 nanometer range [1-3,8,25,26], which is optimal for passively selective transvascular delivery into hyperpermeable pathologies such as solid tumors but not to healthy tissues [2] (Figures 3 through 7; Table 1); (2) Optimizing density by covalent attachment of strongly chelated imageable heavy metals [3,8,25,26], which maintains their compactness and slows proteolytic degradation while in systemic blood circulation [2,7] (Figures 1 and 2); and (3)

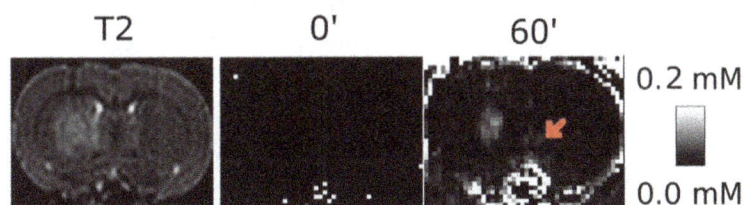

Figure 8 T_2-weighted anatomic MRI scan image of an orthotopic RG-2 malignant brain tumor and T_1-weighted dynamic contrast-enhanced MRI voxel-by-voxel Gd concentration maps at baseline and at 60 minutes following Gd-G5-doxorubicin dendrimer infusion. Red arrow highlights non-selective contrast enhancement in normal brain tissue. The Gd-G5-doxorubicin dendrimer administered intravenously over 2 minutes at a Gd dose of 0.09 mmol Gd/kg animal body weight, which is equivalent to a doxorubicin dose of 8 mg/kg animal body weight. Scale from 0 mM [Gd] to 0.2 mM [Gd]. Adapted from reference [3,8].

Optimizing exterior functionality for anionicity or hydroxylated anionicity via covalent attachment [3,8,25,26], which makes them biocompatible in blood circulation for prolonged duration and maximizes their blood half-life while rendering them free from biophysical interactions with circulatory or interstitial proteins such as serum albumins [2,7] (Figures 1 and 2).

Quantitative dynamic contrast-enhanced imaging for theranostic purpose

In the case of contrast-enhanced CT- and PET-based imaging employing purely hydrophilic contrast agents there is a linear correlation between the observed contrast enhancement signal and concentration of the contrast agent in tissue as these modalities detect either the opacity or the radioopacity, respectively, of the contrast agent. This, however, is not the case for contrast-enhanced MRI where the observed contrast enhancement signal is a function of several factors that must be taken into consideration the concentration of the agent infused and the temperature, the imaging sequence repletion and echo times (T_R, T_E) and the amount of the decrease in the longitudinal relaxation time (T_1) and increase in longitudinal relaxation rate (R_1, 1/ms) of water molecule protons resulting per unit concentration of the contrast agent (r, ms^{-1}/mM) in context of the Larmor precession frequency (ω), which is a product of the gyromagnetic ratio (g) of a charged protons of water molecules and the strength of the magnetic field (B_0) [80]. In magnetic resonance imaging, tissue signal results when energy is applied (E) when a radiofrequency pulse is applied in a static magnetic field to perturb tissue water molecule protons (nuclear spin with 1+ charge) already precessing at the Larmor frequency in alignment with the magnetic field (M vector: M_0, Equilibrium Magnetization), with the rate of re-alignment being detected at the sequence pre-determined time of detection (Echo time: T_E) by a receiving coil. Repetitive firing of radiofrequency pulses (Repetition time: T_R) of a pre-determined strength (flip angle α) results in repetitive deviations from z-axis (Mz longitudinal axis vector) towards the x-y plane (Mx-My plane vectors) that are measured during the return of the longitudinal magnetization (longitudinal re-growth time: T_1 relaxation time), which is the basis for the T_1-weighted MRI image generation following Fourier transforms of the detected signal, the T_1 signal.

In dynamic contrast-enhanced imaging, a small molecule or macromolecular contrast agent is infused while images are acquired sequentially in real-time, these being radiographic images in the case of dynamic CT and PET, and resonance images in the case of dynamic MRI, making it possible to observe the difference in the baseline pre-contrast signal to that of the contrast-enhanced signal (normalized signal), which, in the case of dynamic contrast-enhanced MRI can be further quantified in terms of contrast agent concentration by applying the dual-flip angle methodology and the pre-determined molar relaxivity of a hydrophilic contrast agent (r: ms^{-1}/mM), upon which concentration curves and maps can be generated voxel-by-voxel for the duration of imaging session (All figures except Figure 7). In the case of purely hydrophilic small molecule contrast agents such as Gd-DTPA/DOTA (0.73 kDa; 0.8 nm), which has an overall charge of 2-, a temporal resolution of 30 minutes or less is sufficient to assess the pathologic tissue's pharmacokineticodynamic curve profile; whereas, in the case of small molecule contrast agents of part hydrophilic character such as serum albumin-associating contrast agent Gadofosveset (~0.91 kDa), which is part neutral and part anionically charged and remains in the blood pool for increased duration [81], as well as in the case of hydrophilic macromolecular contrast and theranostic agents greater than 4 nanometers in diameter, a temporal resolution of upwards of 2 hours is often necessary to properly assess the pathologic tissue's pharmacokineticodynamic curve profile. The visualized contrast concentration results from the combination of contrast-enhanced intra-vascular signal, and in the subset of tissues supplied by blood capillaries permeable to the contrast agent, from the pooling of contrast agent within tissue interstitium followed by intracellular uptake [12], processes that can be separated out by visual inspection of the pathologic tissue's pharmacokineticodynamic curve profile, in context of the blood plasma's pharmacokineticodynamic curve profile, for the theranostic dendrimer, with the potential for increased diagnostic imaging sensitivity upon the assessment of the tissue response pharmacokineticodynamic curve profiles for a couple or series of imageable dendrimer-based contrast agents of various sizes (generations).

The sensitivity of dynamic contrast MRI-based detection of hyperpermeable pathologic tissue utilizing a purely hydrophilic contrast agent is primarily a function of, one, hydrophilic contrast agent size, which increases its blood half-life of the agent, and two, the efficiency by which it relaxes water protons per molar concentration, which increases with polyvalency and then plateaus off. The short blood plasma half-lives of hydrophilic small molecule contrast agents and their lower efficiency to relax water protons (low molar relaxivity) are limitations that can be overcome by decreasing renal filtration fraction [12] or increasing the dose of the contrast agent, both of which increase agent blood plasma half-life, but which also increase the risk for non-selective systemic toxicity of small molecule contrast agents of less than 2 nanometers, which can extravasate appreciably across healthy microvascular barriers, and in the case of small molecule chemotherapy, often becomes the treatment dose-limiting toxicity [1,2].

In contrast to hydrophilic small molecule contrast agents, the mid-sized higher generation dendrimer-based theranostic agents possess longer blood half lives and those with neutralized-to-anionic exteriors within the optimal size range of 7 to 10 nanometers are passively selective for solid tumor foci and provide exquisite contrast enhancement of solid tumor foci over several hours as they accumulate over time to 0.20 mM average maximum with respect to Gadolinium concentration in peripheral solid tumors and to 0.15 mM average maximum with respect to Gadolinium concentration in intracranial solid tumors [8,29] at significantly lower doses of administration than in their free small molecule form of Gd-DTPA, whereby, the Gd-G5 DTPA-dendrimer (est at 7.5 nm) provides superior intra-tumoral accumulation and prolonged contrast enhancement upon intravenous administration at 0.09 mmol Gd/kg body weight over 1 minute [3,8,28,29] (Figure 7), as compared to Gd-DTPA administered at the 0.30 mmol Gd/kg body weight dose over one minute (triple dose Gd-DTPA), which provides fleeting contrast enhancement [12]. Furthermore, the dosing of Gd-G5 DTPA/DOTA-dendrimers is on the order of 80–100 mg/kg body weight per dose [3,8] and $1/7^{th}$ to 1/2 of that of hydrophilic small molecule contrast agents such as Gd-DTPA/DOTA administered at triple dose, for which reason the probability for any systemic hypersensitivity associated with MRI imageable dendrimers functionalized biocompatibly with small molecule therapeutics is likely low.

On the applicability of *in vitro* determinations of theranostic dendrimer molar relaxivity to the *in vivo* state

The molar relaxivity of the contrast agent, r (ms^{-1}/mM), which is the amount of increase in the relaxation rate of water protons per unit concentration of agent, has been extensively studied *in vitro* for a variety of paramagnetic contrast agents at various field strengths (T) at various temperatures (°C) including dendrimer-based, ie [82,83], which has been from the basic science perspective of the physical sciences, with the objective of selecting MRI contrast agents with improved proton longitudinal relaxation efficiency per millimolar concentration of the paramagnetic contrast agent (r_1, .here simply r). Based on these *in vitro* studies, it has been determined that paramagnetic contrast agent molar relaxivity increases with increasing exterior polyvalency of chelated Gadolinium to a point after which it plateaus, whereby the Gd-chelated high-generation dendrimers (Gd-DTPA/DOTA G5 dendrimers and higher) have a plateaued r of 20 ms^{-1}/mM at 1.5 T @ 20° [83] and of ~25 ms^{-1}/mM at 1.5 T @ 37° [82,83], and a plateaued r of between 10 and 12 ms^{-1}/mM at 3.0 T @ 37° [3,8,28,29,83], in contrast to monovalent Gd-DTPA, which has a r of ~4 ms^{-1}/mM at 1.5 T @ 37° [81] and a r of 3.8 ms^{-1}/mM at 3.0 T @ 37° [12]. These findings are analogous to those noted with respect to the adsorption of several small molecule contrast agents onto nanoporous surfaces [84].

It is difficult, however, to determine the molar relaxivity *in vivo* as it requires accurate determinations of the actual tissue concentration of the contrast agent at the time of the acquired image, which historically typically has been Gd-DTPA, a hydrophilic contrast agent with a short blood half-life that readily diffuses out of the tissue interstitium [85,86], unlike, for example, 14C-alpha aminoisobutyric acid (14C-AIB) [7,11], a 14C-modified synthetic amino acid that readily localizes intracellularly [7]. In the case of macromoleculars, if the molar relaxivity of a theranostic dendrimer can be determined accurately *in vitro*, then the *in vitro* approach would methodologically useful for application across laboratories and centers due to the ease of reproducibility.

From the translational science perspective, it is important to understand the salient biophysical interactions that alter a theranostic agent's molar relaxivity in the physiologic state *in vivo*. An important observation in this respect is that for a contrast agent with part lipophilic character, the molar relaxivity is much greater in the presence of protein serum albumin, which is the case of Gadofosveset (Vasovist), a Gd-DTPA-based contrast agent of anionic hydro-lipophilic character with serum albumin-associating ability [7] that has a r of 28 ms^{-1}/mM at 1.5 T @ 37° [87], in contrast to Gd-DTPA that is of pure hydrophilic character [7] that has a r of 3.8 ms^{-1}/mM at 3.0 T @ 37° [12], irrespective of the presence of protein. This observation that there is increased contrast agent molar relaxivity in the presence of associative serum albumins, blood serum and interstitial, is consistent with transiently acquired non-covalent associative polyvalency in the presence of serum albumins, and becomes particularly relevant to take into consideration when designing theranostic dendrimers, as exterior functionalization with moieties such as fluorescent dyes or chemotherapeutics of lipophilic character. In the case of functionalized theranostic dendrimers or other such nanoparticles where foreseeable protein interactions *in vivo* not considered *a priori*, the dynamic contrast-enhanced MRI-based Gd concentration maps generated on the basis of molar relaxivity determinations of theranostic nanoparticles made *in vitro* in phosphate buffered saline (PBS) would display greater Gd concentration than actually present intratumorally in the form of Gd-DTPA/DOTA-dendrimer; in the case of theranostic nanoparticles without this exterior introduction of lipophilicity and maintained post-functionalization protruding exterior hydrophilicity (i.e. Gd-DTPA-dendrimers), this effect modifier is unlikely to be much of a factor in introducing inaccuracy into the methodology [7].

Therefore, the most important realization here is that a functionalized theranostic agent's *in vivo* molar relaxivity is only equivalent to it's *in vivo* molar relaxivity if the theranostic agent does not associate with serum proteins: This is only the case for purely hydrophilic theranostic agents of anionically neutralized stable exteriors with covalently bound chelates [2,7]. For theranostic probes without this exterior biophysical character of anionically neutralized exteriors, adjustments would need to be made, and furthermore, the reliability of these adjustments for accurate quantification of theranostic agent concentration *in vivo* must be questioned.

Methodology for the *in vitro* determination of theranostic dendrimer molar relaxivity for *in vivo* application

Purely hydrophilic theranostic agents of anionically neutralized stable exteriors with covalently bound chelates, the molar relaxivity can be measured accurately *in vitro* in phosphate buffered saline at body temperature (37°C) in the 3 T magnet solenoid coil utilized for the *in vivo* dynamic contrast-enhanced imaging [3,8,12,28,29], which approximates that of the *in vivo* state in the absence of any appreciable protein binding, as is the case for pure hydrophiles [7,88]. Theranostic dendrimer nanoparticle molar relaxivity is determined by T_1-weighted Spin-Echo (SE) MRI methodology utilizing different repetition times (SE T_R; ie 100, 300, 600 and 1200 ms) and a constant echo time (SE T_E; ie 10 ms) for a series of diluted Gd-DTPA-dendrimer PBS solutions with respect to Gadolinium concentration (0, 0.25, 0.50, 0.75, 1.0 and 2.0 mM) for the determination of the normalized longitudinal relativity rates $(1/T_1)$ for each Gadolinium concentration via column (m: T_R)-by-row (n: Gadolinium concentration) matrix comparisons of contrast-enhanced T_1 signal to non-contrast PBS T_1 signal by applying Equation 1:

$$S = M_0 \left[1 - 2\exp{-\left(\frac{\frac{T_R - T_E}{2}}{T_1} \right)} + \exp\left(\frac{-T_R}{T_1} \right) \right] \quad (1)$$

The Gd-DTPA/DOTA-dendrimer theranostic nanoparticle molar relaxivity rate is calculated by linear regression of normalized longitudinal relativity rates $(1/T_1)$ plotted on the y-axis versus Gd-DTPA-dendrimer Gadolinium concentration (0, 0.25, 0.50, 0.75, 1.0 and 2.0 mM) plotted on the x-axis, with the slope of this line being the theranostic dendrimer nanoparticle molar relaxivity, r (ms^{-1}/mM), as per the relationship in Equation 2:

$$r = \frac{\frac{1}{T_1} - \frac{1}{T_{10}}}{[C]} \quad (2)$$

Since the increase in measured signal intensity is not linear across SE repetition times particularly at concentrations

greater than 0.50 mM Gadolinium, imaging of concentration dilutions at multiple repetition times assures accuracy of the *in vitro* molar relaxivity determination for the entire range of physiologically relevant concentrations of Gadolinium to be encountered in blood plasma (~1.2 mM) and tumor tissue (~0.1-0.2 mM). The tissue specificity of the spin-echo-based *in vitro* molar relaxivity determination methodology can be further improved by narrowing the range of *in vitro* theranostic dendrimer dilutions to that of the Gadolinium concentrations to be encountered specifically in either blood plasma, or in tumor tissue.

The steps for post-processing of the raw Spin Echo molar relaxivity data include molar relaxivity calculations that are performed directly in Matlab following conversion of .Par scan header parameter information into .Brik file signal data and capturing of ROI mask .Brik file signal data into a single Matlab .1D files and then executing UNIX-based custom scripts to batch process, by calling onto the Matlab suite to apply Matlab-based scripts (.m).

Methodology for the dynamic contrast-enhanced magnetic resonance imaging of theranostic dendrimer nanoparticles

In the case of dynamic contrast-enhanced magnetic resonance imaging, the most applicable methodology for dynamic contrast-enhanced MRI is the T_1-weighted SPoiled Gradient Recall Echo (SPGR, GRE; Fast-Field Echo [FFE]) dual-flip angle methodology for quantification of signal intensity in concentration space, which permits the rapid acquisition of high-resolution dynamic scan images over time [80]. Furthermore, SPGR T_1-weighted imaging sequences generate homogenous signal for small field-of-views without tissue interface artifact and are particularly applicable for the treatment cum imaging while delineating discrete volumes of hyperpermeable pathology and pathology-normal tissue interfaces (ie rodent, primate and human tumor foci) following the intravenous bolus administration of paramagnetic theranostic nanoparticles with long blood half lives and low serum albumin-association potential such as the Gd-DTPA/DOTA-dendrimers in the optimal size range of 7 to 10 nanometers.

Being that the maximum achievable magnetization for a radiofrequency pulse is governed by the duration and intensity of the radiofrequency pulse and that a pulse of greater strength yields a larger flip angle α, while the T_1-weighted signal decays at a constant rate irrespective of applied radiofrequency energy, the following relationship holds the T_1-weighted signal, S, in case of the dual flip-angle methodology, as defined per Equations 3 and 4:

$$S = M_0 \frac{(1-E)\sin\alpha}{1-E\cos\alpha} \quad where \quad E = \exp\left(-\frac{T_R}{T_1} \right) \quad (3)$$

$$\frac{S_1(1-E\cos\alpha 1)}{\sin\alpha 1} = \frac{S_2(1-E\cos\alpha 2)}{\sin\alpha 2} \qquad (4)$$

where $\alpha 1$ = low-flip angle for 1st flip radiofrequency pulse signal S_1 (ie 3 deg).

Where $\alpha 2$ = high=flip angle for 2nd flip radiofrequency pulse signal S_2 (ie 12 deg).

Since the objective is to generate the normalized relative signal pre-contrast map for quantification of contrast agent concentration upon $\alpha 2$ high-flip angle dynamic contrast-enhanced image acquisition, Equation 4 can be solved for the $ES\alpha 2pre/S\alpha 1pre$ value to yield Equation 5:

$$Es_\alpha 2pre/s_\alpha 1pre = \frac{S_2\sin\alpha 1 - S_1\sin\alpha 2}{S_2\cos\alpha 2\sin\alpha 1 - S_1\cos\alpha 1\sin\alpha 2} \qquad (5)$$

The $ES\alpha 2pre/S\alpha 1pre$ value is applied to generate the relative normalized T_1-weighted signal intensity map as defined per Equation 6:

$$S_{relative}'(t) = S(t)/S_1 @ \alpha 1 = \left(\frac{\frac{1-E(t)}{1-E(t)\cos\alpha 2}}{\frac{1-E_{S\alpha 2pre/S\alpha 1pre}}{1-E_{S\alpha 2pre/S\alpha 1pre}\cos\alpha 2}} \right) \qquad (6)$$

The expression for the decay in electromagnetic energy over time over successive pulses in context of contrast agent-induced tissue contrast enhancement is:

$$E_{T_1 post/pre}(t) = \exp\left(-\frac{T_R}{T_{1post/pre(t)}}\right)$$
$$= \exp\left(-\frac{T_R}{T_{10\alpha 2pre/\alpha 1pre}} - rT_R C(t)\right) \qquad (7)$$

Knowledge of the relationships defined by Equations 5, 6 and 7 form the basis for quantification of the amount of contrast enhancement at $\alpha 2$ for each image acquisition in concentration space with respect to the imaging agent moiety (i.e. Gadolinium) or even the agent itself (i.e. Gd-DTPA-dendrimer), where r is the molar relaxivity in $msec^{-1}$ time/mM contrast agent concentration measured *in vitro* (Equations 1 and 2) and substituted into Equation 8, whereby the dynamic MRI concentration map is generated voxel-by-voxel (0.5 mm by 0.3 mm by 0.3 mm) per tissue volume slice with respect to contrast agent Gadolinium concentration to quantify the change in the concentration of theranostic dendrimer nanoparticle in the tissue of interest such as blood plasma and solid tumor over time (All figures except Figure 7), which can also be made for a region-of-interest considered as one large voxel, where applicable (Figure 7). The quantitative dynamic MRI theranostic agent Gd concentration over time is defined as per Equation 8:

For calculation of the change in the agent concentration over time in blood plasma, a few representative voxels are chosen from a small vein or artery, of sufficient diameter including the superior sagittal [venous] sinus (Figure 1) and the common carotid artery (Figure 2): The systemic healthy tissue extraction per circulatory pass in insignificant for optimally sized imageable nanoparticles while the blood transit time from arterial-to-venous circulation is $1/4^{th}$ of that of the temporal resolution (20 s per slice) resulting in similar concentrations in either circulation, whereby it is appropriate to utilize SSS voxels for determining blood concentration of the theranostic agent. It is bit more difficult to select artifact-free voxels in the common carotid artery due to flow artifact on slices that are in the periphery of the field-of-view and requires some training. The tumor tissue fractional blood plasma volume (Vp) is relatively insignificant and on the order of 3-5% and not necessary to factor in for determination of concentrations of interstitial and cellular solid tumor tissue contrast agent concentrations. The concentration of the theranostic dendrimer nanoparticle in the plasma of blood requires knowledge of the red blood cell fraction (Hematocrit: Hct), which is typically around 0.46 in the case of blood-less microsurgery and defined as per Equation 9:

$$C_p = \frac{C_b}{1-Hct} \qquad (9)$$

Native acquired dynamic contrast-enhanced MRI signal data are analyzed using the Analysis of Functional NeuroImages (AFNI; http://afni.nimh.nih.gov/) [89] software suite programs such as 3Dvolreg for motion correction, 3Dautobox for cropping, and 3Droistats and 3Dmaskave for extracting parameters for manually-drawn ROI masks in the UNIX programming environment, called-on by simple commands and in custom-made UNIX scripts (.csh). For the dynamic contrast-enhanced MRI signal data, the dual flip angle dynamic contrast-enhanced MRI signal data files (.Par header information and .Rec files) are extracted and converted to native AFNI format signal data (.Head .Brik files), with the entire hi-flip dynamic signal data set motion corrected, after which the low flip and high flip signal data are co-registered, each dynamic high flip angle volume over time to its corresponding low flip angle volume signal data of a single time point, with alignments made by Fourier interpolation. The signal space to concentration space data conversion is then performed by the application of the custom-made UNIX scripts applying Equations 3 through 9.

$$Dynamic\ MRI\ C(t)\ map = \frac{1}{rT_R}\ln\frac{E_{S\alpha 2pre/S\alpha 1pre}[S'(t)(1-E_{S\alpha 2pre/S\alpha 1pre})\cos\alpha 2 - E_{S\alpha 2pre/S\alpha 1pre}\cos\alpha 2 - 1]}{S'(t)(1-E_{S\alpha 2pre/S\alpha 1pre}) + E_{S\alpha 2pre/S\alpha 1pre}\cos\alpha 2 - 1} \qquad (8)$$

In vivo considerations for theranostic dynamic contrast-enhanced magnetic resonance imaging

Two different variations of the SPoiled Gradient Recall Echo (SPGR) dual-flip methodology have been applied for *in vivo* dynamic contrast-enhanced MRI for the quantitative theranostic imaging of functionalized dendrimer nanoparticle accumulation over time into the interstitium of rat glioma-2 (RG-2) malignant gliomas grown orthotopically and ectopically [3,8,11,12,28,29], which are syngenic to the Fischer rat strain [90,91], and equivalent to astrocytomas of the World Health Organization (WHO) Grades III-to-IV (glioblastoma multiforme [GBM]) [55,90,92-94]. In one variation of the methodology, voxel-by-voxel tumor region of interest concentration and maps have been generated via co-registration of slices over time for tumor imaging over 2 hours under continuous general anesthesia sedation without the need for intubation and without complications, which has enabled the systematic study of MRI imageable dendrimer nanoparticle accumulation voxel-by-voxel over time for theranostic purposes [3,8,12,28,29] (Figures 3 through 6; Figure 8); whereas, in the other variation, whole tumor slice volume ROI concentration maps has been performed for determination of change in whole tumor contrast agent concentration over a more prolonged duration of 10 hours upon re-awakening the rodent for 30 minutes in-between 2 minute dynamic scans, also without complications [3,8,29] (Figure 7).

During the course of these laboratory studies, it has been observed that hemodynamic depression resulting from being under continuous sedation results in less MRI imageable dendrimer and theranostic dendrimer nanoparticle accumulation in orthotopic and ectopic solid tumors of rodents (Figures 3 through 6; Figure 8), which is not the case in orthotopic and ectopic solid tumors of rodents awakened in-between dynamic scans (Figure 7), and furthermore, that there is a more significant effect of anesthesia-induced hemodynamic depression on the accumulation of optimally sized MRI imageable dendrimer nanoparticles in the interstitium of extra-cranial peripheral solid tumors as compared to on intra-cranial malignant gliomas, which underscores the effect of hemodynamic depression-induced decreased perfusion on the intratumoral accumulation of even nanoparticle-sized therapeutics in perfusion-limited hyperpermeable pathologies such as peripheral solid tumors with greater permeability surface area product (*Ktrans*).

Conclusions

The realization that nanoparticle-based formulations could serve as more efficient molecular forms for either the purpose of imaging, or alternatively, for the purpose of the treatment of disease states, is relatively long-standing in the field of translational nanoparticle science, whereby over the years a variety of functionalized nanoparticles over a spectrum of shapes, sizes and exterior biophysical properties have been investigated for their suitability for either imaging or therapeutic applications, but the majority have failed to meet the criterion of passive selectivity for hyperpermeable pathologies cum biocompatibility in the physiologic state. In more recent years, from 2006 to 2009, quantitative high-resolution dynamic contrast-enhanced MRI at a field strength of 3 T has been utilized for the detailed imaging of the accumulation potential of 2 to 14 nanometer-sized imageable gadolinium chelate-conjugated dendrimer nanoparticles in the solid tumor interstitium of rodent malignant gliomas of volumes as small as 20 mm^3, which has been upon bolus intravenous administration over 1 minute; based on the findings of this research, it has been discovered that MRI imageable dendrimers are uniquely biocompatible nanoparticles in that optimally designed MRI imageable dendrimers within the 7 to 10 nanometer size range are applicable for the dynamic contrast-enhanced imaging and concomitant treatment of malignant solid tumors irrespective of tumor permeability surface area product, and importantly, quantitatively, while affording the ability to detect solid tumor tissue with sensitivity and specificity at the translational level.

The translational quantitative dynamic contrast-enhanced MRI imaging methodology that has been applied, and is discussed herein, utilizes the measure of the ability of a paramagnetic MRI imageable dendrimer functionalized with a small molecule therapeutic to contrast enhance water proton signal, its molar relaxivity (r_1), with the realization that this measure, in fact, can be appropriately determined *in vitro* utilizing T$_1$-weighted Spin-Echo and applied for the accurate determination of theranostic agent concentration in blood plasma and in the solid tumor tissue interstitium overtime on a voxel-by-voxel basis for an accurate non-invasive assessment of *in vivo* theranostic pharmacokinetics utilizing T$_1$-weighted Gradient-Recall Echo.

Based on the observations taken together from the findings of these relatively recent research studies, it can be surmised that the optimally functionalized biocompatible theranostic nanoparticle is a non-metal core-based nanoparticle of dendritic architecture in the 7 to 10 nanometer size range with a therapeutic xenobiotic drug covalently bound inwardly via a labile linkage sensitive to pH (i.e. hydrazone type) along with a covalently bound anionic moiety exteriorly such as an imageable chelate, which imparts dense hydrophilic biophysical character to the exterior. A theranostic nanoparticle based on this design will demonstrate favorable drug release kinetics upon passive selective transvascular passage into the hyperpermeable pathology interstitium during its peak blood plasma concentration, while there being minimal risk for systemic or lymphatic hypersensitivity while in systemic circulation.

The future perspective is to apply the translational theranostic quantitative dynamic contrast-enhanced MRI-based methodology discussed herein based on knowledge of the optimal nanoparticle size range of 7 to 10 nanometers, density and exterior functionalization necessary for biocompatible passively selective effective transvascular delivery of small molecule therapeutics into solid tumors while maximizing the effectiveness of the approach by locking in MRI imageable theranostic dendrimer nanoparticle treatments for maximum intratumoral accumulation favoring intratumoral release of small molecule drug at peak intratumoral nanoparticle concentration. The further future objective will be to demonstrate the clinical efficacy of the fine tuned refined approach within a few years.

It is foreseeably envisioned that the translational theranostic methodology for diagnostic imaging and the concomitant treatment of solid malignancies discussed herein will result in the effective treatment of solid malignancies, and will also result in the development of effective transvascular therapies for other disease states of pathologic hyperpermeability and without.

Competing Interests

The author declares that he has no competing interests.

Author's contribution

HS conceptualized and performed the original research, and wrote the article.

Author's information

HS: Freelance Investigator in Translational Science and Medicine (unaffiliated).

Acknowledgements

No funding was acquired for this research. Previous funding entities and authors have been properly acknowledged for their contributions and have been additionally cited herein.

References

1. Sarin H. Physiologic upper limits of pore size of different blood capillary types and another perspective on the dual pore theory of microvascular permeability. Journal of angiogenesis research. 2010;2:14.
2. Sarin H. Permeation thresholds for hydrophilic small biomolecules across microvascular and epithelial barriers are predictable on the basis of conserved biophysical properties: Pharmacotherapeutic implications. Submitted TBD, TBD(TBD):TBD.
3. Sarin H. Recent progress towards development of effective systemic chemotherapy for the treatment of malignant brain tumors. Journal of translational medicine. 2009;7:77.
4. Fung SH, Roccatagliata L, Gonzalez RG, Schaefer PW. MR diffusion imaging in ischemic stroke. Neuroimaging clinics of North America. 2011;21(2):345–77. xi.
5. Habgood MD, Bye N, Dziegielewska KM, Ek CJ, Lane MA, Potter A, et al. Changes in blood–brain barrier permeability to large and small molecules following traumatic brain injury in mice. European Journal of Neuroscience. 2007;25(1):231–8.
6. G P, J M, C S, J P, MA K, K Q, A S. Nephrogenic systemic fibrosis: a review of published cases and results from three prospective observational studies. Insights Imaging 2012, 3 (supp 1):S293.
7. Sarin H. Nanomolecular function is conserved in the physiological state. Journal of Nanotechnology: Nanomedicine & Nanobiotechnology 2015, TBD(TBD):TBD.
8. Essig M, Weber M-A, von Tengg-Kobligk H, Knopp MV, Yuh WTC, Giesel FL. Contrast-Enhanced Magnetic Resonance Imaging of Central Nervous System Tumors: Agents, Mechanisms, and Applications. Topics in Magnetic Resonance Imaging. 2006;17(2):89–106.
9. Sarin H. Effective transvascular delivery of chemotherapy into cancer cells with imageable nanoparticles in the 7 to 10 nanometer size range. In: Current Advances in the Medical Application of Nanotechnology. Volume 1, edn. Bentham Science Publishers Ltd.; 2012: 10–24
10. Tofts PS, Brix G, Buckley DL, Evelhoch JL, Henderson E, Knopp MV, et al. Estimating kinetic parameters from dynamic contrast-enhanced T(1)-weighted MRI of a diffusable tracer: standardized quantities and symbols. J Magn Reson Imaging. 1999;10(3):223–32.
11. Ferrier MC, Sarin H, Fung SH, Schatlo B, Pluta RM, Gupta SN, et al. Validation of dynamic contrast-enhanced magnetic resonance imaging-derived vascular permeability measurements using quantitative autoradiography in the RG2 rat brain tumor model. Neoplasia. 2007;9(7):546–55.
12. Sarin H, Kanevsky AS, Fung SH, Butman JA, Cox RW, Glen D, et al. Metabolically stable bradykinin B2 receptor agonists enhance transvascular drug delivery into malignant brain tumors by increasing drug half-life. Journal of translational medicine. 2009;7:33.
13. Degani H, Gusis V, Weinstein D, Fields S, Strano S. Mapping pathophysiological features of breast tumors by MRI at high spatial resolution. Nature medicine. 1997;3(7):780–2.
14. Tofts PS, Kermode AG. Measurement of the blood–brain barrier permeability and leakage space using dynamic MR imaging. 1. Fundamental concepts. Magn Reson Med. 1991;17(2):357–67.
15. Jackson A, Jayson GC, Li KL, Zhu XP, Checkley DR, Tessier JJ, et al. Reproducibility of quantitative dynamic contrast-enhanced MRI in newly presenting glioma. The British journal of radiology. 2003;76(903):153–62.
16. Padhani AR, Hayes C, Landau S, Leach MO. Reproducibility of quantitative dynamic MRI of normal human tissues. NMR in biomedicine. 2002;15(2):143–53.
17. Yang C, Karczmar GS, Medved M, Oto A, Zamora M, Stadler WM. Reproducibility assessment of a multiple reference tissue method for quantitative dynamic contrast enhanced-MRI analysis. Magnetic resonance in medicine: official journal of the Society of Magnetic Resonance in Medicine/Society of Magnetic Resonance in Medicine. 2009;61(4):851–9.
18. Galbraith SM, Lodge MA, Taylor NJ, Rustin GJ, Bentzen S, Stirling JJ, et al. Reproducibility of dynamic contrast-enhanced MRI in human muscle and tumours: comparison of quantitative and semi-quantitative analysis. NMR in biomedicine. 2002;15(2):132–42.
19. Vincensini D, Dedieu V, Renou JP, Otal P, Joffre F. Measurements of extracellular volume fraction and capillary permeability in tissues using dynamic spin–lattice relaxometry: studies in rabbit muscles. Magnetic resonance imaging. 2003;21(2):85–93.
20. Dedieu V, Bailly C, Vincent C, Achard JL, Le Bouedec G, Penault-Llorca F, et al. Capillary permeability and extracellular volume fraction in uterine cervical cancer as patient outcome predictors: measurements by using dynamic MRI spin–lattice relaxometry. Journal of magnetic resonance imaging: JMRI. 2008;27(4):846–53.
21. Verma S, Turkbey B, Muradyan N, Rajesh A, Cornud F, Haider MA, et al. Overview of dynamic contrast-enhanced MRI in prostate cancer diagnosis and management. AJR American journal of roentgenology. 2012;198(6):1277–88.
22. Turnbull LW. Dynamic contrast-enhanced MRI in the diagnosis and management of breast cancer. NMR in biomedicine. 2009;22(1):28–39.
23. Knopp MV, Weiss E, Sinn HP, Mattern J, Junkermann H, Radeleff J, et al. Pathophysiologic basis of contrast enhancement in breast tumors. Journal of magnetic resonance imaging : JMRI. 1999;10(3):260–6.
24. Su MY, Wang Z, Roth GM, Lao X, Samoszuk MK, Nalcioglu O. Pharmacokinetic changes induced by vasomodulators in kidneys, livers, muscles, and implanted tumors in rats as measured by dynamic Gd-DTPA-enhanced MRI. Magn Reson Med. 1996;36(6):868–77.
25. Sarin H. On the future development of optimally-sized lipid-insoluble systemic therapies for CNS solid tumors and other neuropathologies. Recent patents on CNS drug discovery. 2010;5(3):239–52.
26. Sarin H. Overcoming the challenges in the effective delivery of chemotherapies to CNS solid tumors. Therapeutic delivery. 2010;1(2):289–305.
27. de Lussanet QG, Langereis S, Beets-Tan RG, van Genderen MH, Griffioen AW, van Engelshoven JM, et al. Dynamic contrast-enhanced MR imaging kinetic parameters and molecular weight of dendritic contrast agents in tumor angiogenesis in mice. Radiology. 2005;235(1):65–72.
28. Sarin H, Kanevsky AS, Wu H, Brimacombe KR, Fung SH, Sousa AA, et al. Effective transvascular delivery of nanoparticles across the blood–brain tumor barrier into malignant glioma cells. Journal of translational medicine. 2008;6:80.

29. Sarin H, Kanevsky AS, Wu H, Sousa AA, Wilson CM, Aronova MA, et al. Physiologic upper limit of pore size in the blood-tumor barrier of malignant solid tumors. Journal of translational medicine. 2009;7:51.

30. Gerstner ER, Fine RL. Increased permeability of the blood–brain barrier to chemotherapy in metastatic brain tumors: establishing a treatment paradigm. J Clin Oncol. 2007;25(16):2306–12.

31. Neuwelt E, Abbott N, Abrey L, Banks W, Blakley B, Davis T, et al. Strategies to advance translational research into brain barriers. Lancet Neurol. 2008;7:84–96.

32. Kanal E, Maravilla K, Rowley HA. Gadolinium Contrast Agents for CNS Imaging: Current Concepts and Clinical Evidence. AJNR American journal of neuroradiology. 2014;35(12):2215–26.

33. Soo Choi H, Liu W, Misra P, Tanaka E, Zimmer JP, Itty Ipe B, et al. Renal clearance of quantum dots. Nat Biotech. 2007;25(10):1165–70.

34. Louis C, Bazzi R, Marquette CA, Bridot J-L, Roux S, Ledoux G, et al. Nanosized Hybrid Particles with Double Luminescence for Biological Labeling. Chemistry of Materials. 2005;17(7):1673–82.

35. van de Watering FC, Rijpkema M, Perk L, Brinkmann U, Oyen WJ, Boerman OC. Zirconium-89 labeled antibodies: a new tool for molecular imaging in cancer patients. BioMed research international. 2014;2014:203601.

36. Jarrett BR, Frendo M, Vogan J, Louie AY. Size-controlled synthesis of dextran sulfate coated iron oxide nanoparticles for magnetic resonance imaging. Nanotechnology. 2007;18(3):035603.

37. Muldoon L, Sandor M, Pinkston K, Neuwelt E. Imaging, distribution, and toxicity of superparamagnetic iron oxide magnetic resonance nanoparticles in the rat brain and intracerebral tumor. Neurosurgery 2005, 57

38. Moore A, Marecos E, Bogdanov A, Weissleder R. Tumoral distribution of long-circulating dextran-coated iron oxide nanoparticles in a rodent model. Radiology. 2000;214:568–74.

39. Wagner M, Wagner S, Schnorr J, Schellenberger E, Kivelitz D, Krug L, et al. Coronary MR angiography using citrate-coated very small superparamagnetic iron oxide particles as blood-pool contrast agent: initial experience in humans. Journal of magnetic resonance imaging : JMRI. 2011;34(4):816–23.

40. Misselwitz B, Schmitt-Willich H, Ebert W, Frenzel T, Weinmann HJ. Pharmacokinetics of Gadomer-17, a new dendritic magnetic resonance contrast agent. Magma. 2001;12(2–3):128–34.

41. Venditto VJ, Regino CA, Brechbiel MW. PAMAM dendrimer based macromolecules as improved contrast agents. Molecular pharmaceutics. 2005;2(4):302–11.

42. Kobayashi H, Kawamoto S, Sakai Y, Choyke PL, Star RA, Brechbiel MW, et al. Lymphatic drainage imaging of breast cancer in mice by micro-magnetic resonance lymphangiography using a nano-size paramagnetic contrast agent. Journal of the National Cancer Institute. 2004;96(9):703–8.

43. Barrett T, Kobayashi H, Brechbiel M, Choyke PL. Macromolecular MRI contrast agents for imaging tumor angiogenesis. European Journal of Radiology. 2006;60:353–66.

44. Yordanov AT, Kobayashi H, English SJ, Reijnders K, Milenic D, Krishna MC, et al. Gadolinium-labeled dendrimers as biometric nanoprobes to detect vascular permeability. Journal of Materials Chemistry. 2003;13(7):1523–5.

45. Kobayashi H, Reijnders K, English S, Yordanov AT, Milenic DE, Sowers AL, et al. Application of a macromolecular contrast agent for detection of alterations of tumor vessel permeability induced by radiation. Clinical cancer research: an official journal of the American Association for Cancer Research. 2004;10(22):7712–20.

46. Langer R. Drug delivery and targeting. Nature. 1998;392(6679 Suppl):5–10.

47. Matsumura Y, Maeda H. A new concept for macromolecular therapeutics in cancer chemotherapy: Mechanism of tumoritropic accumulation of proteins and the antitumor agent smancs. Cancer Research. 1986;46(12 I):6387.

48. Tomalia DA, Baker H, Dewald J, Hall M, Kallos G, Martin S, et al. A New Class of Polymers: Starburst-Dendritic Macromolecules. Polym J. 1985;17(1):117–32.

49. Brechbiel M, Gansow O, Atcher R, Schlom J, Esteban J, Simpson D, et al. Synthesis of 1-(p-isothiocyanatobenzyl) derivatives of DTPA and EDTA. Antibody labeling and tumor-imaging studies. Inorganic Chemistry. 1986;25:2772–81.

50. Maeda H. Vascular permeability in cancer and infection as related to macromolecular drug delivery, with emphasis on the EPR effect for tumor-selective drug targeting. Proceedings of the Japan Academy Series B, Physical and biological sciences. 2012;88(3):53–71.

51. Rosier RN, O'Keefe RJ, Teot LA, Fox EJ, Nester TA, Puzas JE, et al. P-glycoprotein expression in cartilaginous tumors. Journal of surgical oncology. 1997;65(2):95–105.

52. Brem H, Mahaley M, Vick N, Black K, Schold S, Burger P, et al. Interstitial chemotherapy with drug polymer implants for the treatment of recurrent gliomas. J Neurosurg. 1991;74:441–6.

53. Campbell RB, Fukumura D, Brown EB, Mazzola LM, Izumi Y, Jain RK, et al. Cationic charge determines the distribution of liposomes between the vascular and extravascular compartments of tumors. Cancer research. 2002;62(23):6831–6.

54. Stylianopoulos T, Soteriou K, Fukumura D, Jain R. Cationic Nanoparticles Have Superior Transvascular Flux into Solid Tumors: Insights from a Mathematical Model. Ann Biomed Eng. 2013;41(1):68–77.

55. Hobbs SK, Monsky WL, Yuan F, Roberts WG, Griffith L, Torchilin VP, et al. Regulation of transport pathways in tumor vessels: role of tumor type and microenvironment. Proc Natl Acad Sci U S A. 1998;95(8):4607–12.

56. Chauhan VP, Stylianopoulos T, Martin JD, Popovic Z, Chen O, Kamoun WS, et al. Normalization of tumour blood vessels improves the delivery of nanomedicines in a size-dependent manner. Nature nanotechnology. 2012;7(6):383–8.

57. Mross K, Niemann B, Massing U, Drevs J, Unger C, Bhamra R, et al. Pharmacokinetics of liposomal doxorubicin (TLC-D99; Myocet) in patients with solid tumors: an open-label, single-dose study. Cancer Chemother Pharmacol. 2004;54(6):514–24.

58. Lotem M, Hubert A, Lyass O, Goldenhersh MA, Ingber A, Peretz T, et al. Skin toxic effects of polyethylene glycol–coated liposomal doxorubicin. Archives of Dermatology. 2000;136(12):1475–80.

59. Taupitz M, Schnorr J, Abramjuk C, Wagner S, Pilgrimm H, Hunigen H, et al. New generation of monomer-stabilized very small superparamagnetic iron oxide particles (VSOP) as contrast medium for MR angiography: preclinical results in rats and rabbits. Journal of magnetic resonance imaging: JMRI. 2000;12(6):905–11.

60. Jackson C, Chanzy H, Booy F, Drake B, Tomalia D, Bauer B, et al. Visualization of dendrimer molecules by transmission electron microscopy (TEM): Staining methods and cryo-TEM of vitrified solutions. Macromolecules. 1998;31:6259–65.

61. Tomalia DA, Frechet JM. Discovery of dendrimers and dendritic polymers: a brief historical perspective. Journal of Polymer Science, Part A: Polymer Chemistry. 2002;40(16):2719–28.

62. Tomalia DA. Dendrons/dendrimers. The convergence of quantized dendritic building blocks/architectures for applications in nanotechnology. Chimica Oggi. 2005;23(6):41.

63. Gillies ER, Dy E, Frechet JMJ, Szoka FC. Biological evaluation of polyester dendrimer: Poly(ethylene oxide) "bow-tie" hybrids with tunable molecular weight and architecture. Molecular Pharmaceutics. 2005;2(2):129.

64. Lee CC, Gillies ER, Fox ME, Guillaudeu SJ, Frechet JMJ, Dy EE, et al. A single dose of doxorubicin-functionalized bow-tie dendrimer cures mice bearing C-26 colon carcinomas. Proceedings of the National Academy of Sciences of the United States of America. 2006;103(45):16649.

65. Kono K, Kojima C, Hayashi N, Nishisaka E, Kiura K, Watarai S, et al. Preparation and cytotoxic activity of poly(ethylene glycol)-modified poly(amidoamine) dendrimers bearing adriamycin. Biomaterials. 2008;29(11):1664–75.

66. Choi Y, Baker Jr JR. Targeting cancer cells with DNA-assembled dendrimers: a mix and match strategy for cancer. Cell cycle. 2005;4(5):669–71.

67. Tekade RK, Dutta T, Tyagi A, Bharti AC, Das BC, Jain NK. Surface-engineered dendrimers for dual drug delivery: a receptor up-regulation and enhanced cancer targeting strategy. Journal of drug targeting. 2008;16(10):758–72.

68. Okuda T, Kawakami S, Akimoto N, Niidome T, Yamashita F, Hashida M. PEGylated lysine dendrimers for tumor-selective targeting after intravenous injection in tumor-bearing mice. J Control Release. 2006;116(3):330–6.

69. Kojima C, Regino CA, Umeda Y, Kobayashi H, Kono K. Influence of dendrimer generation and polyethylene glycol length on the biodistribution of PEGylated dendrimers. International Journal of Pharmaceutics. 2010;383:293–6.

70. Kukowska-Latallo JF, Candido KA, Cao Z, Nigavekar SS, Majoros IJ, Thomas TP, et al. Nanoparticle targeting of anticancer drug improves therapeutic response in animal model of human epithelial cancer. Cancer Research. 2005;65(12):5317.

71. Swanson SD, Kukowska-Latallo JF, Patri AK, Chen C, Ge S, Cao Z, et al. Targeted gadolinium-loaded dendrimer nanoparticles for tumor-specific magnetic resonance contrast enhancement. International Journal of Nanomedicine. 2008;3(2):201.

72. Thomas TP, Huang B, Choi SK, Silpe JE, Kotlyar A, Desai AM, et al. Polyvalent dendrimer-methotrexate as a folate receptor-targeted cancer therapeutic. Molecular pharmaceutics. 2012;9(9):2669–76.

73. Konda SD, Wang S, Brechbiel M, Wiener EC. Biodistribution of a 153 Gd-folate dendrimer, generation = 4, in mice with folate-receptor positive and negative ovarian tumor xenografts. Investigative radiology. 2002;37(4):199–204.

Translational theranostic methodology for diagnostic imaging and the concomitant treatment...

89

74. Li MH, Choi SK, Thomas TP, Desai A, Lee KH, Kotlyar A, et al. Dendrimer-based multivalent methotrexates as dual acting nanoconjugates for cancer cell targeting. Eur J Med Chem. 2012;47(1):560–72.

75. Sousa AA, Aronova MA, Wu H, Sarin H, Griffiths GL, Leapman RD. Determining molecular mass distributions and compositions of functionalized dendrimer nanoparticles. Nanomedicine. 2009;4(4):391–9.

76. Sousa A, Aronova M, Wu H, Sarin H, Griffiths G, Leapman R. Quantitative STEM and EFTEM characterization of dendrimer-based nanoparticles used in magnetic resonance imaging and drug delivery. Microsc Microanal. 2008;14 Suppl 2:694–5.

77. Lee CC, Gillies ER, Fox ME, Guillaudeu SJ, Frechet JM, Dy EE, et al. A single dose of doxorubicin-functionalized bow-tie dendrimer cures mice bearing C-26 colon carcinomas. Proc Natl Acad Sci U S A. 2006;103(45):16649–54.

78. Swanson SD, Kukowska-Latallo JF, Patri AK, Chen C, Ge S, Cao Z, et al. Targeted gadolinium-loaded dendrimer nanoparticles for tumor-specific magnetic resonance contrast enhancement. International journal of nanomedicine. 2008;3(2):201–10.

79. Yue Y, Eun JS, Lee MK, Seo SY. Synthesis and characterization of G5 PAMAM dendrimer containing daunorubicin for targeting cancer cells. Archives of pharmacal research. 2012;35(2):343–9.

80. Haacke EM, Brown RW, Thompson MR, Venkatesan M. Magnetic Resonance Imaging: Physical Principles and Sequence Design. New York: Wiley; 1999.

81. Aime S, Caravan P. Biodistribution of gadolinium-based contrast agents, including gadolinium deposition. Journal of magnetic resonance imaging: JMRI. 2009;30(6):1259–67.

82. Bryant Jr LH, Brechbiel MW, Wu C, Bulte JW, Herynek V, Frank JA. Synthesis and relaxometry of high-generation (G = 5, 7, 9, and 10) PAMAM dendrimer-DOTA-gadolinium chelates. Journal of magnetic resonance imaging: JMRI. 1999;9(2):348–52.

83. Langereis S, de Lussanet QG, van Genderen MH, Meijer EW, Beets-Tan RG, Griffioen AW, et al. Evaluation of Gd(III)DTPA-terminated poly(propylene imine) dendrimers as contrast agents for MR imaging. NMR in biomedicine. 2006;19(1):133–41.

84. Sethi R, Ananta JS, Karmonik C, Zhong M, Fung SH, Liu X, et al. Enhanced MRI relaxivity of Gd(3+) -based contrast agents geometrically confined within porous nanoconstructs. Contrast media & molecular imaging. 2012;7(6):501–8.

85. Orth RC, Bankson J, Price R, Jackson EF. Comparison of single- and dual-tracer pharmacokinetic modeling of dynamic contrast-enhanced MRI data using low, medium, and high molecular weight contrast agents. Magnetic resonance in medicine: official journal of the Society of Magnetic Resonance in Medicine/Society of Magnetic Resonance in Medicine. 2007;58(4):705–16.

86. Landis CS, Li X, Telang FW, Coderre JA, Micca PL, Rooney WD, et al. Determination of the MRI contrast agent concentration time course in vivo following bolus injection: Effect of equilibrium transcytolemmal water exchange. Magnetic Resonance in Medicine. 2000;44(4):563–74.

87. Eldredge HB, Spiller M, Chasse JM, Greenwood MT, Caravan P. Species dependence on plasma protein binding and relaxivity of the gadolinium-based MRI contrast agent MS-325. Investigative radiology. 2006;41(3):229–43.

88. Donahue KM, Burstein D, Manning WJ, Gray ML. Studies of Gd-DTPA relaxivity and proton exchange rates in tissue. Magn Reson Med. 1994;32(1):66–76.

89. Cox RW. AFNI: software for analysis and visualization of functional magnetic resonance neuroimages. Comput Biomed Res. 1996;29(3):162–73.

90. Aas AT, Brun A, Blennow C, Stromblad S, Salford LG. The RG2 rat glioma model. J Neurooncol. 1995;23(3):175–83.

91. Barth R. Rat brain tumor models in experimental neuro-oncology: The 9 L, C6, T9, F98, RG2 (D74), RT-2 and CNS-1 gliomas. Journal of Neuro-Oncology. 1998;36:91–102.

92. Camphausen K, Purow B, Sproull M, Scott T, Ozawa T, Deen DF, et al. Influence of in vivo growth on human glioma cell line gene expression: convergent profiles under orthotopic conditions. Proc Natl Acad Sci U S A. 2005;102(23):8287–92.

93. Wen PY, Kesari S. Malignant Gliomas in Adults. New England Journal of Medicine. 2008;359(5):492–507.

94. Kleinschmidt-DeMasters BK, Lillehei KO, Breeze RE. Neoplasms involving the central nervous system in the older old. Human pathology. 2003;34(11):1137–47.

12

Neurovascular 4DFlow MRI (Phase Contrast MRA): emerging clinical applications

Patrick Turski[1*], Andrew Scarano[1], Eric Hartman[1], Zachary Clark[1], Tilman Schubert[3], Leonardo Rivera[2], Yijing Wu[2], Oliver Wieben[2] and Kevin Johnson[2]

Abstract

Recent advances in 4DFlow MRI (Phase Contrast MRA) acquisition and reconstruction enable high resolution exams to be obtained in practical imaging times. 4DFlow MRI provides images of vascular morphology and quantitative measurements of blood velocity throughout a 3D imaging volume. Hemodynamic parameters such as flow volume, relative wall shear stress, streamlines, vorticity and pressure gradients can be derived from the velocity data. The combination of anatomic vessel wall imaging, lumen visualization and physiologic data derived from accelerated 4DFlow MRI augments the characterization of intracranial arterial stenosis, aneurysms, vascular malformations and dural sinus pathology. This review provides an update for clinicians interested in 4DFlow MRI of the brain.

Background

Blood flow is altered in a variety of diseases; however, clinically viable methods for evaluating intracranial arterial and venous flow have been limited. With recent advances, blood velocities can be measured with transcranial Doppler ultrasound, magnetic resonance imaging (MRI) and potentially by digital subtraction angiography (DSA). Of these modalities, MRI is an appealing imaging option due to its non-invasive nature, ability to image vessels with complex geometry, high spatial resolution and ability to correlate well with other imaging features. The ability to measure velocities by flow encoded MRI was demonstrated by Moran [1] in 1983, shortly after MR was implemented for clinical imaging. Using this strategy flow encoding was implemented for 2D and 3D acquisition by Dumoulin [2, 3] and clinical applications for vascular flow imaging were expanded by Pelc et al [4] and Wigstrom et al [5]. However, general use of the flow imaging was limited by long acquisition times, complex implementation and motion artifacts. Consequently, for several decades flow measurements with MRI played only a minor role in neurovascular assessment.

Recently, substantial technology has been developed which has dramatically expanded the opportunities for flow assessment with MRI. These include faster, stronger and more stable imaging gradients, phased array receiver technology and orders of magnitude increases in reconstruction hardware. Together and as detailed in this article, these technologies have allowed for cardiac cycle time resolved, 3D flow imaging (4DFlow) to be obtained with clinically relevant resolution in relatively short imaging times. 4DFlow acquires a volumetric imaging acquisition which allows the retrospectively visualization and quantification of complex flow fields. Recent interest from the MRI and post-processing software vendors along with promising clinical studies suggest that 4DFlow MRI will likely become widely available in the near future.

Clinical applications of 4DFlow MRI are now expanding and 4DFlow is increasing used to supplement MRI and MRA exams. The ability to quantitatively measure velocity has many applications in neurovascular imaging [6]. However, clinical implementation of 4DFlow MRI requires an understanding of the strengths and limitations of the technique. This overview discusses the basic features of 4DFlow MRI from a clinical perspective. The review outlines the role of 4DFlow MRI in the detection and characterization of arterial stenosis, atherosclerotic disease, aneurysms, vascular malformations and dural sinus pathology.

* Correspondence: pturski@uwhealth.org
[1]Department of Radiology, University of Wisconsin School of Medicine and Public Health, Madison, Wisconsin, USA
Full list of author information is available at the end of the article

Intracranial 4DFlow MRI acquisition

The principles for flow measurement remain similar to those initially proposed by Moran [1]. Briefly, when a spin is moving along the magnetic field gradient its resonance frequency changes whereas for a static spin the resonance frequency would remain constant. Thus, if a gradient is applied for some time and an equal and opposite gradient is applied for the same time (flow encoding gradients) static spins will rotate faster and then slower such that the net change in frequency (rotation speed) is zero. For moving spins, the faster and slow frequency will not cancel. For each spin, this results in a phase shift in the acquired signal which is directly proportional to velocity. If the flow encoding gradients are small enough and the motion is coherent (e.g. blood flow) the phase difference in the detected signal is directly proportional to the average velocity in the voxel of interest. This phase difference is only detectable up to a $\pm180°$ in each direction and the minimum velocity that causes a 180° rotation is the velocity encoding, V_{enc}. Due to this fixed dynamic range, to avoid aliasing, the V_{enc} must be selected to be only slightly higher than the maximum expected velocity. As demonstrated in Fig. 1, for angiograms generated from a 4D flow acquisition, there is a tradeoff between the sensitivity to slow flow and the range of detectable velocities. In some instances, such as in the case of imaging venous flow, the velocity encoding is selected to maximize the signal from slow flow and aliasing of higher velocities is identified and accepted in the images as signal loss.

4DFlow MRI is based on an RF and gradient spoiled 3D gradient echo sequence (i.e. SPGR/FLASH/TFE/Fast FE). Starting from a standard sequence, flow encoding

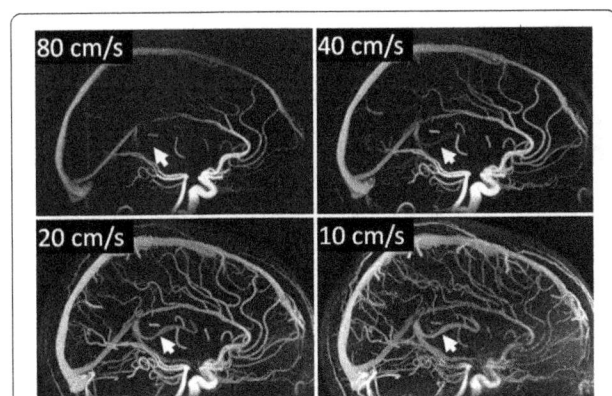

Fig. 1 Limited maximum intensity projections (MIPS) of angiograms generated from 4DFlow acquisitions with V_{enc}'s of 80, 40, 20 and 10 cm/s. As the V_{enc} is reduced to 10 cm/sec the visualization of large arterial vessels is reduced. In these vessels, the measured velocity values will be unreliable due to limited detectable velocity dynamic range. At the same time, the visualization of slow flowing venous structures is improved as the V_{enc} is reduced

gradients are inserted after excitation and before the imaging readout, as shown in Fig. 2. This increases the echo time (TE) and repetition time (TR) by ~1–3 ms depending on the V_{enc} and scanner gradient performance. Further, in order to measure flow in 3 directions at least 4 images must be collected with different flow encoding gradient directions, 1 for background phase and 1 for each direction. Typical implementations interleave these encodings. Finally, cardiac gating is incorporated either though prospective or retrospective triggering. For intracranial applications typically 10–20 cardiac phases are acquired. This results in cardiac time resolved 3D volumes, which are subtracted to produce flow fields (Fig. 3). Considering the increase in TR, the need for at least 4 flow encodings, and a minimum 10 cardiac phases, the acquisition time for a 4D flow exam is ~50-100x longer than a traditional gradient echo scan, such as those used for contrast enhanced angiography.

Fortunately, technologic advances have shorted imaging time and increased spatial and temporal resolution. Current implementation varies from site to site and vendor to vendor but follows similar trends. Nearly all implementation of 4DFlow utilize parallel imaging, most commonly direct techniques such as SENSE or GRAPPA [7–9] but also with indirect methods such as using localized coils. In the case of Cartesian imaging, this reduces the required scan time by a factor of 2–4; and is typically not sufficient to reduce scan times for clinically relevant coverage and spatial resolution (<1 mm) to feasible scan times. One potential method for reducing scan times is to use non-Cartesian sampling trajectories which either collect more data per excitation, as in spiral [10] or allow greater under sampling of the imaging volume without obscuring artifacts, as in radial trajectories. Non-Cartesian imaging additionally allows for a reduction of the echo time [11, 12], allowing improved imaging of complex flow and/or higher spatial resolution [13, 14]. Another method commonly used to reduce scan time is to utilize a reconstruction which harnesses correlation in space and time [9, 15–22]. These techniques make the observation that most signal is from non-moving tissues and thus the same in all the time frames. The amount of the acceleration possible with these techniques is extremely high but requires substantial computational power to fully achieve high levels of acceleration [23]. More modest accelerations can be achieved utilizing lower computational burden of k-t acceleration techniques [19]. With the combination of parallel imaging and k-t acceleration techniques, the major arterial circulation can be imaged with 1 mm isotropic spatial resolution within 5–10 min. The joint combination of parallel imaging, spatiotemporal acceleration and non-Cartesian sampling provides the opportunity to further increase spatial resolution (<0.7 isotropic) and provide whole brain coverage [14]. While vendors'

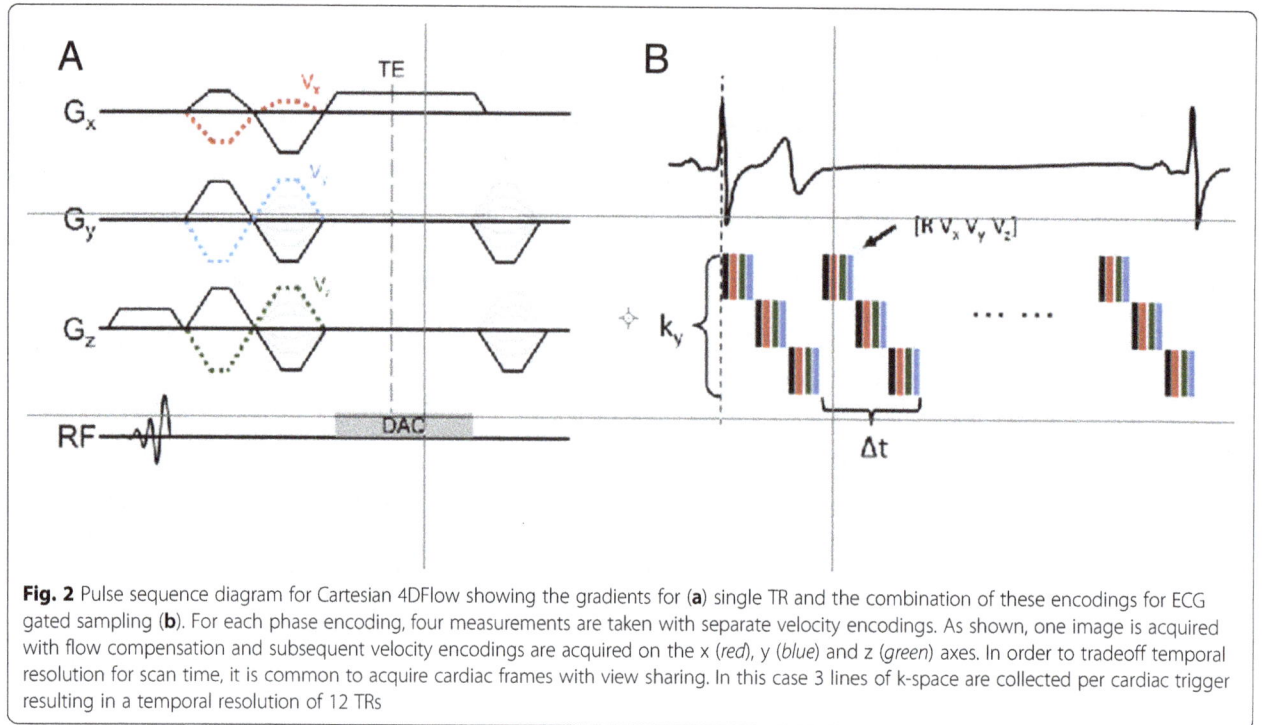

Fig. 2 Pulse sequence diagram for Cartesian 4DFlow showing the gradients for (**a**) single TR and the combination of these encodings for ECG gated sampling (**b**). For each phase encoding, four measurements are taken with separate velocity encodings. As shown, one image is acquired with flow compensation and subsequent velocity encodings are acquired on the x (*red*), y (*blue*) and z (*green*) axes. In order to tradeoff temporal resolution for scan time, it is common to acquire cardiac frames with view sharing. In this case 3 lines of k-space are collected per cardiac trigger resulting in a temporal resolution of 12 TRs

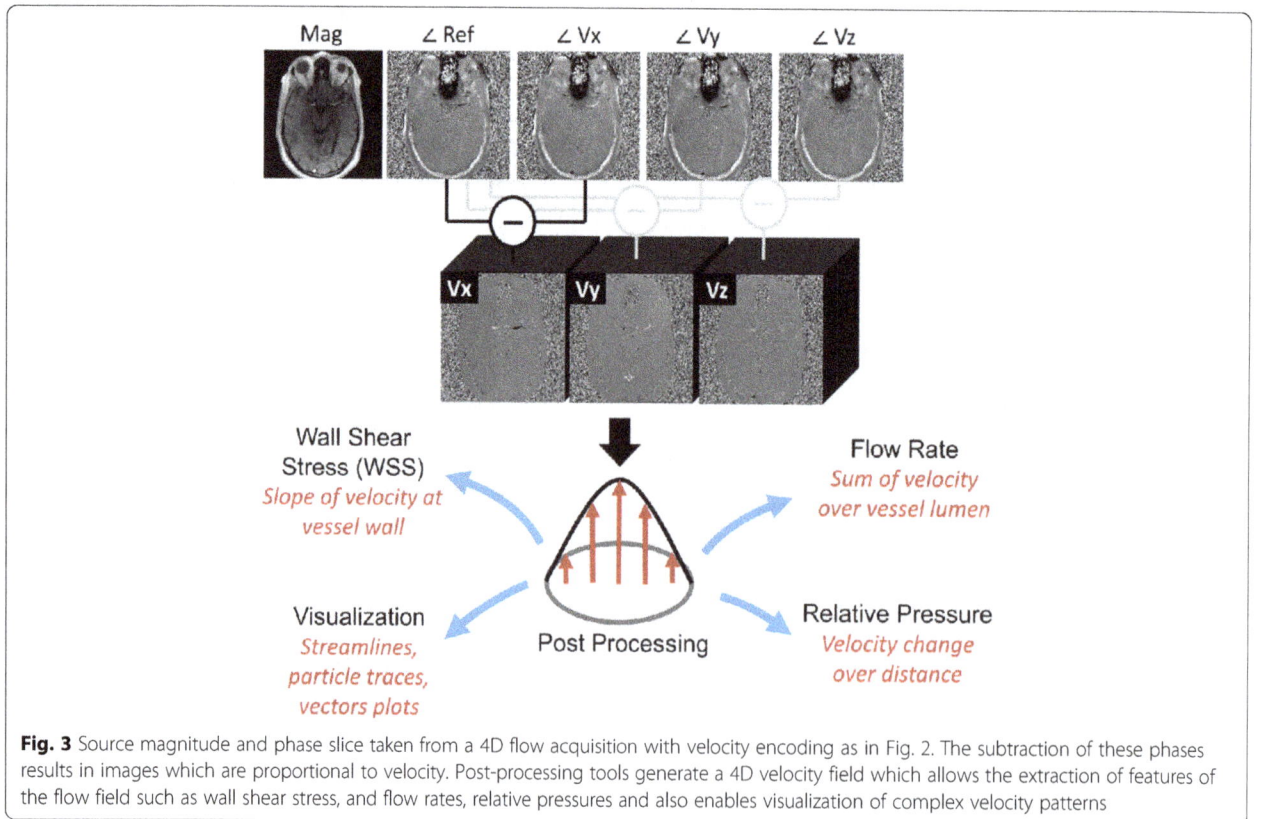

Fig. 3 Source magnitude and phase slice taken from a 4D flow acquisition with velocity encoding as in Fig. 2. The subtraction of these phases results in images which are proportional to velocity. Post-processing tools generate a 4D velocity field which allows the extraction of features of the flow field such as wall shear stress, and flow rates, relative pressures and also enables visualization of complex velocity patterns

have not released specific 4D flow packages, it is most likely that products will be based on simple k-t acceleration, Cartesian sampling and parallel imaging; with computational hurdles existing for advanced constrained reconstructions and non-Cartesian approaches.

4DFlow MRI display and flow analysis

4DFlow imaging acquisitions produce a large number of images which can be challenging to interrogate with standard imaging viewing and analysis platforms. In scenarios where advanced processing is unavailable, there are several components of the 4DFlow MRI data readily available for clinical assessment. The magnitude images display both stationary tissue and flow compensated vascular structures providing the opportunity to precisely related soft tissue abnormalities to the adjacent vessels. Following subtraction of the stationary background tissues, the flow (or speed) images are displayed without specifying the direction of flow. An important feature is that the signal intensity of the flow images is dependent on the velocity encoding selected at the time of the acquisition; flow velocities that closely approximate the velocity encoding will have the highest signal intensity.

Alternatively, each flow encoding direction can be independently displayed. In this instance, the velocity images are reconstructed with velocity displayed in the superior/inferior, anterior/posterior and right/left using a gray scale or color display. Velocity is a vector that has direction and magnitude, if a color display is used, direction is displayed by the chosen color scheme and magnitude is displayed as brightness. Velocity aliasing occurs when the velocities exceed the velocity encoding. In this scenario the pixel signal intensity will flip to display flow in the opposite direction. If a gray scale display is used the pixels change from bright to dark when aliasing occurs incorrectly indicating the direction of velocity and flow.

A more complete and quantitative interrogation of the 4DFlow data is possible with dedicated flow analysis software. This allows the simultaneous visualization of the direction and magnitude of the velocity field and can enable flow measurements of specific vessels. The initial step in flow analysis is the segmentation of the vascular structures from the imaging volume. The resulting vascular and flow data are subsequently analyzed using a 4DFlow package. To date, numerous packages have been adopted most frequently these have been tools developed for generalized visualization of flow fields (e.g. EnSight; CEI, Apex, NC, applications in the aerospace industry); however, FDA approved tools are now available (e.g. Arterys, San Francisco, CA USA). Such flow analysis packages provide software tools allowing for navigation throughout the 3D flow field. The flow field can be transected by 2D planes at the desired location and angle. Velocity and flow rate (flow rate = velocity x cross sectional area of the vessel) can be measured from a 2D plane orthogonal to the vessel of interest. The flow field can also be displayed as color coded velocity vectors representing the magnitude and direction of flow. Streamline displays are virtual instantaneous paths that are tangent to the velocity vectors at the specified point in time. Streamlines are relatively easy to interpret and provide an intuitive sense of the hemodynamics. Particle paths are another option and represent virtual particles that follow the velocity vectors from one time point to another simulating the flow of particles in the flow channels. Many important derivatives of velocity can be calculated. Estimations of wall shear stress can be generated by calculating the velocity gradient perpendicular to the vessel wall, WSS can be thought of as the drag of the flowing blood on the endothelial surface [24]. Measurements of pulsatility can be obtained and expressed as the pulsatility index (PI = (QmaxQmin)/Qmean; Q = flow mL/min) [25]. Vorticity is a curl in the velocity field and measures local rotation, vorticity can be quantified and has the potential to improve characterization of aneurysm flow [26]. Relative pressure variations within the velocity field can be calculated by using the Pressure Poisson Equation derived from the Navier-Stokes equations. For example, relative pressure drop across a stenosis can be determined from the velocity measurements using this approach [27] (Fig. 3). All of these measurements are limited by partial volume effect, phase errors, aliasing and motion. Fortunately, strategies are in development to speed analysis by using automated segmentation, quantification, aliasing corrections and methods to improve streamline, and particle path displays by reducing vector divergence [28–32].

Clinical applications

4DFlow MRI of intracranial atherosclerosis

The current standard of care for treatment of symptomatic intracranial atherosclerotic disease is medical therapy rather than percutaneous endovascular therapy due in large part to the SAMMPRIS trial in 2011 [33]. However, the only imaging parameter utilized in this trial was percent vessel stenosis. Furthermore, about 12 % of the medical therapy group reached the primary endpoint of stroke or death within 1 year of a symptomatic stroke related to an atherosclerotic plaque raising the likelihood that a certain subset of patients could benefit from more advanced risk stratification and treatment options.

Certain hemodynamic conditions predispose patients to the development and progression of atherosclerotic plaques. The most clearly identified relationship of this nature is the development of atherosclerotic disease in regions of low wall shear stress. Wall shear stress (WSS) is detected by the endothelial cell surface mechanoreceptors which signal the cell regarding the presence of elevated, normal or low wall shear stress. Normal or high wall shear stress promotes reorganization of the cell cytoskeleton, tightens endothelial cell junctions and reduced the endothelial cell permeability to lipids. Whereas, low wall shear stress promotes endothelial cell disorganization, reduces tight junctions and increases permeability to lipids [34]. For example, atherosclerotic disease is most often encountered in the bulb of the carotid bifurcation where there is recirculating flow and low wall shear stress demonstrated by 4Dflow MRI [35–37].

Studies of intracranial stenosis hemodynamics using computational fluid dynamic models (CFD) based on 3D CTA data have been performed in patients with stenosis of the proximal middle cerebral artery greater than 70 %. In a study of 32 patients, the risk of recurrent stroke increased as the spatial gradient of the flow velocity increased within the stenosis. Interestingly, the risk of recurrent stroke did not correlate with the degree of stenosis measured by DSA in this group of patients [38].

Intracranial arterial WSS has also been studied with 4Dflow MRI. Large vessel arterial wall shear stress decreases with age, drops significantly during the 5th decade of life, is lower in males than females, and is lowest in the anterior cerebral arteries [39]. These relationships are likely influenced by multiple factors as humans age including increased vessel diameter, decreased blood flow [39], and other contributions such as cardiac output, blood pressure and hormone effects. Other 4DFlow MRI studies have been used to assess vertebrobasilar insufficiency [40], endovascular stenting [41], subclavian steal [42], extracranial-intracranial (EC-IC) bypass [43], and cerebrovascular blood flow reactivity to carbon dioxide inhalation [44].

Recent reports using contrast enhanced 3D T1 weighted black blood arterial wall imaging have demonstrated that intracranial atherosclerotic plaque wall enhancement is associated with an increased likelihood that the plaque is the culprit plaque responsible for the ischemic event [45, 46]. The wall enhancement has been shown to decrease with time after the event [47]. Intracranial plaque morphology including intra-plaque hemorrhage [48, 49] and increased lipid rich necrotic core volume [50] have also been established as stroke risk factors. In addition, carotid artery studies have demonstrated that complex plaque morphology including intra-plaque hemorrhage, thrombus or fibrous cap rupture is located predominantly on the ipsilateral side of stroke [51–53].

4DFlow MRI provides an opportunity to explore wall-flow-lesion interactions utilizing the combination of vessel wall imaging, 4Dflow and vessel lumen morphology. Unfortunately, achieving the high spatial resolution required to quantitatively depict the intracranial vasculature

is challenging due to competing factors including SNR, scan time and artifacts. This is especially true for 4Dflow and CE-MRA. Current investigations of ultrashort echo (UTE) imaging suggest that UTE increases acquisition efficiency while offering improved flow compensation, increased spatial resolution and robustness to artifacts [14] (Fig. 4).

4DFlow MRI of intracranial aneurysms

There is intense investigation into aneurysm hemodynamics and how flow contributes to aneurysm formation, growth and rupture. Although the major of investigations have been based on computation fluid dynamics modeling (CFD) [54–58], it is clear that 4DFlow MRI provides information similar to CFD and can contribute to the hemodynamic assessment of intracranial aneurysms [24, 59–62].

Aneurysm hemodynamic patterns can be grouped into three categories: 1) entry events, 2) intrasaccular flow characteristics and 3) wall/flow interactions. Entry events

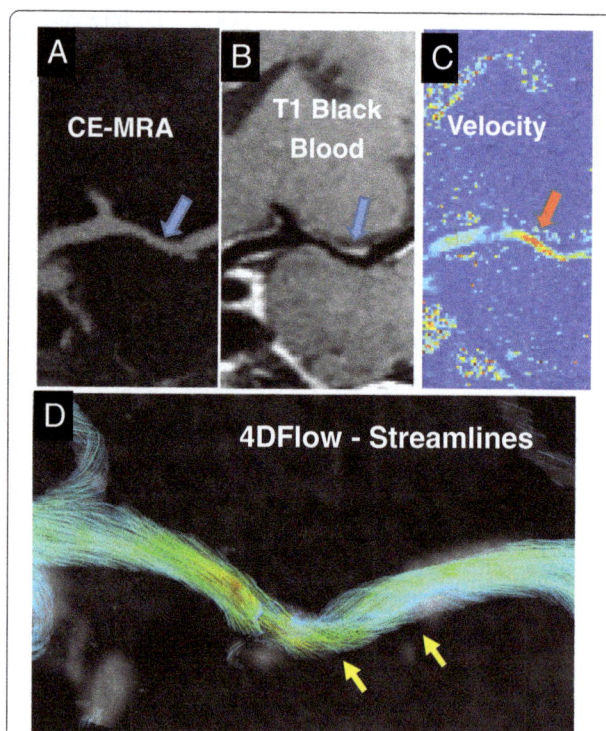

Fig. 4 Left middle cerebral artery stenosis in a patient with diffuse atherosclerotic disease. Images **a**–**c** are displayed as curved vessel reformations. **a** The ultra short echo time CE MRA demonstrates a stenosis of the proximal left middle cerebral artery (*arrow*). **b** Arterial wall enhancement is seen on post contrast T1BB at the location of the stenosis (*arrow*) and distal to the stenosis. **c** Elevated 4Dflow MRI velocities derived from the ultra short echo time acquisition are identified within the stenosis suggesting that the lesion is hemodynamically significant. **d** Streamlines generated through the stenosis demonstrate a helical flow pattern (*arrows*)

are comprised of measured inflow concentration indices related to the inflow jet. Intrasaccular flow characteristics consider features such as vorticity, vortex core line length as well as ratios of kinetic energy, shear strain rate and viscous dissipation. Finally, wall/flow interactions include maximum and minimum WSS measurements, shear concentration index, area of aneurysm exposed to low WSS, and oscillatory shear index [63].

Sforza et al [63] also found that the hemodynamic environment predisposing to aneurysm growth was composed of a concentrated inflow stream leading to complex intrasaccular flow patterns; specifically, patterns characterized by areas of concentrated high WSS accompanied by larger areas of low WSS. They concluded that the concentrated inflow stream disperses into complex intravascular flow streams that produce non-uniform WSS distributions with concentrated areas of high WSS and large areas of low WSS. They propose that these hemodynamic conditions represent the features which promote aneurysm growth. They also noted that the same trends were observed in rupture versus non ruptured aneurysms. As 4DFlow MRI methods evolve, similar measurements of in vivo hemodynamics will be possible and will be able to provide objective criteria to aid in aneurysm risk stratification.

Meng et al. [64] tried to unify conflicting CFD data by proposing that in large aneurysms low WSS promotes wall inflammation through an inflammatory cell mediated pathway leading growth. Whereas, in small aneurysms or blebs high WSS and a positive WSS gradient

promotes a different mural cell mediated inflammation pathway leading to growth and rupture.

Using contrast enhanced 3D T1 black blood wall imaging, several reports have demonstrated an association of aneurysm wall enhancement with aneurysm growth or rupture [65–67]. Additional approaches are being developed that combine 4DFlow MRI and 3D T1 black blood imaging of the aneurysm wall to link aneurysm wall thickness and wall enhancement to specific flow dynamics [68] (Fig. 5).

To provide risk stratification, the flow and wall imaging features will need to be correlated with other known vascular health factors (smoking, hypertension, family history, collagen vascular disease) and individual patient details (size, location, age, gender) to allow further predictability for risk of aneurysm growth and rupture [69].

4DFlow vascular malformations

Imaging cerebrovascular arteriovenous malformations (AVMs) with high flow and rapid arteriovenous shunting presents several challenges. The malformations are often supplied by multiple arterial pedicles and have complex anomalous venous drainage necessitating a large field of view that encompasses the majority of the cerebrovascular system. High spatial resolution for imaging small vessels and high temporal resolution for detecting rapid arteriovenous shunting is needed to adequately characterize AVMs. The classification of AVMs requires description of size, location, arterial supply and venous drainage. This

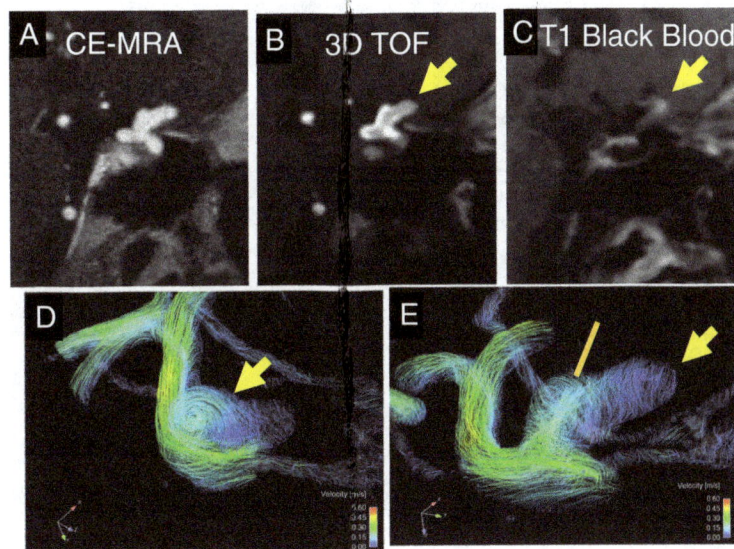

Fig. 5 Aneurysm of the supraclinoid carotid artery. **a** and **b** The CE MRA and 3D TOF MRA demonstrate that the aneurysm has a more spherical proximal component and a distal outpouching (*arrow*). **c** The distal outpouching and apex of the aneurysm enhance on the 3D T1 weighted contrast enhanced black blood image (*arrow*). **d** and **e** The streamline displays reveals vortex flow (*arrow*) and a central vortex core (*line*) in the proximal spherical component of the aneurysm. The distal outpouching has low flow velocity and presumed low wall shear stress

information enables Spetzler-Martin grading [70] which predicts operative morbidity and mortality. DSA has long been considered the gold standard for full characterization of AVMs due to exceptional temporal and spatial resolution. However 4DFlow MRI has emerged as a tool capable of characterizing size, location, arterial supply and drainage noninvasively. A major advantage of 4DFlow MRI is the ability to provide additional physiologic information including velocity, flow volume, wall shear stress, pressure gradients, streamlines and flow path lines [71]. The hemodynamic features combined with the morphological image provide an expanded perspective on the impact of the AVM on global cerebrovascular blood flow (Fig. 6). Selective vessel imaging can be accomplished by vessel segmentation and seeding of streamlines at the origin of the vessels of interest [31, 72] (Fig. 7).

Wu et al [73] demonstrated that there was a relationship between the macrovascular hemodynamics of AVMs and the microvascular effects on tissue perfusion. In this study, higher grade Spetzler-Martin AVMs were associated with higher peak velocity and blood flow in feeding arterial vessels and higher blood flow in draining veins. As postulated previously, these macrovascular parameters lead to a steal phenomenon affecting microvascular tissue perfusion with an inverse relationship between perinidal perfusion measures including cerebral blood flow (CBF) and cerebral blood volume (CBV) with macrovascular arterial and venous blood flow. However,

these parameters did not predict symptomatic presentation and were not associated with other previously described AVM risk factors (deep AVM location, deep venous drainage, associated aneurysm or venous stenosis). Time integrated 3D path lines of the entire cerebrovasculature can be color coded to provide a pre surgical roadmap of large feeding arteries and draining vessels. This approach has been successfully used to select target vessels for staged embolization and to follow the results of embolization [74]. Recent work by Wu et al [75] also demonstrates the value of 4DFlow MRI to precisely define the hemodynamics of a particularly complex AVM guiding surgical intervention.

4DFlow MR Imaging has also proved useful to assess dural arteriovenous fistulas (DAVFs). Delineation of the arterial anatomy and venous drainage is essential for the Cognard classification [76] of DAVFs. Similar to AVMs the 4DFlow data can be used to isolate flow in individual vessels providing selective display of streamline flow. Using this technique it may be possible to classify DAVFs using the Cognard system and provide a vascular roadmap for surgical planning [29, 72].

In contrast to AVMs, DAVFs often present less aggressively with symptoms of pulsatile tinnitus rather than intracranial hemorrhage. Often times the only imaging clue to the presence of a DAVF is asymmetric early venous filling on time resolved contrast enhanced MRA. A new approach called HYPRFlow combines a dynamic

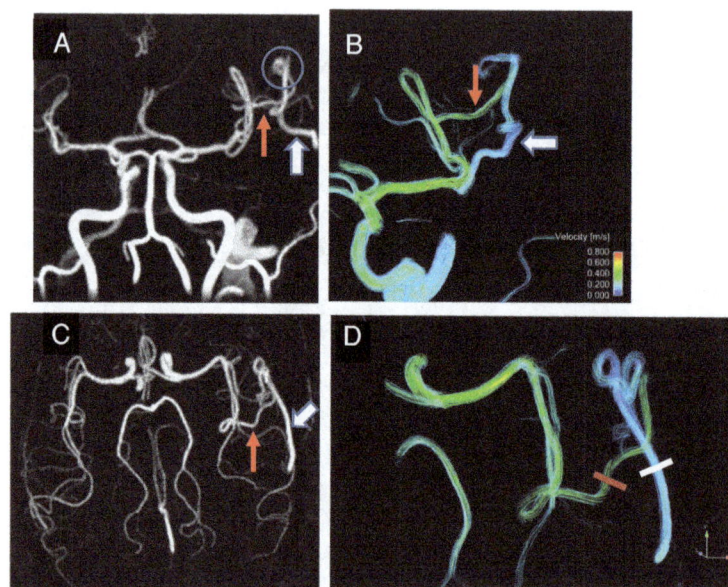

Fig. 6 Left frontal lobe Arteriovenous Malformation. **a** 4D Flow Coronal MIP demonstrates an enlarged Left MCA opercular branch (*red arrow*) supplying a small frontal lobe AVM (*circle*) and a cortical draining vein (*white arrow*). **b** Streamline flow displayed in the coronal plane reveals preferential flow in the feeding artery (*red arrow*) and draining cortical vein (*white arrow*). **c** 4DFlow Axial MIP displaying the main arterial feeder (*red arrow*) and largest draining cortical vein (*white arrow*). **d** Quantitative 4D flow analysis (*axial projection*) reveals moderately elevated flow volume in the arterial feeder of 55 mL/min (measured at the *red lined*) and nearly matching venous outflow of 52 mL/min (measured at the *blue line*)

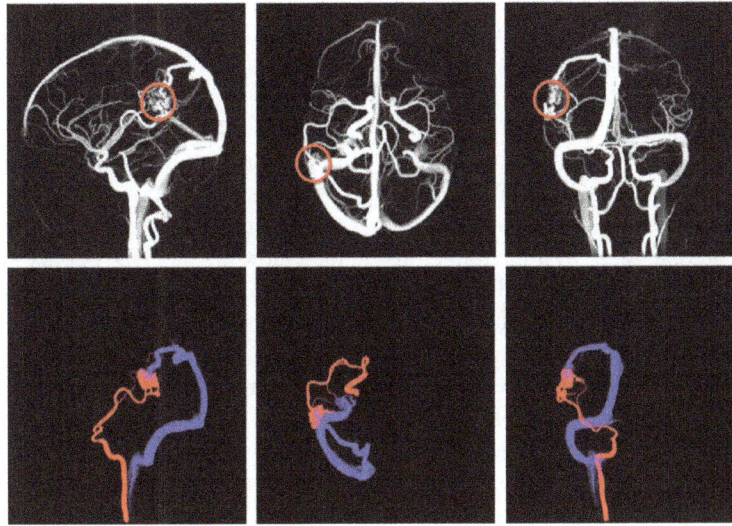

Fig. 7 4DFlow MRI Cartography of a right parietal brain AVM. Top row: Sagittal, axial and coronal 4DFlow MRI MIP images of the AVM. Bottom row: Selective streamline display demonstrates a large MCA branch feeding artery and the dominant draining cortical vein. Images courtesy of Michael Loecher, PhD

time resolved contrast enhanced MRA during the passage of a contrast bolus with a 4DFlow acquisition which is used to improve the image quality of the time series using an innovative reconstruction method (constrained reconstruction) [77]. Initial experience using HYPRFlow MRI with DAVFs demonstrated excellent arteriovenous separation, high resolution vascular images and concordant Cognard classification with DSA [78].

4DFLOW MRI dural sinuses

4DFlow MRI is the only imaging modality that can assess global intracranial venous blood flow and hemodynamics in adults. 4DFlow MRI has been shown to be accurate and reproducible for measuring dural sinus flow velocity, flow rate and demonstrating streamline flow in normal subjects [79]. In the sagittal sinus, blood flow velocity and blood flow rate increases from anterior to posterior as the sagittal sinus increases in size. The transvers sinus velocities and flow rates are dependent on the anatomic configuration of the transverse sinus and torcular herophili. Small venous structures are less reliably assessed due to limitations in spatial resolution and low signal due to very slow flow. Reference values for dural sinus velocity and blood flow rates in normal subjects are available for comparison across age groups and provide a foundation for developing clinical applications [79].

The role of 4DFlow MRI in the diagnosis and follow up of dural sinus thrombosis continues to evolve. Recent comparisons of 4DFlow MRI to contrast enhanced 3D GE T1 weighted imaging demonstrated false positive results for 4DFlow MRI ranging from 4.7 to 8.2 %. This was due to signal loss in regions of complex/turbulent flow, susceptibility artifacts and very slow flow. 4DFlow

MRI also missed 10.4 % of thrombosed segments detected by 3D GE T1 weighted imaging [80, 81]. One limitation of this comparison is that the authors did not include the magnitude images in the review. In the setting of possible dural sinus thrombosis, the 4DFlow MRI exam should be obtained following the administration of a gadolinium contrast agent. In this instance, the magnitude images from the 4DFlow MRI acquisition are the equivalent of contrast enhanced 3D GE T1 weighted images. The contrast enhanced magnitude images are not flow encoded and thus do not suffer from velocity dependent signal loss. Including these images would likely have reduced the number of false positives. In addition to the magnitude images, 4DFlow provides objective blood flow data that allows for qualitative and quantitative assessment of treatment related improvements in dural sinus blood flow [79].

Another important application of 4DFlow MRI is the assessment of dural sinus flow in patients with intracranial hypertension due to venous outflow obstruction. In this population flow velocity and relative pressure measurement can assist in the monitoring of therapy and assess the results in interventions such as dural sinus stenting. Esfahani et al. assessed five patients with intracranial venous hypertension and dural sinus stenosis [81]. The mean pre-stenotic intravenous pressure measured by endovascular catheter placement was 45.2 mm Hg and decreased to 27.4 mm Hg following stenting. In these patients, the total jugular flow measured by 4D Flow MRI increased by 260.2 mL/min. Analysis of changes in intravenous pressure and 4D flow were highly correlated (Pearson correlation $r = 0.926$, Wilcoxon signed rank test $p = 0.4$) and all patients displayed clinical improvement at 6 weeks. The role of 4DFlow MRI may significantly expand in this patient population as post processing methods become more generally available to non-invasively calculate pressure gradients within the dural sinus from the velocity data (Fig. 8).

Alterations in 4DFlow and pulsatility related to dementia

There is increasing evidence that cerebral arteries are often morphologically altered and dysfunctional in Alzheimer's disease (AD) [82]. Cerebral blood flow, arterial pulsation and vasomotion are reduced in AD patients, and thus the normal perivascular transmission of metabolites out of the brain is diminished. The decrease in perivascular drainage may allow beta-amyloid protein to accumulate within the vessel wall. Vessel rigidity due to arteriosclerosis, atherosclerosis and amyloid deposition will ultimately translate into the inability to dissipate the systolic pressure created by the heart. Consequently, there is interest in non-invasive methods to assess cerebrovascular hemodynamics such as mean blood flow rate and pulsatility index (PI = (QmaxQmin)/Qmean; Q = flow) as potential systemic indicators of AD. The PI is a parameter dependent on the cerebrovascular resistance, the pulse amplitude of arterial pressure, and compliance of the cerebral arterial bed, and thus serves to characterize the cerebrovascular health. Due to temporal averaging, 4Dflow MRI mean velocities are approximately 30 % lower compared with transcranial Doppler ultrasound accounting for the differences between the techniques [83].

4Dflow MRI has demonstrated significant differences in the cerebral hemodynamics of an AD group when compared to cognitively healthy age matched controls [84]. There is a significant decrease in arterial mean blood flow in the AD population and a significant increase in PI, particularly the middle cerebral arteries and the cavernous internal carotids. An increased in intracranial PI is an indicator of increased distal resistance to blood flow within the microvasculature which is often related to small vessel disease [85]. These results are in agreement with other studies that have used TCD to determine the effect of AD on blood flow to the brain [82].

Conclusion

The barriers to the routine use of 4DFlow MRI to study cerebrovascular hemodynamics are gradually being overcome. The combination of parallel imaging, spatiotemporal acceleration and non-Cartesian sampling provides increase spatial resolution (<0.7 isotropic) and whole brain coverage in practical imaging times. Commercial packages are in development which will enable the

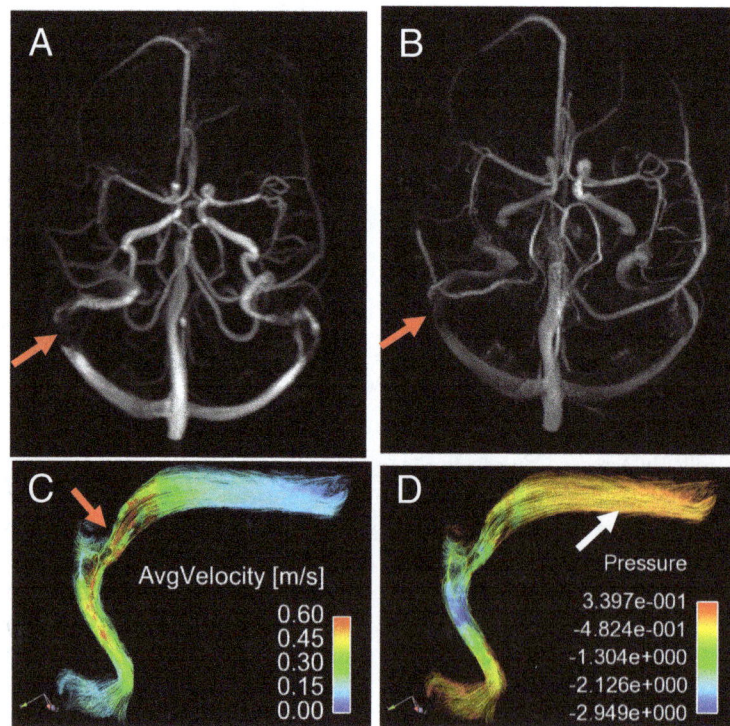

Fig. 8 Idiopathic intracranial hypertension. **a** The axial 4DFlow MRI image demonstrates a stenosis of the right transverse sinus (*arrow*). **b** The CE MRA confirms a stenosis at the junction of the transvers and sigmoid sinus (*arrow*). **c** The 4DFlow MRI velocities are elevated in the stenotic segment (*arrow*). **d** The relative pressure map reveals higher pressure in the transvers sinus (*white arrow*) compared to the stenotic segment and distal sigmoid sinus

clinical implementation of 4Flow and hemodynamic analysis. The physiological parameters derived from 4DFlow MRI will augment anatomical imaging and has the potential to improve characterization of the entire spectrum of cerebrovascular diseases.

Competing interests
The authors declare that they have no competing interests.

Authors' contributions
PT concept, data acquisition, manuscript preparation and editing. Address: Radiology, 600 Highland Ave, Madison 53792 Wisconsin USA. AS manuscript preparation. EH manuscript preparation. ZC manuscript preparation. TS data analysis. LR data analysis. YW data analysis. OW concept, design, development, data acquisition. KJ data acquisition, data analysis, design, manuscript preparation and editing. All authors read and approved the final manuscript.

Author details
[1]Department of Radiology, University of Wisconsin School of Medicine and Public Health, Madison, Wisconsin, USA. [2]Department of Medical Physics, University of Wisconsin School of Medicine and Public Health, Madison, Wisconsin, USA. [3]Department of Clinic of Radiology and Nuclear Medicine, Basel, Switzerland.

References
1. Moran PR. A flow velocity zeugmatographic interlace for NMR imaging in humans. Magn Reson Imaging. 1982;1(4):197–203.
2. Dumoulin CL, Hart Jr HR. Magnetic resonance angiography. Radiology. 1986; 161(3):717–20.
3. Dumoulin CL, Souza SP, Walker MF, Wagle W. Three-dimensional phase contrast angiography. Magn Reson Med. 1989;9(1):139–49.
4. Pelc NJ, Herfkens RJ, Shimakawa A, Enzmann DR. Phase contrast cine magnetic resonance imaging. Magn Reson Q. 1991;7(4):229–54.
5. Wigstrom L, Sjoqvist L, Wranne B. Temporally resolved 3D phase-contrast imaging. Magn Reson Med. 1996;36(5):800–3.
6. Chang W, Huang M, Chien A. Emerging techniques for evaluation of the hemodynamics of intracranial vascular pathology. Neuroradiol J. 2015;28(1):19–27.
7. Bauer S, Markl M, Foll D, et al. K-t GRAPPA accelerated phase contrast MRI: Improved assessment of blood flow and 3-directional myocardial motion during breath-hold. J Magn Reson Imaging. 2013;38(5):1054–62.
8. Bauer S, Markl M, Honal M, Jung BA. The effect of reconstruction and acquisition parameters for GRAPPA-based parallel imaging on the image quality. Magn Reson Med. 2011;66(2):402–9.
9. Stadlbauer A, van der Riet W, Crelier G, Salomonowitz E. Accelerated time-resolved three-dimensional MR velocity mapping of blood flow patterns in the aorta using SENSE and k-t BLAST. Eur J Radiol. 2010;75(1):e15–21.
10. Petersson S, Sigfridsson A, Dyverfeldt P, et al. Retrospectively gated intracardiac 4D flow MRI using spiral trajectories. Magn Reson Med. 2015;76:196–206.
11. Chang W, Frydrychowicz A, Kecskemeti S, et al. The effect of spatial resolution on wall shear stress measurements acquired using radial phase contrast magnetic resonance angiography in the middle cerebral arteries of healthy volunteers. Preliminary results. Neuroradiol J. 2011;24(1):115–20.
12. Wu Y, Chang W, Johnson KM, et al. Fast whole-brain 4D contrast-enhanced MR angiography with velocity encoding using undersampled radial acquisition and highly constrained projection reconstruction: image-quality assessment in volunteer subjects. AJNR Am J Neuroradiol. 2011;32(3):E47–50.
13. Gu T, Korosec FR, Block WF, et al. PC VIPR: a high-speed 3D phase-contrast method for flow quantification and high-resolution angiography. AJNR Am J Neuroradiol. 2005;26(4):743–9.
14. Johnson KM, Markl M. Improved SNR in phase contrast velocimetry with five-point balanced flow encoding. Magn Reson Med. 2010;63(2):349–55.
15. Wetzel S, Meckel S, Frydrychowicz A, et al. In vivo assessment and visualization of intracranial arterial hemodynamics with flow-sensitized 4D MR imaging at 3T. AJNR Am J Neuroradiol. 2007;28(3):433–8.
16. Jung B, Honal M, Ullmann P, et al. Highly k-t-space-accelerated phase-contrast MRI. Magn Reson Med. 2008;60(5):1169–77.
17. Bock J, Frydrychowicz A, Stalder AF, et al. 4D phase contrast MRI at 3T: effect of standard and blood-pool contrast agents on SNR, PC-MRA, and blood flow visualization. Magn Reson Med. 2010;63(2):330–8.
18. Liu J, Dyverfeldt P, Acevedo-Bolton G, et al. Highly accelerated aortic 4D flow MR imaging with variable-density random undersampling. Magn Reson Imaging. 2014;32(8):1012–20.
19. Schnell S, Markl M, Entezari P, et al. k-t GRAPPA accelerated four-dimensional flow MRI in the aorta: effect on scan time, image quality, and quantification of flow and wall shear stress. Magn Reson Med. 2014;72(2):522–33.
20. Stankovic Z, Allen BD, Garcia J, et al. 4D flow imaging with MRI. Cardiovasc Diagn Ther. 2014;4(2):173–92.
21. Callaghan FM, Kozor R, Sherrah AG, et al. Use of multi-velocity encoding 4D flow MRI to improve quantification of flow patterns in the aorta. J Magn Reson Imaging. 2015;42:352–63.
22. Nayak KS, Nielsen JF, Bernstein MA, et al. Cardiovascular magnetic resonance phase contrast imaging. J Cardiovasc Magn Reson. 2015;17(1):71.
23. Hutter J, Schmitt P, Aandal G, et al. Low-rank and sparse matrix decomposition for compressed sensing reconstruction of magnetic resonance 4D phase contrast blood flow imaging (loSDeCoS 4D-PCI). Med Image Comput Comput Assist Interv. 2013;16(Pt 1):558–65.
24. Boussel L, Rayz V, Martin A, et al. Phase-contrast magnetic resonance imaging measurements in intracranial aneurysms in vivo of flow patterns, velocity fields, and wall shear stress: comparison with computational fluid dynamics. Magn Reson Med. 2009;61(2):409–17.
25. Schubert T, Santini F, Stalder AF, et al. Dampening of blood-flow pulsatility along the carotid siphon: does form follow function? AJNR Am J Neuroradiol. 2011; 32(6):1107–12.
26. Kim GB, Ha H, Kweon J, et al. Post-stenotic plug-like jet with a vortex ring demonstrated by 4D flow MRI. Magn Reson Imaging. 2015;34:371–5.
27. Krittian SB, Lamata P, Michler C, et al. A finite-element approach to the direct computation of relative cardiovascular pressure from time-resolved MR velocity data. Med Image Anal. 2012;16(5):1029–37.
28. Bustamante M, Petersson S, Eriksson J, et al. Atlas-based analysis of 4D flow CMR: automated vessel segmentation and flow quantification. J Cardiovasc Magn Reson. 2015;17:87.
29. Loecher M, Schrauben E, Johnson KM, Wieben O. Phase unwrapping in 4D MR flow with a 4D single-step laplacian algorithm. J Magn Reson Imaging. 2015;43:833–42.
30. von Spiczak J, Crelier G, Giese D, et al. Quantitative Analysis of Vortical Blood Flow in the Thoracic Aorta Using 4D Phase Contrast MRI. PLoS One. 2015;10(9):e0139025.
31. Santelli C, Loecher M, Busch J, et al. Accelerating 4D flow MRI by exploiting vector field divergence regularization. Magn Reson Med. 2016;75(1):115–25.
32. Frydrychowicz A, Francois CJ, Turski PA. Four-dimensional phase contrast magnetic resonance angiography: potential clinical applications. Eur J Radiol. 2011;80(1):24–35.
33. Chimowitz MI, Lynn MJ, Derdeyn CP, et al. Stenting versus aggressive medical therapy for intracranial arterial stenosis. N Engl J Med. 2011; 365(11):993–1003.
34. Traub O, Berk BC. Laminar shear stress: mechanisms by which endothelial cells transduce an atheroprotective force. Arterioscler Thromb Vasc Biol. 1998;18(5):677–85.
35. Harloff A, Albrecht F, Spreer J, et al. 3D blood flow characteristics in the carotid artery bifurcation assessed by flow-sensitive 4D MRI at 3T. Magn Reson Med. 2009;61(1):65–74.
36. Markl M, Wegent F, Zech T, et al. In vivo wall shear stress distribution in the carotid artery: effect of bifurcation geometry, internal carotid artery stenosis, and recanalization therapy. Circ Cardiovasc Imaging. 2010;3(6):647–55.
37. Harloff A, Zech T, Wegent F, et al. Comparison of blood flow velocity quantification by 4D flow MR imaging with ultrasound at the carotid bifurcation. AJNR Am J Neuroradiol. 2013;34(7):1407–13.
38. Leng X, Scalzo F, Ip HL, et al. Computational fluid dynamics modeling of symptomatic intracranial atherosclerosis may predict risk of stroke recurrence. PLoS One. 2014;9(5):e97531.
39. Zhao X, Zhao M, Amin-Hanjani S, et al. Wall shear stress in major cerebral arteries as a function of age and gender–a study of 301 healthy volunteers. J Neuroimaging. 2015;25(3):403–7.
40. Amin-Hanjani S, Pandey DK, Rose-Finnell L, et al. Effect of hemodynamics on stroke risk in symptomatic atherosclerotic vertebrobasilar occlusive disease. JAMA Neurol. 2015;73:178–85.

41. Amin-Hanjani S, Du X, Zhao M, et al. Use of quantitative magnetic resonance angiography to stratify stroke risk in symptomatic vertebrobasilar disease. Stroke. 2005;36(6):1140–5.

42. Bauer AM, Amin-Hanjani S, Alaraj A, Charbel FT. Quantitative magnetic resonance angiography in the evaluation of the subclavian steal syndrome: report of 5 patients. J Neuroimaging. 2009;19(3):250–2.

43. Sekine T, Takagi R, Amano Y, et al. 4D flow MRI assessment of extracranial-intracranial bypass: qualitative and quantitative evaluation of the hemodynamics. Neuroradiology. 2015;58:237–44.

44. Kellawan JM, Harrell JW, Schrauben EM, et al. Quantitative cerebrovascular 4D flow MRI at rest and during hypercapnia challenge. Magn Reson Imaging. 2015;34:422–8.

45. Qiao Y, Zeiler SR, Mirbagheri S, et al. Intracranial plaque enhancement in patients with cerebrovascular events on high-spatial-resolution MR images. Radiology. 2014;271(2):534–42.

46. Dieleman N, van der Kolk AG, Zwanenburg JJ, et al. Imaging intracranial vessel wall pathology with magnetic resonance imaging: current prospects and future directions. Circulation. 2014;130(2):192–201.

47. Skarpathiotakis M, Mandell DM, Swartz RH, et al. Intracranial atherosclerotic plaque enhancement in patients with ischemic stroke. AJNR Am J Neuroradiol. 2013;34(2):299–304.

48. Xu WH, Li ML, Gao S, et al. Middle cerebral artery intraplaque hemorrhage: prevalence and clinical relevance. Ann Neurol. 2012;71(2):195–8.

49. Turan TN, Bonilha L, Morgan PS, et al. Intraplaque hemorrhage in symptomatic intracranial atherosclerotic disease. J Neuroimaging. 2011;21(2):e159–61.

50. Xu WH, Li ML, Gao S, et al. In vivo high-resolution MR imaging of symptomatic and asymptomatic middle cerebral artery atherosclerotic stenosis. Atherosclerosis. 2010;212(2):507–11.

51. Sun J, Yuan C. Seeking culprit lesions in cryptogenic stroke: The utility of vessel wall imaging. J Am Heart Assoc. 2015;4(6):002207.

52. Freilinger TM, Schindler A, Schmidt C, et al. Prevalence of nonstenosing, complicated atherosclerotic plaques in cryptogenic stroke. JACC Cardiovasc Imaging. 2012;5(4):397–405.

53. Gupta A, Gialdini G, Lerario MP, et al. Magnetic resonance angiography detection of abnormal carotid artery plaque in patients with cryptogenic stroke. J Am Heart Assoc. 2015;4(6):e002012.

54. Oeltze-Jafra S, Cebral JR, Janiga G, Preim B. Cluster analysis of vortical flow in simulations of cerebral aneurysm hemodynamics. IEEE Trans Vis Comput Graph. 2016;22(1):757–66.

55. Chung B, Cebral JR. CFD for evaluation and treatment planning of aneurysms: review of proposed clinical uses and their challenges. Ann Biomed Eng. 2015;43(1):122–38.

56. Cebral JR, Vazquez M, Sforza DM, et al. Analysis of hemodynamics and wall mechanics at sites of cerebral aneurysm rupture. J Neurointerv Surg. 2015;7(7):530–6.

57. Cebral JR, Duan X, Chung BJ, et al. Wall mechanical properties and hemodynamics of unruptured intracranial aneurysms. AJNR Am J Neuroradiol. 2015;36(9):1695–703.

58. Berg P, Roloff C, Beuing O, et al. The computational fluid dynamics rupture challenge 2013-phase II: Variability of hemodynamic simulations in two intracranial aneurysms. J Biomech Eng. 2015;137(12):121008.

59. Schnell S, Ansari SA, Vakil P, et al. Three-dimensional hemodynamics in intracranial aneurysms: influence of size and morphology. J Magn Reson Imaging. 2014;39(1):120–31.

60. Meckel S, Stalder AF, Santini F, et al. In vivo visualization and analysis of 3-D hemodynamics in cerebral aneurysms with flow-sensitized 4-D MR imaging at 3T. Neuroradiology. 2008;50(6):473–84.

61. Isoda H, Hirano M, Takeda H, et al. Visualization of hemodynamics in a silicon aneurysm model using time-resolved, 3D, phase-contrast MRI. AJNR Am J Neuroradiol. 2006;27(5):1119–22.

62. van Ooij P, Schneiders JJ, Marquering HA, et al. 3D cine phase-contrast MRI at 3T in intracranial aneurysms compared with patient-specific computational fluid dynamics. AJNR Am J Neuroradiol. 2013;34(9):1785–91.

63. Sforza DM, Kono K, Tateshima S, et al. Hemodynamics in growing and stable cerebral aneurysms. J Neurointerv Surg. 2015;8:407–12.

64. Meng H, Tutino VM, Xiang J, Siddiqui A. High WSS or low WSS? Complex interactions of hemodynamics with intracranial aneurysm initiation, growth, and rupture: toward a unifying hypothesis. AJNR Am J Neuroradiol. 2014;35(7):1254–62.

65. Matouk CC, Mandell DM, Gunel M, et al. Vessel wall magnetic resonance imaging identifies the site of rupture in patients with multiple intracranial aneurysms: proof of principle. Neurosurgery. 2013;72(3):492–6. discussion 6.

66. Nagahata S, Nagahata M, Obara M, et al. Wall Enhancement of the Intracranial Aneurysms Revealed by Magnetic Resonance Vessel Wall Imaging Using Three-Dimensional Turbo Spin-Echo Sequence with Motion-Sensitized Driven-Equilibrium: A Sign of Ruptured Aneurysm? Clin Neuroradiol. 2014 [Epub ahead of print].

67. Edjlali M, Gentric JC, Regent-Rodriguez C, et al. Does aneurysmal wall enhancement on vessel wall MRI help to distinguish stable from unstable intracranial aneurysms? Stroke. 2014;45(12):3704–6.

68. Blankena R, Kleinloog R, Verweij BH, et al. Thinner regions of intracranial aneurysm wall correlate with regions of higher wall shear stress: A 7T MRI Study. AJNR Am J Neuroradiol. 2016 [Epub ahead of print].

69. Greving JP, Wermer MJ, Brown Jr RD, et al. Development of the PHASES score for prediction of risk of rupture of intracranial aneurysms: a pooled analysis of six prospective cohort studies. Lancet Neurol. 2014;13(1):59–66.

70. Spetzler RF, Martin NA. A proposed grading system for arteriovenous malformations. J Neurosurg. 1986;65(4):476–83.

71. Chang W, Loecher MW, Wu Y, et al. Hemodynamic changes in patients with arteriovenous malformations assessed using high-resolution 3D radial phase-contrast MR angiography. AJNR Am J Neuroradiol. 2012;33(8):1565–72.

72. Edjlali M, Roca P, Rabrait C, et al. MR selective flow-tracking cartography: a postprocessing procedure applied to four-dimensional flow MR imaging for complete characterization of cranial dural arteriovenous fistulas. Radiology. 2014;270(1):261–8.

73. Wu C, Ansari SA, Honarmand AR, et al. Evaluation of 4D vascular flow and tissue perfusion in cerebral arteriovenous malformations: influence of Spetzler-Martin grade, clinical presentation, and AVM risk factors. AJNR Am J Neuroradiol. 2015;36(6):1142–9.

74. Markl M, Wu C, Hurley MC, et al. Cerebral arteriovenous malformation: complex 3D hemodynamics and 3D blood flow alterations during staged embolization. J Magn Reson Imaging. 2013;38(4):946–50.

75. Wu C, Schnell S, Markl M, Ansari SA. Combined DSA and 4D flow demonstrate overt alterations of vascular geometry and hemodynamics in an unusually complex cerebral AVM. Clin Neuroradiol. 2015 [Epub ahead of print].

76. Cognard C, Gobin YP, Pierot L, et al. Cerebral dural arteriovenous fistulas: clinical and angiographic correlation with a revised classification of venous drainage. Radiology. 1995;194(3):671–80.

77. Chang W, Wu Y, Johnson K, et al. Fast contrast-enhanced 4D MRA and 4D flow MRI using constrained reconstruction (HYPRFlow): potential applications for brain arteriovenous malformations. AJNR Am J Neuroradiol. 2015;36(6):1049–55.

78. Clark Z, Johnson KM, Wu Y, et al. Accelerated time-resolved contrast-enhanced magnetic resonance angiography of dural arteriovenous fistulas using highly constrained reconstruction of sparse cerebrovascular data sets. Invest Radiol. 2015 [Epub ahead of print].

79. Schrauben EM, Johnson KM, Huston J, et al. Reproducibility of cerebrospinal venous blood flow and vessel anatomy with the use of phase contrast-vastly undersampled isotropic projection reconstruction and contrast-enhanced MRA. AJNR Am J Neuroradiol. 2014;35(5):999–1006.

80. Sari S, Verim S, Hamcan S, et al. MRI diagnosis of dural sinus - Cortical venous thrombosis: Immediate post-contrast 3D GRE T1-weighted imaging versus unenhanced MR venography and conventional MR sequences. Clin Neurol Neurosurg. 2015;134:44–54.

81. Esfahani DR, Stevenson M, Moss HE, et al. Quantitative Magnetic Resonance Venography is Correlated With Intravenous Pressures Before and After Venous Sinus Stenting: Implications for Treatment and Monitoring. Neurosurgery. 2015;77(2):254–60.

82. Roher AE. Cardiovascular system participation in Alzheimer's disease pathogenesis. J Intern Med. 2015;277(4):426–8.

83. Chang W, Landgraf B, Johnson KM, et al. Velocity measurements in the middle cerebral arteries of healthy volunteers using 3D radial phase-contrast HYPRFlow: comparison with transcranial Doppler sonography and 2D phase-contrast MR imaging. AJNR Am J Neuroradiol. 2011;32(1):54–9.

84. Rivera-Rivera LA, Turski P, Johnson KM, et al. 4D flow MRI for intracranial hemodynamics assessment in Alzheimer's disease. J Cereb Blood Flow Metab. 2015 [Epub ahead of print].

85. Peng X, Haldar S, Deshpande S, et al. Wall stiffness suppresses Akt/eNOS and cytoprotection in pulse-perfused endothelium. Hypertension. 2003; 41(2):378–81.

13

Association between carotid artery and abdominal aortic aneurysm plaque

Eytan Raz[1]*, Michele Anzidei[2], Michele Porcu[3], Pier Paolo Bassareo[4], Michele di Martino[2], Giuseppe Mercuro[4], Luca Saba[3] and Jasjit S. Suri[5,6,7]

Abstract

Background: The correlation between AAA and carotid artery plaque is unknown and a common etiology and pathophysiology is suspected by some authors. The purpose of this work was to explore the association between the features of a) carotid artery plaque and b) abdominal aortic aneurysm (AAA) plaques using multi-detector-CT Angiography (MDCTA).

Methods: Forty-eight (32 males; median age 72 years) patients studied using a 16-detectors CT scanner were retrospectively analyzed. A region of interest (ROI) ≥ 2 mm^2 was used to quantify the HU value of the plaque by two readers independently. Inter-observer reproducibility was calculated and Pearson correlation analysis was performed.

Results: The Bland-Altman plots showed the inter-observer reproducibility to be good. The Pearson correlation was 0.224 (95 % CI = 0.071 to 0.48), without statistically significant association between HU measured in the carotid artery plaque and in the AAA plaques ($p = 0.138$); after exclusion of the calcified plaques from the analysis, the rho values resulted 0.494 (95 % CI = 0.187 to 0.713) with a statistically significant association ($p = 0.003$).

Conclusion: In this study, we found an association between the features of the non calcific carotid plaque and the features of AAA plaque.

Keywords: Carotid, Aneurysm, Plaque, CTA

Background

Atherosclerotic disease of carotid artery is considered the most important cause of cerebrovascular events [1, 2]; imaging techniques in the last years focused their attention in finding those parameters that are associated with an increased risk of stroke and transitory ischemic attacks (TIA) [3, 4]. The concept of "vulnerable plaque" has thus been introduced, focusing on those atherosclerotic plaques with a high likelihood to cause thrombotic complications [5, 6]. However, atherosclerosis is a process that may affect all the arterial vessels in the body [7] and, commonly, a significant target of this pathology is the abdominal aorta [8, 9].

The most prevalent pathology of the aorta is the abdominal aortic aneurysm (AAA), whose rupture has been recognized to be a significant cause of mortality for adults aged >60 years in the developed world [10]. The pathogenesis of AAA is still poorly understood with some studies suggesting the importance of inflammatory pathways, hemodynamic forces, matrix degradation and thrombosis [11, 12]. Subjects with AAAs have frequently atherosclerosis: Cornuz et al. [13] showed the association of peripheral atherosclerosis with AAAs. Whether the association between atherosclerosis and AAA is simply due to common risk factors or is causal is unknown [14].

In the last few years MDCTA has emerged as an outstanding technique to explore the vascular system [15–18], and by using the Hounsfield Units (HU) sampling it is possible to have quantitative and reproducible information of the analyzed tissue [19].

The purpose of this work was to explore the association between plaques in the carotid artery and abdominal aortic aneurysm by using quantitative data obtained with MDCTA.

* Correspondence: eytan.raz@gmail.com
[1]Department of Radiology, New York University School of Medicine, 660 First Avenue, New York, NY 10016, USA
Full list of author information is available at the end of the article

Methods

Patient population

Forty-eight (32 males; median age 72 ± 14 years) patients studied between August 2005 and May 2011 by using a 16-detector CT scanner (Philips Brilliance, Rotterdam, Netherlands) were retrospectively analyzed. Patients with medical history of cardiac output failure, or any contra-indications to iodinated contrast media did not undergo MDCTA exams. Criteria to be included in this study were: 1) Patients underwent MDCTA of carotid and abdominal aorta for AAA. 2) The time interval between the carotid and the AAA studies was not more than 3 months. Each examination was performed when clinically indicated and was ordered by the patient's physician as part of routine clinical care. The patients were all neurologically asymptomatic, without history of TIA or stroke. In accordance with the applicable National Research Ethics Service guidance, ethical approval for the study was not required because the study was performed retrospectively on routinely acquired images and specimens.

MDCTA technique

All patients underwent MDCTA of the supra-aortic vessels using a technique previously described [blinded for peer review].

In our protocol for the analysis of carotid arteries, the angiographic phase is obtained by injecting 80-110 mL of contrast using a power injector at a flow rate of 5 mL/s. A bolus tracking technique is used to calculate the correct timing of the scan. Dynamic monitoring scanning begins 6 s after the beginning of the intravenous injection of contrast material. The trigger threshold inside the ROI is set at + 90 HU above the baseline. The delay between the acquisitions of each monitoring scan is 1 s. CT technical parameters include: matrix 512x512, field of view (FOV) 14–19 cm; mAs 180–220; kV 120–140.

For the analysis of AAA, the angiographic phase is obtained by injecting 80-110 mL of contrast medium into a cubital vein (usually the left side was used), using a power injector at a flow rate of 4-5 mL/s and an 18-gauge intravenous catheter. The scan starts at the level of the diaphragm up to the pubic symphysis. For the study of AAA a bolus tracking technique similar to the procedure described for the carotid arteries is used.

Image analysis

In the first phase two experienced radiologists independently measured the HU value of the carotid artery plaques. A region of interest (ROI) ≥ 2 mm^2 was used to quantify the HU value of the plaque. After two weeks, the same radiologists independently measured the HU value of the AAA plaque (Fig. 1). Images were blinded and randomized. MDCTA images were analysed with a varying magnification from 120 to 400 % in comparison to the acquisition.

Window parameters (width and level) were freely modifiable but the parameters from another article [20] were followed. To quantifiy the HU value, a circular or elliptical region of interest cursor in the predominant area of plaque was used. Regions of beam hardening in calcified areas were excluded and areas showing contamination by contrast material or calcification were avoided.

Statistical analysis

Continuous data were described as the mean value $\pm$ standard deviation (SD). In order to evaluate the inter-observer reproducibility in HU quantification, Bland-Altman analysis with 95 % limits of agreement (mean difference ± 1.96 SDs) was performed and the differences between the measured values were plotted against the mean of the 2 measurements to assess the relationship between the difference and the magnitude of the measurement. Mann-Whitney test was used to test the differences between groups. For the analysis of correlation (Pearson Rho correlation) between HU measured in the carotid artery and AAA plaques, the HU values between the 2 observers were averaged. R software (www.r-project.org) was employed for statistical analyses.

Results

General results

Three patients were excluded from the final analysis because of sub-optimal image quality due to movement artifact. Therefore the final number of analyzed patients was 45 (29 males; median age 72 ± 13 years). Demographic characteristics are summarized in Table 1. The total number of carotid artery plaque measured were 79 because in 11 carotid arteries no evidence of plaque was found. The ROI value was between 2 mm^2 and 5 mm^2 (mean value 2.56 mm^2).

Bland-Altman analysis

We analyzed the inter-observer reproducibility of HU measurement of the plaque in the 79 carotid arteries and in the 45 patients with AAA and the plots are given in the Fig. 2. The plots showed that the inter-observer reproducibility is good for both analysis and the best agreement is obtained in the carotid artery plaque HU quantification (with 95 % CI from −25.5 % to 20.3 %.

Mann-Whitney analysis

We tested the differences between HU values in carotid arteries and AAA also by using the Mann-Whitney test and we found that there were no differences in HU analysis between the two observers in the carotids ($p = 0.836$)

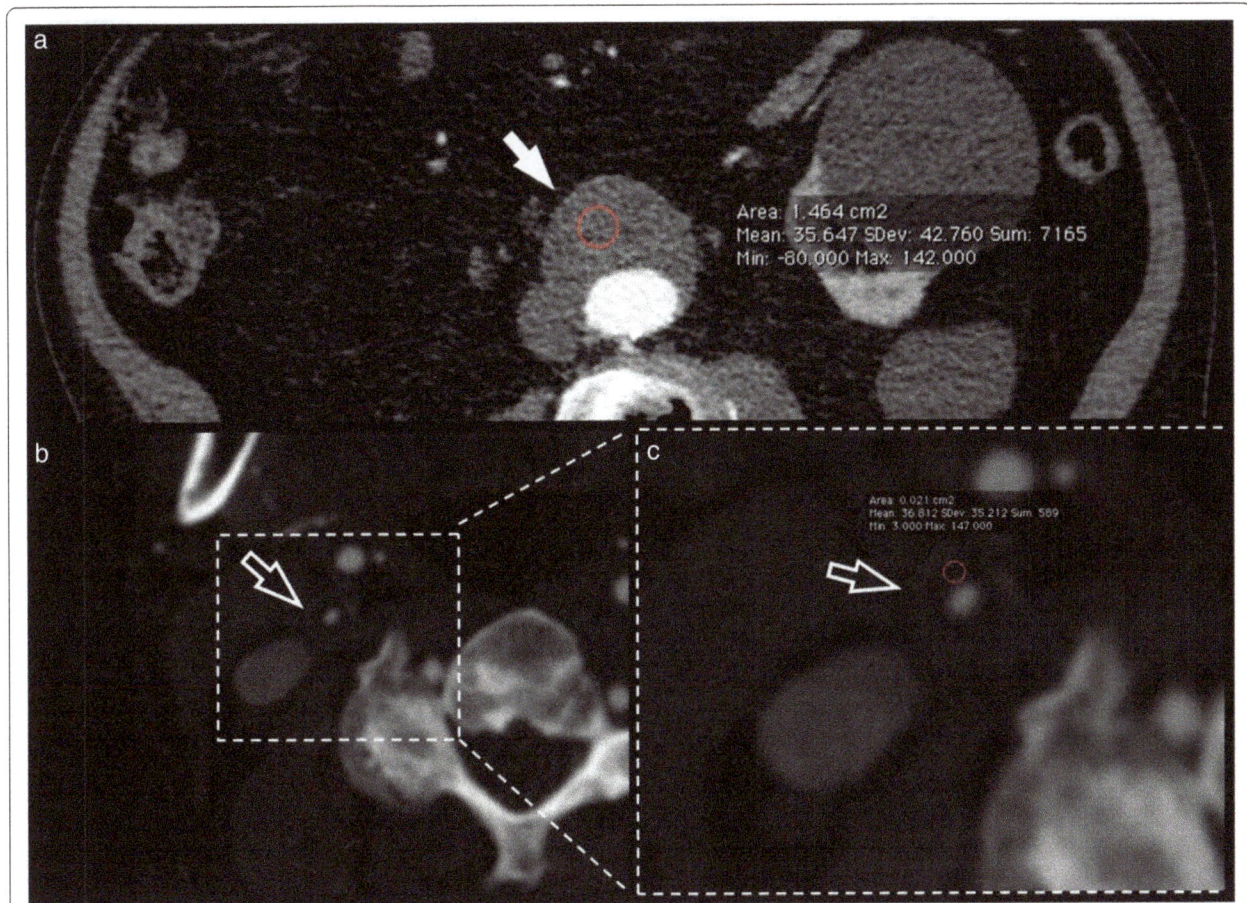

Fig. 1 MDCTA axial images of AAA (**a**) and carotid arteries (**b**, **c**). The AAA is indicated by the white arrow (**a**) and the circle represents the analyzed ROI. The carotid artery plaques is indicated by the open white arrow (**b**, **c**) and the circle represents the analyzed ROI. Panel **c** represent the 200 % zoom of the panel **b**

and in the AAA ($p = 0.353$). Summary statistic is given in Table 2. These results demonstrate that the HU measurement performed by the 2 observers in the carotid and AAA plaques are not statistically different.

Pearson correlation analysis

The correlation coefficient rho was 0.224 (95 % CI = 0.071 to 0.48) and there was no statistically significant association between HU measured in the carotid artery plaque

and HU measured in the AAA plaque ($p = 0.138$). The scatter-plot with 95 % confidence interval is shown in Fig. 3. We analyzed also the correlation between carotid and AAA plaques by excluding the calcified plaques (namely those plaques with HU value > 130 HU) and we performed a further analysis by obtaining a coefficient rho of 0.494 (95 % CI = 0.187 to 0.713) with a statistically significant association ($p = 0.003$).

Discussion

In the last few years several papers demonstrated that the plaque composition of the carotid arteries plays a significant role in the "vulnerability" of the plaque and in the risk of develop cerebrovascular events.

In the carotid artery (as well as in the coronary arteries), it is possible to find different types of plaque [3, 4] and the very hypodense regions (<30 HU) in the center of atherosclerotic carotid plaque are associated with the presence of a lipid core (i.e., lipid, hemorrhage, or necrotic debris) [21, 22]; this kind of plaques are associated with the development of cerebrovascular events [19].

Table 1 Patients characteristics

Age[a]	72 y (SD[b] 13 y)
Sex (male)	65 % (n = 31)
Hypertension	53 % (n = 25)
Smoker	62 % (n = 30)
CAD	59 % (n = 28)
Diabetes	15 % (n = 7)
Dyslipidemia	61 % (n = 29)

[a]Mean age
[b]SD standard deviation

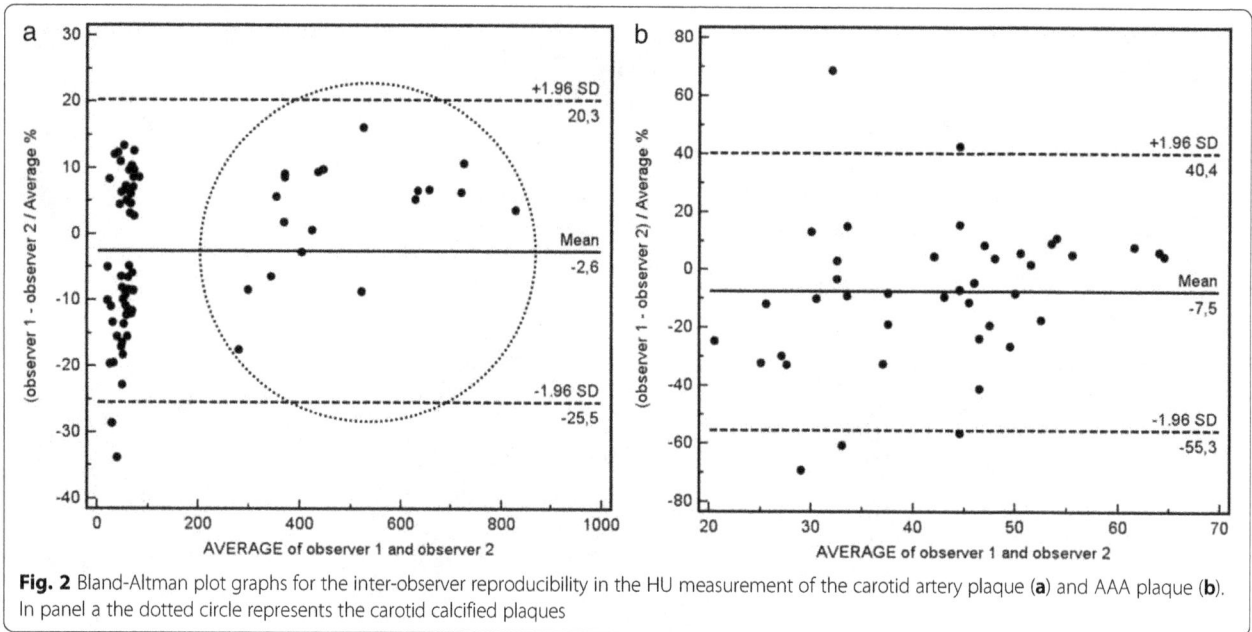

Fig. 2 Bland-Altman plot graphs for the inter-observer reproducibility in the HU measurement of the carotid artery plaque (**a**) and AAA plaque (**b**). In panel a the dotted circle represents the carotid calcified plaques

The presence of atherosclerotic pathology and plaque development in the AAA is well described but if this association is simply due to common risk factors or is causal, is still unknown [14]. In this study, our purpose was to evaluate whether there was an association between the HU values measured in the carotid artery plaque and the HU values measured in the AAA plaque.

By analyzing the correlation between HU values in carotid plaques and AAA plaques a rho value of 0.224 (95 % CI = 0.071 to 0.48) was found with the absence of significant p-value ($p = 0.138$). We analyzed the morphology of the scatter-plot and we found that the calcified plaques of carotid plaques represent, for this kind of analysis, a confounding factor. In the Fig. 3a the calcified plaques of carotid are clearly visible (dotted circle) and by excluding this kind of plaques the coefficient rho changed to 0.494 (95 % CI = 0.187 to 0.713) with the presence of a statistically significant association ($p = 0.003$). This is an interesting point to discuss because the presence of carotid calcified plaques are considered a protective factor for the development of cerebrovascular events [23, 24].

Nandalur et al. [23], demonstrated that calcified plaques are 21 times less likely to be symptomatic than non-calcified plaques ($p = 0.030$) whereas no significant predictive value was found between fatty ($p = 0.23$) or mixed ($p = 0.18$) plaque type for the occurrence of symptoms. The results of this study were further confirmed by Saba et al. [19] that showed that carotid calcified plaques are less frequently associated with cerebrovascular symptoms. In that paper the non calcified plaques were found to be associated with the presence of stroke-TIA.

Previous studies have attributed the development of AAA to atherosclerosis [25] because these conditions share risk factors, such as hypertension, smoking, and hypercholesterolemia [26, 27]. The presence of atherosclerotic process in the aneurismal wall is a common finding in AAA patients but several patients with advanced atherosclerosis do not develop AAA [28, 29].

The results of this study suggest that the atherosclerotic process involved in the carotid artery plaques and in the wall of the AAA is of a different nature: in fact in the carotid plaques may show a calcified type (HU value > 130)

Table 2 Mann-Whitney analysis

	HU carotid artery plaque		HU AAA plaque	
	Observer 1	Observer 2	Observer 1	Observer 2
Sample size	79	79	45	45
Lowest value	19	21	18	21
Highest value	843	812	66	63
Median	62	63	43	45
95 % CI for the median	54.88 to 67	57 to 66.12	35.27 to 46.1	40 to 49
Interquartile range	45 to 82.75	49.5 to 76.75	32 to 49	34.5 to 52

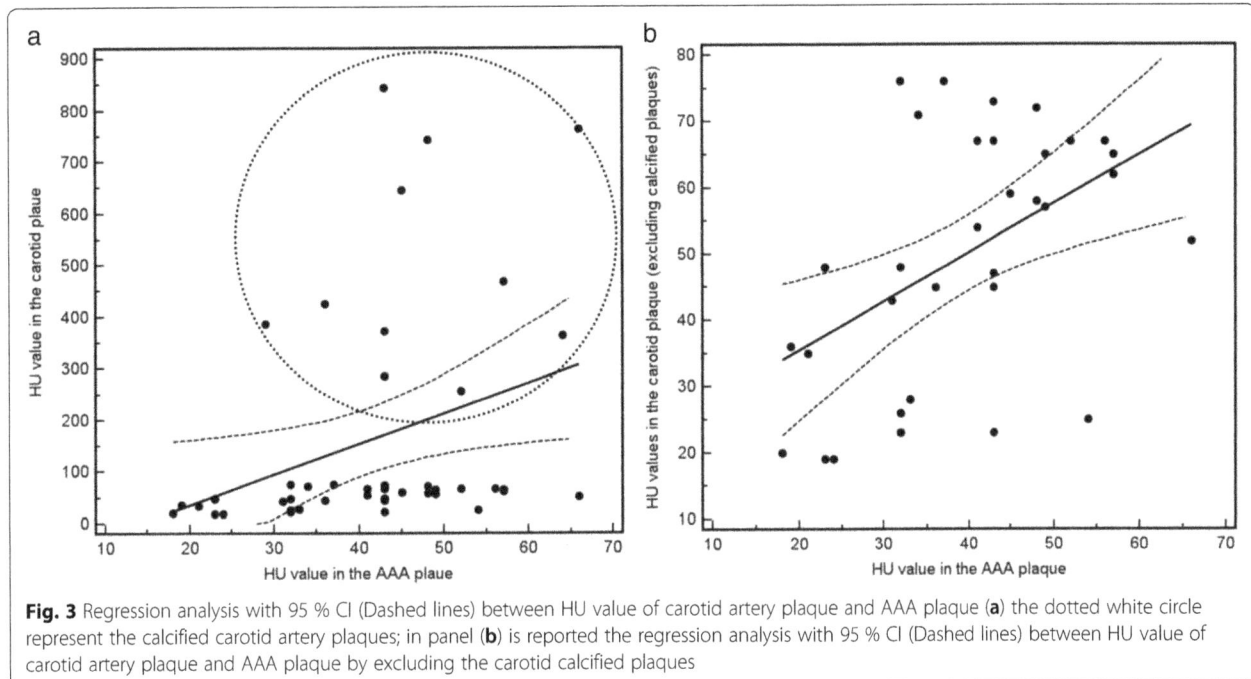

Fig. 3 Regression analysis with 95 % CI (Dashed lines) between HU value of carotid artery plaque and AAA plaque (**a**) the dotted white circle represent the calcified carotid artery plaques; in panel (**b**) is reported the regression analysis with 95 % CI (Dashed lines) between HU value of carotid artery plaque and AAA plaque by excluding the carotid calcified plaques

that is not present in the AAA. Nonetheless, when the carotid calcified plaques are excluded, a significant correlation is found between the HU values in the carotid and in the AAA.

From a pathological point of view authors reported that AAA is characterized by transmural infiltration of lymphocytes and macrophages and by the destruction of elastin and collagen in the media and adventitia loss of medial smooth muscle cells with thinning of the vessel wall [30, 31] and these pathological elements are quite similar in those found in the carotid (and coronary) artery "vulnerable" plaques [3, 4, 32, 33]. A study by Zweig et al., demonstrated that the calcifications of the abdominal aorta correlated with the presence of calcifications in the coronary arteries and even suggested abdominal aortic as a possible tool to help exclude obstructive coronary disease and improve the selection of patients that may benefit from further risk stratification [34].

In this type of study the analysis of reproducibility in the HU measurement is important and Bland-Altman plot analysis showed that the inter-observer reproducibility is good for both analysis and the best agreement is obtained in the carotid artery plaque HU quantification (with 95 % CI from −25.5 % to 20.3 %. In the HU quantification of the carotid artery plaque our results are concordant with previous observations [35, 36] whereas, on the best of our knowledge no previous analysis of concordance in the HU quantification of AAA plaque was found. These results were also confirmed by the Mann-Whitney test where we found no differences in HU analysis between the two

observers in the carotids ($p = 0.836$) and in the AAA ($p = 0.353$).

In this paper there are some limitations. First, we quantified the HU values in the carotid and AAA by using a circular ROI; a more precise system like manual drawing of the plaque would be more reliable and this fact may introduce a bias in the data analysis: however we think that this can be considered a minor limitation because the predominant area of the plaque was selected. Second, the total number of analysed patients was forty-five and this represents a relative small population: therefore the obtained results should be further verified in larger cohort.

Conclusion

In this study, we found an association between the features of the non calcific carotid plaque and the features of AAA plaque.

Competing interests
The authors declare that they have no competing interests.

Authors' contributions
All authors read and approved the final manuscript.

Author details
[1]Department of Radiology, New York University School of Medicine, 660 First Avenue, New York, NY 10016, USA. [2]Departments of Radiological Sciences, University of Rome La Sapienza, Viale Regina Elena 324, Rome 00161, Italy. [3]Department of Imaging, Azienda Ospedaliero Universitaria (A.O.U.), di Cagliari – Polo di Monserrato, s.s. 554 Monserrato, Cagliari 09045, Italy. [4]Department of Cardiology, Azienda Ospedaliero Universitaria (A.O.U.), di Cagliari – Polo di Monserrato, s.s. 554 Monserrato, Cagliari 09045, Italy. [5]Monitoring and Diagnostic Division, AtheroPoint(TM) LLC, Roseville, CA, USA. [6]Point of Care Devices, Global Biomedical Technologies, Inc, Roseville,

CA, USA. [7]Electrical Engineering Department (Affl.), U of Idaho, Moscow, ID, USA.

References

1. Sadat U, Teng Z, Young VE, Graves MJ, Gaunt ME, Gillard JH. High-resolution magnetic resonance imaging-based biomechanical stress analysis of carotid atheroma: a comparison of single transient ischaemic attack, recurrent transient ischaemic attacks, non-disabling stroke and asymptomatic patient groups. Eur J Vasc Endovasc Surg. 2011;41(1):83–90.

2. U-King-Im JM, Young V, Gillard JH. Carotid-artery imaging in the diagnosis and management of patients at risk of stroke. Lancet Neurol. 2009;8(6):569–80.

3. Naghavi M, Libby P, Falk E, Casscells SW, Litovsky S, Rumberger J, et al. From vulnerable plaque to vulnerable patient: a call for new definitions and risk assessment strategies: Part I. Circulation. 2003;108(14):1664–72.

4. Naghavi M, Libby P, Falk E, Casscells SW, Litovsky S, Rumberger J, et al. From vulnerable plaque to vulnerable patient: a call for new definitions and risk assessment strategies: Part II. Circulation. 2003;108(15):1772–8.

5. Naghavi M, Falk E, Hecht HS, Shah PK. The first SHAPE (Screening for Heart Attack Prevention and Education) guideline. Crit Pathw Cardiol. 2006;5(4):187–90.

6. Casscells W, Naghavi M, Willerson JT. Vulnerable atherosclerotic plaque: a multifocal disease. Circulation. 2003;107(16):2072–5.

7. Curtiss LK. Reversing atherosclerosis? N Engl J Med. 2009;360(11):1144–6.

8. Biros E, Norman PE, Jones GT, van Rij AM, Yu G, Moxon JV, et al. Meta-analysis of the association between single nucleotide polymorphisms in TGF-β receptor genes and abdominal aortic aneurysm. Atherosclerosis. 2011;219(1):218–23.

9. Desai MY, Lima JA. Imaging of atherosclerosis using magnetic resonance: state of the art and future directions. Curr Atheroscler Rep. 2006;8(2):131–9.

10. U.S. Department of Health and Human Services Centers for Disease Control and Prevention National Center for Health Statistics. MD LCWK1. Deaths, percent of total deaths, and death rates for the 15 leading causes of death in 5-year age groups, by race and sex: United States, 2006, 2009:7–9. http://www.cdc.gov/nchs/data/dvs/LCWK1_2006.pdf.

11. Golledge J, Muller J, Daugherty A, Norman P. Abdominal aortic aneurysm: pathogenesis and implications for management. Arterioscler Thromb Vasc Biol. 2006;26:2605–13.

12. Golledge J, Norman PE. Pathophysiology of abdominal aortic aneurysm relevant to improvements in patients' management. Curr Opin Cardiol. 2009;24:532–8.

13. Cornuz J, Sidoti Pinto C, Tevaearai H, Egger M. Risk factors for asymptomatic abdominal aortic aneurysm: systematic review and meta-analysis of population-based screening studies. Eur J Public Health. 2004;14:343–9.

14. Golledge J, Norman PE. Atherosclerosis and abdominal aortic aneurysm: cause, response, or common risk factors? Arterioscler Thromb Vasc Biol. 2010;30(6):1075–7.

15. Saba L, Pascalis L, Sanfilippo R, Anzidei M, Bura R, Montisci R, et al. Carotid artery wall thickness and leukoaraiosis: preliminary results using multidetector row CT angiography. AJNR Am J Neuroradiol. 2011;32(5):955–61.

16. Saba L, Sanfilippo R, Montisci R, Mallarini G. Associations between carotid artery wall thickness and cardiovascular risk factors using multidetector CT. AJNR Am J Neuroradiol. 2010;31(9):1758–63.

17. Fraioli F, Catalano C, Napoli A, Francone M, Venditti F, Danti M, et al. Low-dose multidetector-row CT angiography of the infra-renal aorta and lower extremity vessels: image quality and diagnostic accuracy in comparison with standard DSA. Eur Radiol. 2006;16(1):137–46.

18. Catalano C, Fraioli F, Laghi A, Napoli A, Bezzi M, Pediconi F, et al. Infrarenal aortic and lower-extremity arterial disease: diagnostic performance of multi-detector row CT angiography. Radiology. 2004;231(2):555–63.

19. Saba L, Montisci R, Sanfilippo R, Mallarini G. Multidetector row CT of the brain and carotid artery: a correlative analysis. Clin Radiol. 2009;64(8):767–78.

20. Saba L, Mallarin G. Window settings for the study of calcified carotid plaques with multidetector CT angiography. AJNR Am J Neuroradiol. 2009;30(7):1445–50.

21. Saba L, Caddeo G, Sanfilippo R, Montisci R, Mallarini G. CT and US in the study of ulcerated carotid plaque compared with surgical results.

22. Saba L, Caddeo G, Sanfilippo R, Montisci R, Mallarini G. Efficacy and Sensitivity of axial scans and different reconstruction methods in the study of the ulcerated carotid plaque by using multi-detector-row CT angiography. Comparison with surgical results. Am J Neuroradiol AJNR. 2007;28:716–23.

23. Nandalur KR, Baskurt E, Hagspiel KD, Phillips CD, Kramer CM. Calcified carotid atherosclerotic plaque is associated less with ischemic symptoms than is noncalcified plaque on MDCT. AJR Am J Roentgenol. 2005;184(1):295–8.

24. Nandalur KR, Hardie AD, Raghavan P, Schipper MJ, Baskurt E, Kramer CM. Composition of the stable carotid plaque: insights from a multidetector computed tomography study of plaque volume. Stroke. 2007;38(3):935–40.

25. Tilson MD. Atherosclerosis and aneurysm disease. J Vasc Surg. 1990;12:371–2.

26. Forsdahl SH, Singh K, Solberg S, Jacobsen BK. Risk factors for abdominal aortic aneurysms: a 7-year prospective study: the Tromsø study, 1994–2001. Circulation. 2009;119:2202–8.

27. Blanchard JF, Armenian HK, Friesen PP. Risk factors for abdominal aortic aneurysm: results of a case-control study. Am J Epidemiol. 2000;151:575–83.

28. Reed D, Reed C, Stemmermann G, Hayashi T. Are aortic aneurysms caused by atherosclerosis? Circulation. 1992;85:205–11.

29. Sterpetti AV, Feldhaus RJ, Schultz RD, Blair EA. Identification of abdominal aortic aneurysm patients with different clinical features and clinical outcomes. Am J Surg. 1988;156:466–9.

30. Davies MJ. Aortic aneurysm formation: lessons from human studies and experimental models. Circulation. 1998;98:193–5.

31. Freestone T, Turner RJ, Coady A, Higman DJ, Greenhalgh RM, Powell JT. Inflammation and matrix metalloproteinases in the enlarging abdominal aortic aneurysm. Arterioscler Thromb Vasc Biol. 1995;15:1145–51.

32. Redgrave JN, Lovett JK, Gallagher PJ, Rothwell PM. Histological assessment of 526 symptomatic carotid plaques in relation to the nature and timing of ischemic symptoms: the Oxford plaque study. Circulation. 2006;113(19):2320–8.

33. Redgrave JN, Lovett JK, Rothwell PM. Histological features of symptomatic carotid plaques in relation to age and smoking: the oxford plaque study. Stroke. 2010;41(10):2288–94.

34. Zweig BM, Sheth M, Simpson S, Al-Mallah MH. Association of abdominal aortic calcium with coronary artery calcium and obstructive coronary artery disease: a pilot study. Int J Cardiovasc Imaging. 2012;28(2):399–404.

35. Saba L, Mallarini G. Carotid Plaque Enhancement and Symptom Correlations: An Evaluation by Using Multidetector Row CT Angiography. AJNR Am J Neuroradiol. 2011;32(10):1919–25.

36. de Weert TT, de Monyé C, Meijering E, Booij R, Niessen WJ, Dippel DW, et al. Assessment of atherosclerotic carotid plaque volume with multidetector computed tomography angiography. Int J Cardiovasc Imaging. 2008;24(7):751–9.

14

Incremental value of carotid intraplaque hemorrhage for discriminating prior coronary events

Jie Sun[1*], Daniel S. Hippe[1], Hunter R. Underhill[2], Baocheng Chu[1], Tobias Saam[3], Norihide Takaya[4], Jianming Cai[5], Minako Oikawa-Wakayama[6], Wei Yu[7], Li Dong[7], Chun Yuan[1] and Thomas S. Hatsukami[8*]

Abstract

Background: The value of noninvasive assessment of carotid plaque composition in identifying patients with high coronary risk remains elusive. We sought to determine whether and which carotid plaque components are associated with prior coronary events independent of traditional risk factors and plaque burden.

Methods: Asymptomatic subjects with 50-79 % carotid stenosis by ultrasound were imaged with a multi-contrast carotid MRI protocol at 1.5 T. The independent associations between plaque components (fibrous tissue, calcification, lipid-rich necrotic core [LRNC] and intraplaque hemorrhage [IPH]) and prior coronary events, including myocardial infarction and coronary revascularization, were evaluated by controlling for traditional risk factors and plaque burden metrics.

Results: A total of 159 subjects (69.7 ± 9.0 years, 84 % males) were included. Prior coronary events were documented in 66 (42 %) subjects, and were associated with a larger carotid plaque burden consisting of more LRNC and calcification. Additionally, a higher prevalence of IPH was observed in subjects with prior coronary events (32 % vs. 15 %, $p = 0.019$). In multivariate analysis, the percent wall volume was an independent discriminator among plaque burden metrics after accounting for traditional risk factors (odds ratio per 1-SD increase: 1.7 [1.2, 2.6]); the presence of IPH remained as a significant discriminator after accounting for traditional risk factors and percent wall volume (odds ratio: 2.9 [1.1, 7.6]) while other compositional metrics did not.

Conclusions: IPH in the carotid artery was independently associated with prior coronary events. IPH imaging may provide incremental information on patients' coronary risk beyond traditional risk factors and carotid plaque burden assessment.

Keywords: Carotid artery, Coronary artery disease, Intraplaque hemorrhage, Magnetic resonance imaging

Background

Because of the systemic nature of atherosclerosis, subclinical carotid disease has long been used as a surrogate of coronary artery disease (CAD). Measurements on carotid plaque burden have been shown to predict the extent and clinical risk of underlying CAD [1-4], whereas the value of carotid plaque composition, although widely believed to indicate lesion instability, remains elusive for the evaluation of CAD risk.

Assessment of carotid plaque composition has been available via noninvasive imaging, which potentially can provide clinicians with incremental information on patients' coronary risk. Recently, the echolucent carotid plaques by ultrasound [5] and those with high-intensity signals by T1-weighted magnetic resonance imaging (MRI) [6] were shown to predict future coronary events independent of clinical risk factors. However, compositional features are known to have positive relationships with plaque burden [7, 8], and their added value will not be clear unless tested against plaque morphological metrics.

In this study, we sought to test whether and which carotid plaque compositional metrics confer incremental values for discriminating prior coronary events in

---
* Correspondence: sunjie@u.washington.edu; tomhat@u.washington.edu
[1]Department of Radiology, University of Washington, 850 Republican St, WA, Seattle 98109, USA
[8]Department of Surgery, Univeristy of Washington, 850 Republican St, WA, Seattle 98109, USA
Full list of author information is available at the end of the article

subjects with subclinical carotid disease. While all subjects in this study had imaging evidence of atherosclerosis, those with prior coronary events were considered to be at a much higher risk for future events [9]. We hypothesized that specific markers on carotid plaque composition could help identify subjects with prior coronary events and thus serve as novel markers for vulnerable patients. Carotid MRI provides comprehensive plaque morphological measurements, and is a validated tool for detecting major plaque components in vivo [10–12].

Methods
Study population
Subjects in a previously-established cohort were included in this retrospective study [13]. Briefly, asymptomatic subjects with substantial carotid plaques were recruited in this exploratory study to include a wide spectrum of compositional phenotypes. Specific criteria were: 1) 50-79 % stenosis by duplex ultrasound in at least one carotid artery; 2) neurologically asymptomatic defined as no cerebrovascular symptoms in the 6 months prior to enrollment; 3) no prior carotid endarterectomy (CEA), neck radiation or contraindications for MRI (e.g. metal implants, claustrophobia). Enrolled subjects completed a standardized health questionnaire covering demographics and cardiovascular risk factors (smoking, hypertension, hypercholesterolemia, and diabetes mellitus) [13]. Smoking was self-reported and included former smoking and current smoking. Hypertension was defined as systolic blood pressure ≥ 140 mmHg and/or diastolic blood pressure ≥ 90 mmHg, or taking anti-hypertensive agents. Diabetes was defined as previously confirmed diagnosis and/or use of anti-diabetic agents. Hypercholesterolemia was defined as a history of total cholesterol > 5 mmol/l and/or low-density lipoprotein cholesterol (LDL-C) > 3 mmol/l, or taking lipid-lowering medications. Prior coronary events were collected and verified by chart review. A positive history of coronary events was defined as having one or more of the following events: 1) hospitalization for myocardial infarction; 2) coronary revascularization including angioplasty, stenting and coronary artery bypass graft (CABG). All study procedures were reviewed and approved by the institutional review board. Subjects provided informed consent before enrollment.

MRI Protocol
All scans were performed on a 1.5 T scanner (Signa Horizon EchoSpeed, GE Healthcare, Milwaukee, Wisconsin, USA) using phased-array surface coils (Pathway, Seattle, Washington, USA). A previously published standardized protocol [14, 15] was used to acquire cross-sectional, multi-contrast images (3-dimensional time-of-flight [TOF], T1-weighted, proton density-weighted [PD], and T2-weighted) that were centered at the carotid bifurcation of the side with 50-79 % stenosis. No contrast agent was used to increase patient recruitment and compliance. Previous studies have shown that this non-contrast protocol was able to characterize major plaque components [10, 13]. All images were obtained with field-of-view of 13 to 16 cm, matrix size of 256 × 256, and slice thickness of 2 mm. Scan coverage was 40 mm for TOF, 20–24 mm for T1-weighted, and 30 mm for proton density-weighted and T2-weighted sequences. Total acquisition time was approximately 30 min.

Image analysis
Eight reviewers with at least 1-year experience in MR plaque imaging participated in image analysis while blinded to clinical data using a custom-designed image analysis software package (CASCADE, University of Washington, Seattle, Washington, USA) [16]. Only the index artery, defined as the side with 50-70 % stenosis by ultrasound, was analyzed. The four contrast weightings (TOF, T1, PD, and T2) were registered using the carotid bifurcation as a landmark. Lumen and outer wall boundaries were outlined on each cross-sectional slice as well as plaque components that were determined using previous published criteria (Figure 1) [10, 12]. Briefly, calcification appears hypointense on all weightings; intraplaque hemorrhage (IPH) appears hyperintense on TOF and T1-weighted images; lipid-rich necrotic core (LRNC) usually appears hypointense on T2- and PD-weighted images but may have variations if it contains IPH [12]. Remaining wall areas were classified as fibrous tissue. Subsequently, maximum wall thickness, maximum percent wall area (100 % × wall area/total vessel area), percent wall volume (100 % × wall volume/total vessel volume), were calculated. Percent volumes of calcification and LRNC and the presence/absence of IPH were also calculated and/or recorded. All imaging data were based on consensus opinion of at least two reviewers.

Statistical analysis
All data are presented as mean ± standard deviation (SD) for continuous variables and count with percentage for categorical variables. Subjects were stratified according to a positive or negative history of prior coronary events. Clinical and imaging characteristics were compared between the two groups using the independent t-test, Mann–Whitney test, and Fisher's exact test, as appropriate. The incremental values of: 1) carotid plaque morphological metrics over clinical variables; and 2) compositional metrics over clinical variables and morphological metrics, for discriminating prior coronary events, were examined using multivariate logistic regression analysis and presented as odds ratios (OR) with 95 % confidence interval (CI). To examine the influence of plaque burden on the ability of

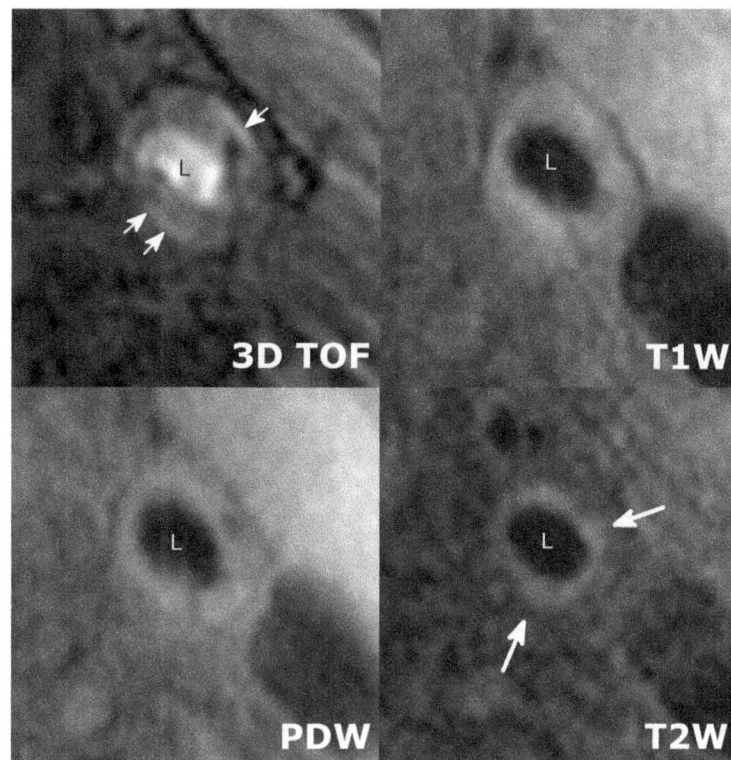

Fig. 1 Carotid plaque burden and composition detected by combined use of multiple MR weightings at 1.5 T. Arrows indicate lipid-rich necrotic core as hypointense areas on T2W images. Arrowheads indicate intraplaque hemorrhage as hyperintense areas on TOF images. PDW = proton-density-weighted; T1W = T1-weighted; T2W = T2-weighted; TOF = time-of-flight

compositional metrics for discriminating prior coronary events, interactions between plaque morphological and compositional metrics were also tested. All data analyses were performed using R 2.15.2 (R Foundation for Statistical Computing, Vienna, Austria). Statistical significance was defined as P < 0.05.

Results

Clinical and imaging characteristics

Table 1 summarizes the clinical and imaging characteristics of the study population ($N = 159$). Prior coronary events were documented in 66 (42 %) subjects. Compared to subjects without prior coronary events, those with prior coronary events had a higher prevalence of hypercholesterolemia (92 % vs. 70 %, $p = 0.001$), and were more frequently on statin therapy (82 % vs. 52 %, $p < 0.001$), but otherwise had similar clinical profiles (Table 1). Observed differences in carotid plaques included larger plaques, less fibrous tissue, and a higher prevalence of IPH in subjects with prior coronary events (Table 1).

Incremental value of carotid plaque morphology

All three morphological metrics of plaque burden were significantly associated with prior coronary events (Table 2).

Table 1 Clinical and imaging characteristics stratified by history of prior coronary events

	Negative (n = 93)	Positive (n = 66)	p value
Clinical characteristics			
Age, years	69.3 ± 8.9	70.2 ± 9.2	0.52
Male sex	75 (81)	59 (89)	0.19
Smoker	79 (85)	61 (92)	0.22
Hypertension	68 (73)	54 (82)	0.25
Hypercholesterolemia	65 (70)	61 (92)	0.001
Diabetes mellitus	25 (27)	18 (27)	0.99
Statin use	48 (52)	54 (82)	<0.001
Imaging characteristics			
Maximum wall thickness, mm	4.1 ± 1.4	4.6 ± 1.7	0.035
Maximum percent wall area	71.5 ± 13.4	76.0 ± 11.0	0.028
Percent wall volume	60.2 ± 10.1	65.4 ± 8.9	0.003
% calcification	3.9 ± 5.0	5.5 ± 6.5	0.098
% lipid-rich necrotic core	9.2 ± 11.1	12.8 ± 12.6	0.13
% fibrous tissue	84.6 ± 11.0	78.7 ± 11.9	0.003
Presence of IPH	14 (15)	21 (32)	0.019

Data are presented as mean ± SD or count (percentage)
% = percent volume; IPH = intraplaque hemorrhage; SD = standard deviation

Table 2 Associations between carotid plaque morphological metrics and prior coronary events

	Unadjusted		Adjusted[b]	
	OR (95 % CI)[a]	p value	OR (95 % CI)[a]	p value
Maximum wall thickness	1.4 (1.0, 2.0)	0.034	1.4 (1.0, 2.0)	0.092
Maximum percent wall area	1.4 (1.0, 2.0)	0.030	1.4 (0.9, 1.9)	0.105
Percent wall volume	1.8 (1.2, 2.5)	0.002	1.7 (1.2, 2.6)	0.005

[a]Data are presented as odds ratios per 1-SD higher values
[b]Adjusted for clinical risk factors (age, gender, smoking status, hypertension, hypercholesterolemia, diabetes mellitus and statin use)
CI = confidence interval; OR = odds ratio; SD = standard deviation

The OR for prior coronary events ranged from 1.4 to 1.8 per 1-SD increase in maximum wall thickness, maximum percent wall area, and percent wall volume. Percent wall volume not only appeared to be the strongest discriminator amongst the plaque morphological metrics for prior coronary events, but also remained significant after adjusting for demographics and clinical risk factors (OR: 1.7 [1.2, 2.6] per 1-SD increase, $p = 0.005$).

Incremental value of carotid plaque composition

Among carotid plaque compositional metrics, a lower percent volume of fibrous tissue and presence of IPH were associated with a positive history of coronary events (Table 3). After adjusting for clinical risk factors, as well as percent wall volume, the presence of IPH remained as a significant discriminator for prior coronary events (OR: 2.9 [1.1, 7.6], $p = 0.033$).

Plaque burden did not appear to influence the ability of IPH to discriminate subjects with prior coronary events (p-value ranged from 0.40 to 0.99 for interactions). Fig. 2 shows the association between IPH and prior coronary events in different subgroups defined by carotid plaque morphological metrics. Of note, all subjects in the lower half of maximum wall thickness and with IPH had prior coronary events.

Discussion

By using carotid MRI, we were able to evaluate and compare carotid plaque morphological and compositional metrics in relation to coronary plaque vulnerability, defined as having prior coronary events in this study. The most pronounced difference in carotid plaque morphology between subjects with and without prior coronary events was shown in percent wall volume. Furthermore, the incremental value of carotid plaque composition for discriminating prior coronary events, specifically the presence of IPH, was demonstrated by accounting for clinical risk factors as well as percent wall volume. In addition to some pathophysiological insights, our findings indicate that a combination of three-dimensional plaque characterization and IPH detection in the assessment of subclinical carotid atherosclerosis may offer the most promising information on patients' coronary risk.

Carotid plaque detection by B-mode ultrasound has been shown to improve individual risk assessment compared to the intima-media thickness [4]. The introduction of novel ultrasound techniques provides additional opportunities to optimize this approach through improved plaque characterization [17, 18]. This concept is further supported by autopsy findings showing that vulnerable features tend to be present at multiple arterial beds within the same individual [19, 20]. To determine what information embedded in carotid plaque tissue composition are relevant to coronary risk, we used carotid MRI to compare carotid plaque compositional metrics between subjects with and without prior coronary events. Carotid MRI gives a comprehensive assessment of local plaque burden by capturing both luminal stenosis and outward remodeling. Additionally, combining MRI contrast weightings has been shown to be able to characterize plaque components [10, 11]. Therefore, multiple morphological and compositional metrics can be compared head-to-head in a single study.

The presence of IPH in the carotid artery was found to be an additional indicator for coronary vulnerability, with an odds ratio of 2.9 (95 % CI: 1.1-7.6) for prior coronary events after adjustment for clinical variables and percent wall volume. The observation is consistent with a previous histopathological study by Hellings et al. [21] in which carotid IPH identified by post-surgical examination of carotid endarterectomy specimens was associated with systemic cardiovascular outcomes. It was noted that the observed relationship between carotid IPH and

Table 3 Associations between carotid plaque compositional metrics and prior coronary events

	Unadjusted		Adjusted[b]	
	OR (95 % CI)[a]	p value	OR (95 % CI)[a]	p value
% calcification	1.3 (1.0, 1.8)	0.083	1.2 (0.8, 1.7)	0.40
% LRNC	1.4 (1.0, 1.9)	0.052	1.2 (0.8, 1.8)	0.40
% fibrous tissue	0.6 (0.4, 0.8)	0.002	0.7 (0.4, 1.1)	0.13
Presence of IPH	2.6 (1.2, 5.7)	0.014	2.9 (1.1, 7.6)	0.033

[a]Data are presented as odds ratios per 1-SD higher values for continuous variables
[b]Adjusted for age, gender, smoking status, hypertension, hypercholesterolemia, diabetes mellitus, statin use and percent wall volume
% = percent volume; CI = confidence interval; IPH = intraplaque hemorrhage; OR = odds ratio; SD = standard deviation

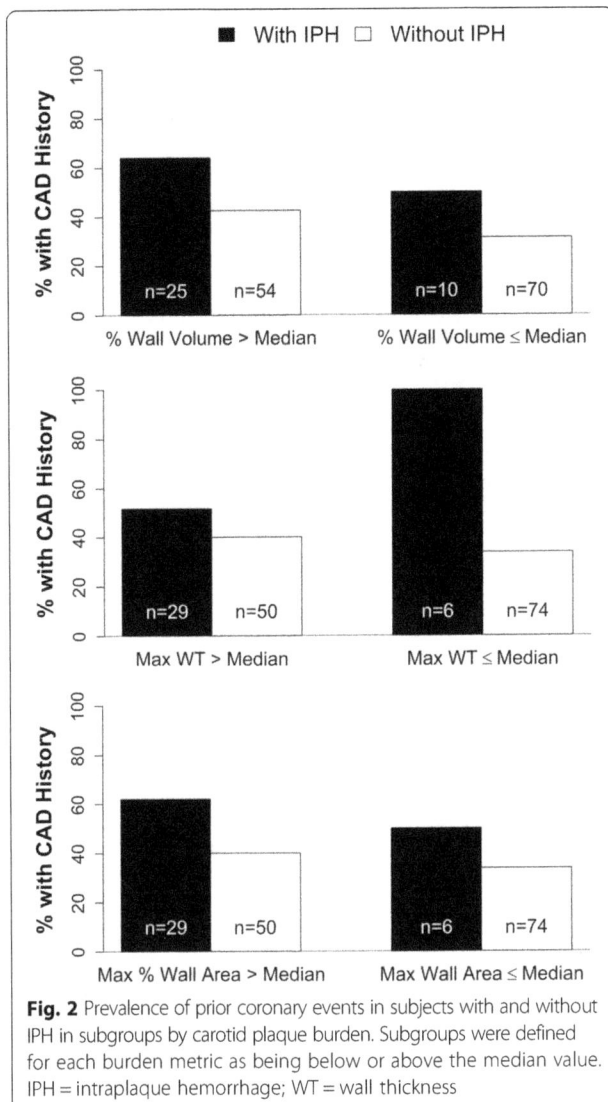

Fig. 2 Prevalence of prior coronary events in subjects with and without IPH in subgroups by carotid plaque burden. Subgroups were defined for each burden metric as being below or above the median value. IPH = intraplaque hemorrhage; WT = wall thickness

due to increase in both calcification and lipid core. However, such an association was largely accounted for by clinical risk factors and concomitantly larger percent wall volume.

Natural history studies have revealed that most coronary events were preceded by rapid plaque expansion that was unusual and unrelated to baseline plaque burden [22–24]. IPH, with the capability to induce changes in plaque behavior [25], may play a critical role in the pathogenesis of coronary events. In a postmortem study, Fleiner et al. described that the hyperplasia of vasa vasorum was a systemic feature of symptomatic patients [20]. As adventitial vasa vasorum is a major source of IPH [26], the finding by Fleiner et al. supports the conjecture that carotid IPH indicates increased probability of coronary IPH. Another study by Moreno et al. also sheds light by showing that genotypes related to hemoglobin clearance may determine one's susceptibility to IPH-induced detrimental effects [27]. It is possible that the presence of carotid IPH by MRI indicates certain genetic vulnerabilities related to IPH metabolism. Nonetheless, given the limited understanding of the pathophysiology of IPH in the current literature, although IPH in the carotid artery appears to indicate additional systemic factors that contribute to plaque instability, the exact mechanisms remain to be investigated.

Singh et al. [28] also noted a higher prevalence of carotid IPH in patients with prior coronary events. That study included subjects referred for carotid MRI due to suspected neurovascular disease, so the study population appears to be a mixture of symptomatic and asymptomatic subjects. It is conceivable that there would be a wider range of carotid plaque burden in the previous report compared to the present data. As IPH is known to be associated with a larger plaque burden [29], a wider range of plaque burden in study population makes it difficult to argue that the observed relationship is not due to the higher plaque burden associated with IPH but related to the unique pathophysiology of IPH. In the present study, by including subjects with similar extent of carotid disease and quantifying plaque burden in a three-dimensional fashion, we were able to test the independent association between carotid IPH and coronary events rigorously. In this study, plaque morphological measurements were derived from MRI rather than ultrasound which is more widely used in clinical practice. However, MRI provides multiple plaque morphological metrics, and therefore the incremental value of carotid plaque composition could be rigorously tested. The maximum wall thickness measures plaque burden at a single location. The maximum percent wall area measures a single slice and essentially indicates luminal narrowing after taking into account outward remodeling, which is similar to stenosis measurement on black-blood carotid MRI proposed by Babiarz et al. [30]. The percent wall volume, as a

coronary events alone was more marginal (hazard ratio: 1.6, 95 % CI: 0.9-3.0) [21]. Surgical patients have end-stage plaques and are frequently symptomatic whereas our study included only asymptomatic subjects with moderate carotid disease. After stratifying our study population by plaque size, there appeared to be no evidence that the relationship between IPH and prior coronary events varied in those with high or low plaque burden. Nonetheless, subjects with IPH but not much wall thickening may represent a unique group for further investigations (Fig. 2). Collectively, existing evidence suggests clinicians to note the increased coronary risk if IPH is detected in the carotid artery, particularly in those with asymptomatic carotid lesions.

In contrast to IPH, other plaque components did not show incremental discriminative power over plaque morphological assessment. Subjects with prior coronary events had significantly less fibrous tissue in the carotid plaque,

3-dimensional metric, is similar to the percent atheroma volume that is used in intravascular ultrasound studies of coronary vasculature [31]. Among the three morphological metrics, the percent wall volume was the best discriminator for prior coronary events, supporting the pursuit of 3-dimensional carotid plaque characterization as a future tool in CAD management [32].

Implications

Findings from this study have implications both for understanding the pathophysiology of vulnerable patients and for optimizing clinical management in individuals. Although atherosclerosis becomes highly prevalent as people get older, certain patients are at a particular high risk for clinical events. Our data suggest that carotid IPH was associated with increased risk for coronary events and the association was not explained by differences in traditional risk factors and plaque burden. Thus, it is conceivable that additional systemic factors that relate to the pathogenesis of IPH may be the underlying players, such as the hyperplasia of vasa vasorum and haptoglobin genotype [20, 27]. Accordingly, there is potential for using carotid IPH as a novel marker for high coronary risk in developing medical treatment strategies, which may include more stringent treatment goals for lipid-lowering and anti-hypertensive agents as well as novel agents that can target IPH and its detrimental effects on plaque progression.

Study limitations

There are several limitations of the present study. Our study population is selective in that it only included neurologically asymptomatic subjects with 50-79 % carotid stenosis by ultrasound. Despite the relatively narrow range in stenosis, a wide range in plaque composition was observed and offered a good opportunity to test the incremental value of plaque composition in discriminating prior coronary events. However, it remains to be seen whether the independent association of IPH with coronary events applies to the general population. Due to the retrospective nature of the design, patients with severe coronary events such as coronary death could not be included. We do not expect this selection bias that is present in most clinical research to affect our study findings. But the prevalence of carotid IPH in those with more severe coronary events could be higher than what was seen in this study. In addition, circulating biomarkers, such as C-reactive protein, which have been shown to improve risk appraisal in individuals [33], were not examined in the present study. Therefore, we could not exclude the possibility that the association between IPH and coronary events may be mediated by biomarkers. It is worth mentioning that epidemiological studies using carotid MRI are still sparse, and no biomarkers have been linked with IPH to date.

Conclusions

In conclusion, subjects with prior coronary events had a high prevalence of IPH. The association could not be explained by differences in traditional risk factors and plaque burden. IPH may provide incremental information on patients' coronary risk, possibly by indicating additional systemic factors that contribute to plaque instability.

Competing interests
DSH reports grants from GE Healthcare and Philips Healthcare. CY receives research grants from the NIH and Philips Healthcare, and serves as a Member of Radiology Advisory Network, Philips. TSH receives research grants from the NIH and Philips Healthcare. The other authors declare that they have no competing interests.

Authors' contributions
JS performed the design of the study, analyzed the data, interpreted the data, and drafted the manuscript. DSH participated in study design, contributed to statistical analysis, data interpretation, and revised the manuscript. HRU, BC, TS, NT, JC, MW, WY, LD participated in image analysis, data interpretation, and manuscript revision. CY assisted in the study design, data interpretation, and manuscript revision. TSH carried out the design of the study, interpreted the data and revised the manuscript. All authors read and approved the final manuscript.

Acknowledgements
None.

Author details
[1]Department of Radiology, University of Washington, 850 Republican St, WA, Seattle 98109, USA. [2]Department of Pediatrics, Univeristy of Utah, Salt Lake City, UT, USA. [3]Institute for Clinical Radiology, Ludwig-Maximilians-Univeristy Hospital Munich, Munich, Germany. [4]Department of Cardiology, Juntendo Univeristy, Tokyo, Japan. [5]Department of Radiology, PLA General Hospital, Beijing, China. [6]Department of Radiology, Japanese Red Cross Sendai Hospital, Sendai, Japan. [7]Department of Radiology, Beijing Anzhen Hospital, Beijing, China. [8]Department of Surgery, Univeristy of Washington, 850 Republican St, WA, Seattle 98109, USA.

References
1. Kallikazaros I, Tsioufis C, Sideris S, Stefanadis C, Toutouzas P. Carotid artery disease as a marker for the presence of severe coronary artery disease in patients evaluated for chest pain. Stroke. 1999;30:1002–7.
2. Sabeti S, Schlager O, Exner M, et al. Progression of carotid stenosis detected by duplex ultrasonography predicts adverse outcomes in cardiovascular high-risk patients. Stroke. 2007;38:2887–94.
3. Rundek T, Arif H, Boden-Albala B, Elkind MS, Paik MC, Sacco RL. Carotid plaque, a subclinical precursor of vascular events: the Northern Manhattan Study. Neurology. 2008;70:1200–7.
4. Brook RD, Bard RL, Patel S, et al. A Negative Carotid Plaque Area Test Is Superior to Other Noninvasive Atherosclerosis Studies for Reducing the Likelihood of Having Underlying Significant Coronary Artery Disease. Arterioscler Thromb Vasc Biol. 2006;26:656–62.
5. Honda O, Sugiyama S, Kugiyama K, et al. Echolucent carotid plaques predict future coronary events in patients with coronary artery disease. J Am Coll Cardiol. 2004;43:1177–84.
6. Noguchi T, Yamada N, Higashi M, Goto Y, Naito H. High-Intensity Signals in Carotid Plaques on T1-Weighted Magnetic Resonance Imaging Predict Coronary Events in Patients With Coronary Artery Disease. J Am Coll Cardiol. 2011;58:416–22.
7. AbuRahma AF, Wulu JT, Crotty B. Carotid Plaque Ultrasonic Heterogeneity and Severity of Stenosis. Stroke. 2002;33:1772–5.
8. Turc G, Oppenheim C, Naggara O, et al. Relationships between recent intraplaque hemorrhage and stroke risk factors in patients with carotid stenosis: the HIRISC study. Arterioscler Thromb Vasc Biol. 2012;32:492–9.

9. Cho E, Rimm EB, Stampfer MJ, Willett WC, Hu FB. The impact of diabetes mellitus and prior myocardial infarction on mortality from all causes and from coronary heart disease in men. J Am Coll Cardiol. 2002;40:954–60.

10. Saam T, Ferguson MS, Yarnykh VL, et al. Quantitative evaluation of carotid plaque composition by in vivo MRI. Arterioscler Thromb Vasc Biol. 2005;25:234–9.

11. Cappendijk VC, Cleutjens KBJM, Kessels AGH, et al. Assessment of Human Atherosclerotic Carotid Plaque Components with Multisequence MR Imaging: Initial Experience1. Radiology. 2005;234:487–92.

12. Yuan C, Mitsumori LM, Ferguson MS, et al. In vivo accuracy of multispectral magnetic resonance imaging for identifying lipid-rich necrotic cores and intraplaque hemorrhage in advanced human carotid plaques. Circulation. 2001;104:2051–6.

13. Takaya N, Yuan C, Chu BC, et al. Association between carotid plaque characteristics and subsequent ischemic cerebrovascular events: a prospective assessment with MRI - initial results. Stroke. 2006;37:818–23.

14. Cai JM, Hatsukami TS, Ferguson MS, Small R, Polissar NL, Yuan C. Classification of human carotid atherosclerotic lesions with in vivo multicontrast magnetic resonance imaging. Circulation. 2002;106:1368–73.

15. Yarnykh VL, Yuan C. High-Resolution Multi-Contrast MRI of the Carotid Artery Wall for Evaluation of Atherosclerotic Plaques, in Current Protocols in Magnetic Resonance Imaging. Wiley: New York; 2004.

16. Kerwin WS, Xu D, Liu F, et al. Magnetic resonance imaging of carotid atherosclerosis: plaque analysis. Top Magn Reson Imaging. 2007;18:371–8.

17. Landry A, Spence JD, Fenster A. Measurement of Carotid Plaque Volume by 3-Dimensional Ultrasound. Stroke. 2004;35:864–9.

18. Kim K, Huang SW, Hall TL, Witte RS, Chenevert TL, O'Donnell M. Arterial vulnerable plaque characterization using ultrasound-induced thermal strain imaging (TSI). IEEE Trans Biomed Eng. 2008;55:171–80.

19. Vink A, Schoneveld AH, Richard W, et al. Plaque burden, arterial remodeling and plaque vulnerability: determined by systemic factors? J Am Coll Cardiol. 2001;38:718–23.

20. Fleiner M, Kummer M, Mirlacher M, et al. Arterial neovascularization and inflammation in vulnerable patients: early and late signs of symptomatic atherosclerosis. Circulation. 2004;110:2843–50.

21. Hellings WE, Peeters W, Moll FL, et al. Composition of carotid atherosclerotic plaque is associated with cardiovascular outcome: a prognostic study. Circulation. 2010;121:1941–50.

22. Glaser R, Selzer F, Faxon DP, et al. Clinical progression of incidental, asymptomatic lesions discovered during culprit vessel coronary intervention. Circulation. 2005;111:143–9.

23. Stone GW, Maehara A, Lansky AJ, et al. A prospective natural-history study of coronary atherosclerosis. N Engl J Med. 2011;364:226–35.

24. Narula J, Nakano M, Virmani R, et al. Histopathologic characteristics of atherosclerotic coronary disease and implications of the findings for the invasive and noninvasive detection of vulnerable plaques. J Am Coll Cardiol. 2013;61:1041–51.

25. Sun J, Underhill HR, Hippe DS, Xue Y, Yuan C, Hatsukami TS. Sustained acceleration in carotid atherosclerotic plaque progression with intraplaque hemorrhage: a long-term time course study. J Am Coll Cardiol Img. 2012;5:798–804.

26. Virmani R, Kolodgie FD, Burke AP, et al. Atherosclerotic plaque progression and vulnerability to rupture: angiogenesis as a source of intraplaque hemorrhage. Arterioscler Thromb Vasc Biol. 2005;25:2054–61.

27. Moreno PR, Purushothaman KR, Purushothaman M, et al. Haptoglobin genotype is a major determinant of the amount of iron in the human atherosclerotic plaque. J Am Coll Cardiol. 2008;52:1049–51.

28. Singh N, Moody AR, Rochon-Terry G, Kiss A, Zavodni A. Identifying a high risk cardiovascular phenotype by carotid MRI-depicted intraplaque hemorrhage. Int J Cardiovasc Imaging. 2013;29:1477–83.

29. Zhao X, Underhill HR, Zhao Q, et al. Discriminating Carotid Atherosclerotic Lesion Severity by Luminal Stenosis and Plaque Burden: A Comparison Utilizing High-Resolution Magnetic Resonance Imaging at 3.0 Tesla. Stroke. 2011;42:347–53.

30. Babiarz LS, Astor B, Mohamed MA, Wasserman BA. Comparison of gadolinium-enhanced cardiovascular magnetic resonance angiography with high-resolution black blood cardiovascular magnetic resonance for assessing carotid artery stenosis. J Cardiovasc Magn Reson. 2007;9:63–70.

31. Nicholls SJ, Hsu A, Wolski K, et al. Intravascular ultrasound-derived measures of coronary atherosclerotic plaque burden and clinical outcome. J Am Coll Cardiol. 2010;55:2399–407.

32. Sillesen H, Muntendam P, Adourian A, et al. Carotid plaque burden as a measure of subclinical atherosclerosis: comparison with other tests for subclinical arterial disease in the High Risk Plaque BioImage study. JACC Cardiovasc Imaging. 2012;5:681–9.

33. Koenig W, Lowel H, Baumert J, Meisinger C. C-reactive protein modulates risk prediction based on the Framingham Score: implications for future risk assessment: results from a large cohort study in southern Germany. Circulation. 2004;109:1349–53.

15

Permeability imaging in cerebrovascular diseases: applications and progress in research

Hui Chen, Nan Liu, Ying Li, Fei Chen and Guangming Zhu*

Abstract

Cerebrovascular disease is currently the second most common cause of death after ischemic heart disease. In this article, we mainly focus on the application of permeability imaging in cases of ischemic and hemorrhagic stroke, and cerebral small vessel disease. In this review, we discuss the application of permeability imaging in ischemic stroke from two aspects: 1) for the prediction of hemorrhagic transformation after infarction, and 2) for the evaluation of newborn secondary and tertiary collateral circulations. Quantitative measurements of blood–brain barrier (BBB) disruption by the Dynamic Contrast Enhance MR (DCE-MR) can reveal the severity of intracranial hemorrhage (ICH)-induced brain damage, and that the technique has the potential to be used for testing the efficacy of interventions aimed at reducing tissue damage around the hematoma. Currently, DCE-MR is mostly applied for the assessment of tumors in patients. There is less research focused on the evaluation of mild BBB defects in normal or abnormal aging brains, dementia, or cerebral small vessel disease. More work needs to be done to select the appropriate contrast agents and decide their doses, as well as to identify methods for parameter collection and data analysis.

Keywords: Permeability imaging, Blood–brain barrier, K^{trans}, Dynamic Contrast Enhance MR, ischemic stroke, Hemorrhagic transformation, Collateral circulation, Hemorrhagic stroke, Cerebral small vessel disease

Background

Cerebrovascular disease is currently the second most common cause of death after ischemic heart disease, and a leading cause of disability [1]. Every year, 15 million people worldwide experience ischemic or hemorrhagic stroke [2]. Modern imaging techniques not only clarify the nature of the stroke within minutes, but also play critical roles in identifying the cause of the stroke, guiding the late-stage treatment, and evaluating the prognosis [2]. Large numbers of molecular imaging techniques, including permeability imaging, have gradually entered clinical practice, and help physicians who are involved in neurosurgery and neuroimaging, gain a deeper understanding of the pathophysiological changes in nervous system disorders.

Permeability imaging is often used in the diagnosis and prognosis of brain tumors, as well as in the blood–brain barrier permeability (BBBP) assessment for ischemic cerebrovascular disease, spontaneous intracerebral hemorrhage (ICH), cerebral small vessel disease, cognitive dysfunction, multiple sclerosis, and brain trauma [3–6]. In this article, we mainly focus on the application of permeability imaging in cases of ischemic and hemorrhagic stroke, and cerebral small vessel disease.

Review

Neurovascular unit, BBB, and BBB permeability

The process of tissue damage after stroke is highly complex, involving changes in brain vasculature and parenchyma that are regulated by the interactions of a variety of mechanisms. More and more studies suggest that the treatment of cerebrovascular diseases must go beyond the concept of cell damage alone. It is important to pay more attention to the dynamic changes in the neurovascular units (NVU), which are the integrative microunits of structure and function of the nervous system. Thus, neurons, endothelial cells, astrocytes, and the extracellular

* Correspondence: zhugmdc@aliyun.com
Department of Neurology, Military General Hospital of Beijing PLA, Beijing 100700, China

matrix that maintains the integrity of the brain tissue need to be viewed comprehensively, with the BBB acting as the core of the NVU [7]. The negative results from clinical trials of neuro-protective drugs also support this idea, making the NVU an important therapeutic target in future clinical research. The extent of damage and the late-stage recovery of the NVU determine the clinical outcome of patients. However, no ideal method can assess NVU dysfunction accurately or quantitatively.

Some researchers quantify the damage to the NVU by examining specific markers, such as Matrix Metalloproteinases (MMPs), Vascular Endothelial Growth Factor (VEGF), Platelet Derived Growth Factor (PDGF), and Fibroblast Growth Factor (FGF), in blood or cerebrospinal fluid [8]. However, the specificity of this method is low, spatially, as it cannot distinguish the location and the extent of NVU damage in different brain regions. Double-photon laser-scanning microscopy, which can detect the dynamic relationship between the microvasculature and the surrounding structure in living tissue, is the ideal imaging method for examining the NVU. However, due to the complicated scanning procedure involved and the need for a craniotomy in order to expose the areas of interest, Double-photon microscopy is currently used only in animal models [9].

The BBB, which is composed of capillary endothelial cells, basement membrane, pericytes located outside the basement membrane, and the perivascular end-feet of astrocytes, is the most important protective structure in the brain. It can reduce the passive movement of water molecules and restrict the passage of soluble substances from the blood, thereby preventing brain cells from being exposed to neurotoxins or other harmful blood-borne substances. The BBB is considered as the core structure of the NVU, and the defects in structure and function can be found in most neurological diseases.

Disorders of the BBB are particularly evident in ischemic cerebrovascular disease, and show dynamic changes under different states of tissue damage and reperfusion. After ischemic brain damage, BBB leakage occurs not only during the acute and subacute phases of stroke [10], but also at the early stage of angiogenesis during stroke recovery [11]. In addition, studies have found that BBB disruption is most significant at the edges of the hematoma, 1 week after spontaneous ICH, and quantitative measurement of the BBB damage can reflect the extent of ICH-induced brain damage. Damage to the BBB can also be found in the early stage of lacunar infarction, white matter osteoporosis, and other cerebral small vessel diseases [12].

The severity of BBB damage is positively correlated with the degree of brain tissue damage or hypoxia and ischemia, and therefore quantitative assessment of the disruption of the BBB (i.e., the BBBP) can be used for quantitative evaluation of the severity of the NVU damage [13].

Principles of permeability imaging

Permeability imaging uses classic pharmacokinetic theory to quantitatively assess the rate at which a contrast agent passes through the BBB [14]. The increase in BBBP reflects BBB-relevant pathophysiological changes, and therefore the quantitative description of the BBBP has important clinical significance [15]. Common parameters include volume transfer constant (K^{trans}) and permeability-surface area product (PS). Between the two, K^{trans} is generally believed to represent permeability.

Though there are multiple methods to obtain permeability parameters, such as first pass data of perfusion CT and Dynamic Susceptibility Contrast MR, the standard method for BBB permeability assessments are based on Dynamic contrast-enhanced MR (DCE-MR). The DCE-MR scanning process begins with multiple flip-angle T1 sequences, followed by intravenous injection of contrast agent, after which the T1-weighted GRE sequence is acquired over several minutes. The observation of a linear relationship between the MR signal intensity and the scan time indicates that the slope is associated with BBB permeability [2]. In patients with subsequent hemorrhagic transformation (HT), even an enhanced T1 sequence does not exhibit a visually identifiable enhanced effect. However, the increase in BBB permeability at this stage can be observed in DCE-MR [16]. Studies have indicated that the DCE acquisition time should be at least 210 s [17] in order to distinguish between patients with HT from those without HT.

Currently, the tracer kinetics model used in most permeability imaging is the corrected single-capillary model proposed by Larsson and Tofts [18, 19]. However, this model requires hemodynamic balance, which calls for relatively long scan times. The Patlak model [20] only analyzes the first-pass data of the contrast agent. Requiring lesser amounts of data, it has been successfully used to analyze permeability data and obtain relevant parameters such as K^{trans}. Multiple studies using Patlak data analysis have correctly assessed the permeability parameter K^{trans} in stroke patients [21]. However, this approach can only be used in cases with moderate BBB leakage. When there is severe BBB leakage, data collection takes a longer time and the results are biased.

In the future, quantitative assessment of BBB leakage needs to mainly focus on reducing errors, particularly on optimizing the assessment of arterial input function to reduce errors caused by different tracers.

Application in ischemic brain injury

The defect of BBB occurs rapidly after acute cerebral infarction and is accompanied by a significant increase in

BBBP. Studies have shown that the average time to BBB defect after the onset of cerebral ischemia is 3.8 h, which is similar to the time at which irreversible brain damage occurs [13].

Here, we discuss the application of permeability imaging in two aspects: 1) for the prediction of HT after infarction, and 2) for the evaluation of newborn secondary and tertiary collateral circulations.

Symptomatic HT is one of the most serious complications of acute ischemic stroke and is closely related to clinical outcomes [22]. Currently, the commonly used imaging techniques cannot directly assess the risk of HT. A number of studies have demonstrated that enhanced MR is highly capable of predicting HT [23, 24]. However, the methods described above can only provide indirect evidence of increased permeability resulting from BBB disruption. They cannot provide quantification data and require highly experienced evaluators for correct interpretation [23]. Using the DCE-MR to quantitatively evaluate the BBB, the K^{trans} has proved to be the most sensitive imaging marker for the prediction of early (within 2–3 h) fibrin leakage in the brain tissue [24]. Kassner et al. added the DCE sequence in the conventional MR of 33 patients within 4 h of the onset of acute cerebral infarction and found progressive increase in the BBBP in the acute phase of nine patients (five patients received tPA thrombolytic therapy), all of whom presented with HT within 48 h [25]. However, due to the long scan time of the DCE-MR, its application in the ultra-early stage of acute cerebral infarction is limited. Thus, some studies obtained BBBP values from first-pass perfusion CT (PCT) data. For example, Wintermark and Lee et al. applied different mathematical models to measure the absolute values of BBBP and proposed that the increase in the BBBP can be utilized to predict HT [26]. Permeability imaging can systematically assess BBB integrity and make personalized predictions regarding the risk of hemorrhage in patients with acute ischemic stroke, which should help realize the transformation from the "time-window" to the "tissue-window" approach. Thus, patients who have a high risk of HT with active treatments even within the 4.5-h therapeutic time window, as well as those who have a relatively low risk of HT and relatively good prognosis even beyond the 4.5-h window, can be screened out. That is, it will be possible to move away from the fixed time-window treatment model and develop more rational therapies based on the evaluation of individualized risks [27].

The intracranial collateral circulation plays a critical role in the occurrence, development, treatment, and prognosis of ischemic stroke. The collateral circulation is capable of maintaining perfusion and stabilizing cerebral blood flow, which in turn, determines the tissue outcomes. Studies have reported that, in the patients with severe carotid artery stenosis, a good collateral circulation could reduce the incidence of long-term stroke, perioperative risk, and transient ischemic attack [28, 29]. Regardless of the success of recanalization of occluded vessels after thrombolytic therapy, the long-term prognosis of patients with leptomeningeal collateral vessels is better than that of other patients [30].

Methods for assessing intracranial collaterals include transcranial Doppler (TCD) ultrasound, computed tomography angiography (CTA), MR angiography (MRA), and digital subtraction angiography (DSA), each of which has its own advantages and disadvantages. For the assessment of secondary collaterals, permeability imaging has sufficient theoretical basis. The dynamic contrast-enhanced sequence itself contains perfusion information. In a study on the assessment of the collateral circulation in patients with acute stroke, Chen et al. [30] used first-pass data of perfusion images to obtain the permeability parameter K^{trans} map, and found that the K^{trans} map can assess collateral circulation in the acute ischemic state. The corresponding collateral circulation score is most consistent with that of DSA. Chen et al. also found that the K^{trans} map can predict clinical outcomes after stroke.

K^{trans}, as well as measurements from other sequences in MR, also confirmed the location and the size of the area of revascularization and angiogenesis [31]. Similar to its usefulness in detecting tumor angiogenesis, K^{trans} is a sensitive parameter for the detection of early brain angiogenesis in post-stroke patients. Although previous research on the detection of angiogenesis by DCE-MR had only revealed that increased intensity of the K^{trans} signal corresponds to increased density of newborn vessels, it was not clear whether secondary and tertiary cerebral collaterals could be evaluated through the assessment of angiogenesis. In a recent study, Chen et al. [32] collected 21 patients with severe intracranial arterial stenosis or occlusion caused by chronic artery atherosclerosis. The patients all presented with severe stenosis or occlusion of the middle cerebral artery and the intracranial segment of the internal carotid artery. The study used the corrected Alberta Stroke Program Early CT Score (ASPECTS) segmentation standard to evaluate collateral circulations in each of the vasculature segments and used K^{trans} maps, Arterial Spin Labeling (ASL), CTA, and DSA to score collaterals. The authors found good agreement between the DSA and K^{trans} map, especially in the assessment of the meningeal collateral circulation. The agreement between the CTA-source image (CTA-SI) and DSA was moderate, while the agreement between the ASL and DSA was the least favorable. However, the sample size in this study was too small to draw definite conclusions.

Although K^{trans} has been applied in cancer patients [33], it is rarely used in stroke patients. This may be due to the lack of awareness regarding the usefulness of K^{trans} measurements. Between perfusion imaging and permeability imaging, physicians usually prefer the former. In fact, permeability imaging itself already contains perfusion information. With optimization of the software, a good perfusion sequence can also be obtained during permeability imaging.

Application in hemorrhagic stroke

Hypertensive ICH is the deadliest and most disabling form of stroke and affects nearly a million people worldwide each year [34]. Studies using animal models have shown that the toxic effects of hemoglobin degradation products can cause increases in the BBB permeability and lead to the formation of edema around the hematoma [35]. Studies have speculated that disruption of the BBB can lead to angiogenesis in the vicinity of the hematoma, which further promotes the formation of vasogenic edema [36]. Therefore, BBB disruption may be an important pathophysiological factor involved in hypertensive ICH–induced brain damage, and is a potential target for therapeutic intervention [35].

The study by Didem et al. showed that the DCE-MR could demonstrate an increase in BBB permeability in the boundary region of the hematoma 8 days after cerebral hemorrhage. However, no contrast agent was found in the hematoma itself, and BBBP was not increased in the contralateral hemisphere [37]. Research on spontaneous ICH in humans has shown that contrast enhancement can be observed around the hematoma in 60 % of patients 5 days after the occurrence of the ICH [38]. No contrast enhancement can be found in the hematoma itself, possibly due to blood clots preventing the leakage of contrast agents. In an ICH rat model, Yang et al. observed increased BBB permeability both in the core and at the edge of the hematoma 7 days after the ICH [36]. However, their ICH model was created by direct injection of autologous blood instead of blood vessel rupture and can therefore not reflect the real pathophysiological changes of ICH in humans.

A study by Didem et al. revealed the relationship between BBB leakage and the size of the hematoma using DCE-MR. BBB leakage is more severe around large hematomas (i.e., ≥30 mL), and a higher increase in the BBBP, as well as its variability, occurred more often in larger hematomas than in smaller ones [37]. This is consistent with the observation that edema volume in bigger hematomas is greater than that in smaller hematomas [39]. BBB leakage varies depending on hemorrhage location. Regardless of the size of the hematoma, BBB permeability and variability is higher in lobar than in deep hemorrhages [37].

Animal studies have indicated that the BBB permeability starts to increase only hours after ICH, and continues until 48–72 h [36]. In these models, the amount of BBB leakage gradually declined after the peak, which occurred in the first few days after the onset of ICH. However, the increase in BBBP was sustained for up to 14 days [36]. One animal study found that the measurements of the BBBP were similar between 1 week and 1-day post-ICH [40].

Taken together, the evidence suggests that quantitative measurements of BBB disruption by the DCE-MR can reveal the severity of ICH-induced brain damage, and that the technique has the potential to be used for testing the efficacy of interventions aimed at reducing tissue damage around the hematoma [37].

Application in cerebral small vessel disease

Cerebral small vessel disease can cause dementia and stroke. The most characteristic imaging manifestations include lacunar infarction [41], leukoaraiosis, enlarged perivascular spaces, and cerebral microbleeds [42]. Studies have demonstrated that endothelial injuries can cause BBB leakage at multiple sites, which leads to ongoing damage of the vessel wall and eventually to blood vessel ruptures and microbleeds [43]. These microbleeds together with reactive small-vessel occlusions induce cystic infarcts of the surrounding parenchyma. Schreiber et al. reported that in spontaneously hypertensive stroke-prone rats, the vascular system reacts with an activated coagulation state after the early endothelial injuries and induces stasis formation and the accumulation of erythrocytes, which represent the earliest detectable histological characteristics of small vessel disease [43].

Many studies have reported that increased BBB permeability occurs in the aging brain, dementia, and leukoaraiosis in humans. However, it must be noted that the sample size of the study on leukoaraiosis was small and the results are unreliable [44]. Most of the studies examined the BBBP using biochemical methods, such as measurement of the cerebrospinal fluid (CSF) albumin/serum albumin ratio. Several studies have used imaging techniques to examine the BBB, mostly through intravenous injection of the MR contrast agent gadolinium, a relatively nonspecific marker for detection of the BBB disruption [44]. Topakian et al. studied 24 patients with lacunar infarction and compared them with controls. They found that in leukoaraiosis patients, DCE-MR revealed increased BBBP even in regions of the white matter that appeared normal [3]. Rosenberg et al. studied patients with vascular cognitive impairment and confirmed the disruption of the BBB in the areas of leukoaraiosis [45].

Overall, BBB integrity deteriorates slowly with aging, with the decline being more severe in patients with dementia and small vessel disease. BBB damage plays an important role in lacunar infarction, leukoaraiosis, other brain small vessel diseases, and age-related diseases (such as Alzheimer disease). Preliminary reports suggest that the BBB defect is present even before the clinical and imaging manifestations arise. The enlarged perivascular space is an important marker for cerebral small vessel disease, and brain damage caused by inflammation and other pathological processes is a marker for the initial damage to the BBB [12].

Long-term follow-up studies are required to determine the role of BBB damage in the pathology of cerebral small vessel disease. The BBB can be quantitatively evaluated by DCE-MR, which can be combined with pathology methods to identify the major mechanisms of BBB damage and further explore its pathogenesis. Currently, DCE-MR is mostly applied for the assessment of tumors in patients. There is less research focused on the evaluation of mild BBB defects in normal or abnormal aging brains, dementia, or cerebral small vessel disease. More work needs to be done to select the appropriate contrast agents and decide their doses, as well as to identify methods for parameter collection and data analysis [46].

Conclusions

This review discusses the applications of DCE-MR-based permeability imaging techniques in cerebrovascular diseases. With regard to the methods, T1-weighted DCE-MR is more developed. However, due to the lack of a unified standard for the image acquisition, data models, and study reports, it is difficult to compare and analyze DCE data between different studies. Further improvements for enhancing the reliability and stability of the DCE-MR are needed for its application in the assessment of subtle changes in the permeability of the BBB. Future research should attempt to establish a unified data collection and analysis method, which should help improve the comparability between studies and promote the wide application of DCE-MR in clinical practice and research [46].

Abbreviations
ASL: Arterial Spin Labeling; BBB: Blood–Brain Barrier; BBBP: blood–brain barrier permeability; CTA: computed tomography angiography; CTA: SI-CTA source image; DCE: Dynamic Contrast Enhance; DSA: digital subtraction angiography; FGF: Fibroblast Growth Factor; HT: hemorrhagic transformation; ICH: intracranial hemorrhage; MMPs: Matrix MetalloProteinases; MRA: MR angiography; NVU: neurovascular units; PDGF: Platelet Derived Growth Factor; PS: surface area product; PCT: perfusion CT; TCD: transcranial Doppler; VEGF: Vascular Endothelial Growth Factor.

Competing interests
The authors declare that they have no competing interests.

Authors' contributions
HC consulted literatures and wrote the review. NL, YL and FC carried out the reference collection. GZ conceived of the idea, and participated in its design and coordination and helped to draft the manuscript. All authors read and approved the final manuscript.

Acknowledgements
This review was supported by the National Natural Science Foundation of China (Grant No. 81371286 and No. 81501024).

References
1. Panchal HB, Ladia V, Amin P, Patel P, Veeranki SP, Albalbissi K, et al. A meta-analysis of mortality and major adverse cardiovascular and cerebrovascular events in patients undergoing transfemoral versus transapical transcatheter aortic valve implantation using edwards valve for severe aortic stenosis. Am J Cardiol. 2014;114:1882–90.
2. Hoffmann A, Zhu G, Wintermark M. Advanced neuroimaging in stroke patients: prediction of tissue fate and hemorrhagic transformation. Expert Rev Cardiovasc Ther. 2012;10:515–24.
3. Topakian R, Barrick TR, Howe FA, Markus HS. Blood–brain barrier permeability is increased in normal-appearing white matter in patients with lacunar stroke and leucoaraiosis. J Neurol Neurosurg Psychiatry. 2010;81: 192–7.
4. van de Haar HJ, Burgmans S, Hofman PA, Verhey FR, Jansen JF, Backes WH. Blood–brain barrier impairment in dementia: current and future in vivo assessments. Neurosci Biobehav Rev. 2015;49:71–81.
5. Alluri H, Wiggins-Dohlvik K, Davis ML, Huang JH, Tharakan B. Blood–brain barrier dysfunction following traumatic brain injury. Metab Brain Dis. 2015; 30:1093–104.
6. Cramer SP, Larsson HB. Accurate determination of blood–brain barrier permeability using dynamic contrast-enhanced T1-weighted MRI: a simulation and in vivo study on healthy subjects and multiple sclerosis patients. J Cereb Blood Flow Metab. 2014;34:1655–65.
7. Muoio V, Persson PB, Sendeski MM. The neurovascular unit - concept review. Acta Physiol (Oxf). 2014;210:790–8.
8. Amtul Z, Hepburn JD. Protein markers of cerebrovascular disruption of neurovascular unit: immunohistochemical and imaging approaches. Rev Neurosci. 2014;25:481–507.
9. Tran CH, Gordon GR. Acute two-photon imaging of the neurovascular unit in the cortex of active mice. Front Cell Neurosci. 2015;9:11.
10. Leigh R, Jen SS, Hillis AE, Krakauer JW, Barker PB, Stir, et al. Pretreatment blood–brain barrier damage and post-treatment intracranial hemorrhage in patients receiving intravenous tissue-type plasminogen activator. Stroke. 2014;45:2030–5.
11. Sun FL, Wang W, Cheng H, Wang Y, Li L, Xue JL, et al. Morroniside improves microvascular functional integrity of the neurovascular unit after cerebral ischemia. PLoS One. 2014;9, e101194.
12. Wardlaw JM. Blood–brain barrier and cerebral small vessel disease. J Neurol Sci. 2010;299:66–71.
13. Chassidim Y, Vazana U, Prager O, Veksler R, Bar-Klein G, Schoknecht K, et al. Analyzing the blood–brain barrier: the benefits of medical imaging in research and clinical practice. Semin Cell Dev Biol. 2015;38:43–52.
14. Tofts PS, Brix G, Buckley DL, Evelhoch JL, Henderson E, Knopp MV, et al. Estimating kinetic parameters from dynamic contrast-enhanced T(1)-weighted MRI of a diffusable tracer: standardized quantities and symbols. J Magn Reson Imaging. 1999;10:223–32.
15. Nagaraja TN, Keenan KA, Aryal MP, Ewing JR, Gopinath S, Nadig VS, et al. Extravasation into brain and subsequent spread beyond the ischemic core of a magnetic resonance contrast agent following a step-down infusion protocol in acute cerebral ischemia. Fluids Barriers CNS. 2014;11:21.
16. Kassner A, Roberts T, Taylor K, Silver F, Mikulis D. Prediction of hemorrhage in acute ischemic stroke using permeability MR imaging. AJNR Am J Neuroradiol. 2005;26:2213–7.
17. Vidarsson L, Thornhill RE, Liu F, Mikulis DJ, Kassner A. Quantitative permeability magnetic resonance imaging in acute ischemic stroke: how long do we need to scan? Magn Reson Imaging. 2009;27:1216–22.
18. Tofts PS, Kermode AG. Measurement of the blood–brain barrier permeability and leakage space using dynamic MR imaging. 1. Fundamental concepts. Magn Reson Med. 1991;17:357–67.
19. Larsson HB, Stubgaard M, Frederiksen JL, Jensen M, Henriksen O, Paulson OB. Quantitation of blood–brain barrier defect by magnetic resonance imaging and gadolinium-DTPA in patients with multiple sclerosis and brain tumors. Magn Reson Med. 1990;16:117–31.

20. Patlak CS, Blasberg RG. Graphical evaluation of blood-to-brain transfer constants from multiple-time uptake data. Generalizations. J Cereb Blood Flow Metab. 1985;5:584–90.

21. Nagaraja TN, Knight RA, Ewing JR, Karki K, Nagesh V, Fenstermacher JD. Multiparametric magnetic resonance imaging and repeated measurements of blood–brain barrier permeability to contrast agents. Methods Mol Biol. 2011;686:193–212.

22. Asuzu D, Nystrom K, Amin H, Schindler J, Wira C, Greer D, et al. Modest Association between the Discharge Modified Rankin Scale Score and Symptomatic Intracerebral Hemorrhage after Intravenous Thrombolysis. J Stroke Cerebrovasc Dis. 2015;24:548–53.

23. Knight RA, Barker PB, Fagan SC, Li Y, Jacobs MA, Welch KM. Prediction of impending hemorrhagic transformation in ischemic stroke using magnetic resonance imaging in rats. Stroke. 1998;29:144–51.

24. Jiang Q, Ewing JR, Ding GL, Zhang L, Zhang ZG, Li L, et al. Quantitative evaluation of BBB permeability after embolic stroke in rat using MRI. J Cereb Blood Flow Metab. 2005;25:583–92.

25. Adraktas DD, Brasic N, Furtado AD, Cheng SC, Ordovas K, Chun K, et al. Carotid atherosclerosis does not predict coronary, vertebral, or aortic atherosclerosis in patients with acute stroke symptoms. Stroke. 2010;41: 1604–9.

26. Dankbaar JW, Hom J, Schneider T, Cheng SC, Bredno J, Lau BC, et al. Dynamic perfusion-CT assessment of early changes in blood brain barrier permeability of acute ischaemic stroke patients. J Neuroradiol. 2011;38:161–6.

27. Kassner A, Mandell DM, Mikulis DJ. Measuring permeability in acute ischemic stroke. Neuroimaging Clin N Am. 2011;21:315–25. x-xi.

28. Winship IR, Armitage GA, Ramakrishnan G, Dong B, Todd KG, Shuaib A. Augmenting collateral blood flow during ischemic stroke via transient aortic occlusion. J Cereb Blood Flow Metab. 2014;34:61–71.

29. Kobayashi J, Uehara T, Toyoda K, Endo K, Ohara T, Fujinami J, et al. Clinical significance of fluid-attenuated inversion recovery vascular hyperintensities in transient ischemic attack. Stroke. 2013;44:1635–40.

30. Chen H, Wu B, Liu N, Wintermark M, Su Z, Li Y, et al. Using standard first-pass perfusion computed tomographic data to evaluate collateral flow in acute ischemic stroke. Stroke. 2015;46:961–7.

31. Li L, Jiang Q, Zhang L, Ding G, Wang L, Zhang R, et al. Ischemic cerebral tissue response to subventricular zone cell transplantation measured by iterative self-organizing data analysis technique algorithm. J Cereb Blood Flow Metab. 2006;26:1366–77.

32. Chen H, Wu B, Zhu G, Wintermark M, Wu X, Su Z, et al. Permeability Imaging as a Biomarker of Leptomeningeal Collateral Flow in Patients with Intracranial Arterial Stenosis. Cell Biochem Biophys. 2014

33. Franiel T, Hamm B, Hricak H. Dynamic contrast-enhanced magnetic resonance imaging and pharmacokinetic models in prostate cancer. Eur Radiol. 2011;21:616–26.

34. Roger VL, Go AS, Lloyd-Jones DM, Adams RJ, Berry JD, Brown TM, et al. Heart disease and stroke statistics–2011 update: a report from the American Heart Association. Circulation. 2011;123:e18–209.

35. Silva-Candal AD, Vieites-Prado A, Gutierrez-Fernandez M, Rey RI, Argibay B, Mirelman D, et al. Blood glutamate grabbing does not reduce the hematoma in an intracerebral hemorrhage model but it is a safe excitotoxic treatment modality. J Cereb Blood Flow Metab. 2015

36. Yang D, Knight RA, Han Y, Karki K, Zhang J, Ding C, et al. Vascular recovery promoted by atorvastatin and simvastatin after experimental intracerebral hemorrhage: magnetic resonance imaging and histological study. J Neurosurg. 2011;114:1135–42.

37. Aksoy D, Bammer R, Mlynash M, Venkatasubramanian C, Eyngorn I, Snider RW, et al. Magnetic resonance imaging profile of blood–brain barrier injury in patients with acute intracerebral hemorrhage. J Am Heart Assoc. 2013;2, e000161.

38. Kidwell CS, Burgess R, Menon R, Warach S, Latour LL. Hyperacute injury marker (HARM) in primary hemorrhage: a distinct form of CNS barrier disruption. Neurology. 2011;77:1725–8.

39. Venkatasubramanian C, Mlynash M, Finley-Caulfield A, Eyngorn I, Kalimuthu R, Snider RW, et al. Natural history of perihematomal edema after intracerebral hemorrhage measured by serial magnetic resonance imaging. Stroke. 2011;42:73–80.

40. Wu G, Li C, Wang L, Mao Y, Hong Z. Minimally invasive procedures for evacuation of intracerebral hemorrhage reduces perihematomal glutamate content, blood–brain barrier permeability and brain edema in rabbits. Neurocrit Care. 2011;14:118–26.

41. Potter GM, Doubal FN, Jackson CA, Chappell FM, Sudlow CL, Dennis MS, et al. Counting cavitating lacunes underestimates the burden of lacunar infarction. Stroke. 2010;41:267–72.

42. Doubal FN, MacLullich AM, Ferguson KJ, Dennis MS, Wardlaw JM. Enlarged perivascular spaces on MRI are a feature of cerebral small vessel disease. Stroke. 2010;41:450–4.

43. Schreiber S, Bueche CZ, Garz C, Braun H. Blood brain barrier breakdown as the starting point of cerebral small vessel disease? - New insights from a rat model. Exp Transl Stroke Med. 2013;5:4.

44. Farrall AJ, Wardlaw JM. Blood–brain barrier: ageing and microvascular disease–systematic review and meta-analysis. Neurobiol Aging. 2009;30:337–52.

45. Rosenberg GA. Inflammation and white matter damage in vascular cognitive impairment. Stroke. 2009;40:S20–3.

46. Heye AK, Culling RD, Valdes Hernandez Mdel C, Thrippleton MJ, Wardlaw JM. Assessment of blood–brain barrier disruption using dynamic contrast-enhanced MRI. A systematic review. Neuroimage Clin. 2014;6:262–74.

16

Longitudinal follow up of coiled intracranial aneurysms: the impact of contrast enhanced MRA in comparison to 3DTOF MRA at 3T

Nicoletta Anzalone[*], C. De Filippis, F. Scomazzoni, G. Calori, A. Iadanza, F. Simionato and C. Righi

Abstract

Background: The role of 3DTOF MRA in the follow up (FU) of coiled cerebral aneurysms is well established. Though CEMRA (Contrast Enhanced Magnetic Resonance Angiography) has demonstrated to be superior to 3DTOF MRA in showing aneurysms residual patency, its role is still debated. The aim of this study was to verify if there is an added value of CEMRA in the long term follow up of coiled treated aneurysms.

Methods: Sixty-four cerebral aneurysms treated with GDC coils regularly followed up with 3DTOF and CEMRA at 3T every year for at least four years were included in the study. Both MR exams were evaluated and scored according to Montreal scale. Residual patency rates and modifications during follow up as depicted by the two techniques on the three item score of the Montreal scale (TO = total occlusion, NR = neck remnant and AR = aneurysm remnant) were registered along with management decisions. Intertechnique agreement was evaluated with respect to patency scoring in earlier and later stages of FU. Moreover the predictive value of earlier scores for both acquisitions with respect to management decision was assessed.

Results: At 1 year FU, TO to NR to AR score ratios were 31/23/10 and 22/31/11 for 3DTOF and CEMRA respectively, whereas at 4 years FU they evolved to 28/22/14 and 19/28/17 respectively. Fifteen patencies (all AR) out of 64 aneurysms were judged suitable of retreatment evaluation during FU and 8 retreatments were effectively performed after overall benefit/risk ratio considerations. All 15 reopenings were equally depicted by both techniques except one that was depicted earlier on CEMRA. Among the 9 TO at TOF MRA and NR at CEMRA at 1 year, 3 cases enlarged to NR at TOF at 4 years, most remained stable. Among the 22 cases judged NR at 1 years with both techniques, 3 cases showed enlargement at both techniques, while in other 3 cases AR was evident only at 3DCEMRA and they were not retreated.

Conclusions: CEMRA superiority in depiction of intracranial aneurysms recanalization is confirmed by our data. Nevertheless a clear impact in patient management is apparently not evident. Evidence of occlusion at 3DTOF FU may not need the addition of a CEMRA study.

* Correspondence: anzalone.nicoletta@hsr.it
Neuroradiology Department, Biostatistic Department, S Raffaele Hospital, Milan, Italy

Background

The role of Magnetic Resonance Angiography (MRA) in the follow up of coiled cerebral aneurysms is well recognized. Many papers have reported the high accuracy of 3DTOF MRA in depicting aneurysms recanalization when compared to DSA (Digital Subtraction Angiography) [1]. Moreover the use of higher field has shown to improve accuracy [2, 5].

Contrast enhanced MRA (CEMRA) has been proposed in the follow up of coiled aneurysms with the aim to reduce the impact of coils artifacts on the evaluation of aneurysm recanalization. Data from the literature are partly incoherent in showing the advantage of CEMRA in aneurysms patency depiction, partly due to the small sample size in the series [3, 4, 6, 7, 9, 10, 12]; nevertheless there is a general agreement in recognizing the advantage of contrast acquisitions in the better depiction of aneurysm remnant either small or large.

A higher sensitivity of CEMRA has been particularly proved in the evaluation of small type 1 patencies (NR), often not evident at 3DTOF where the aneurysm is judged occluded [5, 12]. Nevertheless a clear advantage of this finding, relative to patient treatment is not known; generally such remnants are not considered to be worth a retreatment by most endovascular therapists and we do not know if they will grow to become treatable. Consequently a clear advantage of CEMRA on a clinical perspective is unknown.

No real data on the longitudinal follow up of coiled aneurysms with the aim to compare unenhanced with enhanced acquisitions are available. Pierot L et al. [8] have reported a series of cases with coiled cerebral aneurysms followed up with 3DTOF and CEMRA with a mean interval time from treatment of 22.7 months. They came to the conclusion that 3DTOF MRA was equivalent to CEMRA in the detection of occlusion and better in showing coils. Nevertheless, their data do not cover the span of a longitudinal FU monitoring and therefore no predictiveness test is available of previous to subsequent stages of FU monitoring data. Our aim was to compare 3DTOF MRA and CEMRA in the longitudinal follow up of a series of coiled cerebral aneurysms and verify wether or not a higher depiction of neck remnants at CEMRA at earlier stages of FU is predictive of subsequent growth and if it played a significant impact on management decisions.

Methods

According to internal procedure all patients with ruptured or unruptured cerebral aneurysms treated with coils are followed up with MRA at 3T within one year from the procedure and then once a year for at least 5 years. DSA is performed when retreatment is considered in the presence of aneurysm recanalization.

From June 2004 to December 2010 all coiled aneurysms that were regularly followed up with 3DTOF and 3DCEMRA at 3T for at least 4 years were included in this retrospective evaluation.

MRA

Magnetic resonance angiography exams were performed on 3T Philips equipment (Intera from 2004 upgraded to Achieva in December 2012, Philips, Best, The Netherlands); the parameters are shown in Table 1. 3DTOF acquisition was acquired first, followed by 3DCEMRA after bolus injection of 0.2-0.1 ml/kg of gadolinium (GDBOPTA, Bracco - Gadobutrol, Bayer Healthcare) at 2 ml/sec followed by 20 ml of saline with a bolus track technique.

Data collection

Clinical data regarding patients (age and gender), aneurysm size, location and history (ruptured and unruptured) were collected.

Aneurysm location was classified in four groups: anterior communicating artery (AcoA), middle cerebral artery (MCA), internal carotid artery (ICA), vertebro-basilar system (VB).

Aneurysm size was classified into: small < 10 mm (separated in smaller and larger than 5 mm), large between 10 mm and 25 mm, giant > 25 mm.

During follow up retreated cases were registered; moreover cases judged suitable for retreatment on the MRA results, but not retreated due to clinical-technical unfavourable conditions were also registered as "intention to treat" group.

Data analysis

MRA datasets included source images, MIP reconstructions and volume rendering reconstructions from both acquisitions for all the four years follow up.

Table 1 Parameters of 3DTOF and 3DCEMRA at 3T

	3D-TOF	CEMRA
TE (ms)	3.5	1.8
TR (MS)	23	5.9
FOV	250	220
Matrix	1024 x 1024	304 (ric. 512)
SENSE factor	2.5	3
Slices	180	180
Voxel size	0.5x0.5x1 mm	0.72x0.72x0.80 mm (ric 0.4x0.4x0.4)
Time acquisition	7 min	24 sec

All images were evaluated by a senior neuroradiologist dedicated to MRA. 3DTOF and 3DCEMRA were evaluated blindly and separately in a random order. In all the cases the pre-treatment and end of procedure DSA exams were also evaluated to have notion of aneurysm location, shape, end procedure results and coil position. This is of particular importance in the evaluation of neck remnants.

Aneurysm status was evaluated using the three grade score on the Montreal scale [14, 15]: 0 (Total Occlusion:TO), 1 (Neck Remnant:NR), 2 (Aneurysm Remnant:AR).

Then, Montreal score was assigned to each aneurysm both by 3DTOF and CEMRA acquisitions for each year of follow up.

Statistical analysis

Kappa statistics were used to obtain intertechnique agreement at year 1 and year 4 for each investigation. The interpretation of K was as follow, according to Landis and Koch: k < 0 indicated no agreement; k = 0-0.19 poor agreement; k = 0.20-0.39 fair agreement; k = 0.40-0.59 moderate agreement; K = 0.60-0.79 substantial agreement; and k = 0.80-1.00 almost perfect agreement [16].

McNemar –Bowker test was calculated for each MRA technique to investigate score modifications during the entire length of follow up.

Area under receiver –operating characteristics (ROC) curves were calculated in order to compare the predictive role of 3DTOF and 3DCEMRA at 1 year on the judgement of suitableness to retreatment.

Analysis were performed with SPSS 18 version.

Results

A total of 64 cases satisfied the inclusion criteria and were included in the retrospective evaluation. The population consisted of 14 males and 50 women, age: 33–74 years, mean 56,2 + – 11,1 years, median 55 years.

Thirthy aneurysms were ruptured (46,8 %) and 34 (53,12 %) unruptured. Aneurysms location was ACA/AcomA in 35, ICA in 15,VB in 14. According to pre-treatment aneurysms size, 50 aneurysms measured <5 mm, 12 between 5 and 10 mm, and 2 > 10 mm. Montreal scale score at the end of procedure was: 33 aneurysms TO, 28 NR, 3 AR.

A total of 512 MRA datasets were evaluated.

Aneurysm occlusion/patency

AT 1 year FU, TO to NR to AR Montreal scale scores ratios were 31/23/10 (48/36/16 %) and 22/31/11 (34/49/17 %) at 3DTOF and CEMRA respectively, whereas at 4 years FU they evolved to 28/22/14 (44/34/22 %) and 19/28/17 (30/44/26 %) respectively.

Among 22 cases scored TO in both techniques at 1 year FU, only 3 evolved to NR only at CEMRA. Among the 22 cases scored NR in both techniques at 1 year FU, 3 evolved to AR at 4 year FU in both techniques and 3 additional cases evolved to AR only at CEMRA. In 9 cases scored NR only at CEMRA, none evolved further and 3DTOF ended up scoring NR as well at 4 years FU in 3 of them (Fig. 1).

Fifteen patencies (all AR) out of 64 aneurysms (23 %) were judged suitable of retreatment evaluation during FU and 8 (12,5 %) retreatments were effectively performed after overall benefit/risk ratio considerations. All 15 reopenings were equally depicted by both techniques

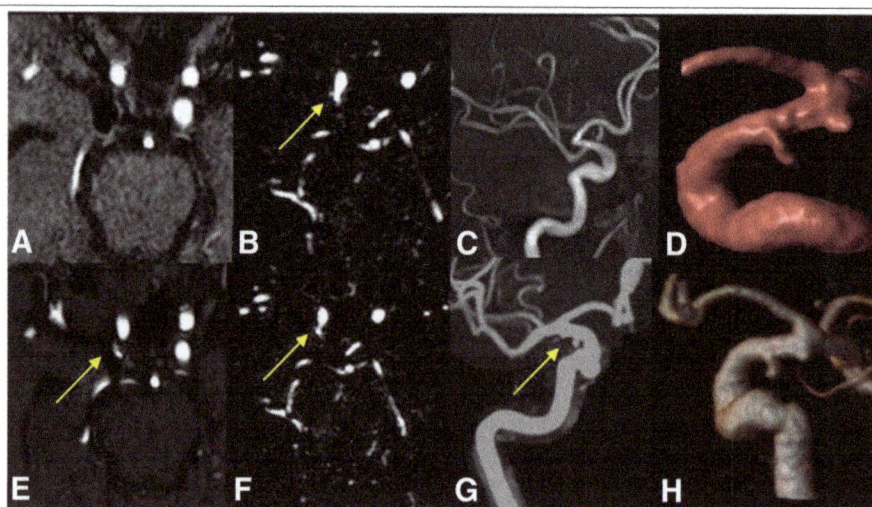

Fig. 1 Internal carotid artery treated aneurysm at 1 year (above) and 4 years (below) FU. At early follow up the remnant is not evident at 3DTOF MRA (**a** and **c**) while it is evident at 3D CEMRA (**b** and **d**, arrow)). At late follow-up the neck remnant is evident at both 3DTOF (**e**, **g**, arrows) and 3DCEMRA (**f**, **h**, arrow), stable

(Fig. 2) except one that was depicted earlier on CEMRA (Fig. 3).

Intermodality agreement and aneurysms grade modification during follow up according to MRA technique

3DTOF/CEMRA intertechnique agreement in Montreal scale scoring was 0.75 (E.S.: 0,07) at 1 year and 0.72 (E.S.: 0,07) at 4 years FU, showing a substantial agreement for both exams.

Both 3DTOF score (p = 0.030) and 3DCEMRA score (p = 0.011) significantly changed at 4 years compared to 1 year; three out of 31 and 3 out of 22 cases rated TO at 1 year FU in 3DTOF and CEMRA respectively evolved to NR at 4 years FU, while 4 out of 23 and 6 out of 31 cases rated NR at 1 year FU in 3DTOF and CEMRA respectively evolved to AR at 4 years FU (Fig. 4).

Aneurysm recanalization and retreatment according to MRA techniques

Area under ROC curves indicated that the performance of 3DTOF and 3DCEMRA in predicting retreatment was very good and very similar, being 0.94 (95 % CI: 0.88; 1) and 0.93 (95 % CI: 0.84; 1) respectively.

Discussion

Our data confirm the higher prevalence of aneurysm recanalization together with better depiction of residual patency in favour of 3DCEMRA that has been already reported in previous studies [5, 12, 13]. Though most of the recanalizations, as known, occur within the first year from treatment, score changes according to Montreal scale are also evident in longer follow up [15]. Longitudinal evaluation of unenhanced and enhanced MRA

available from our data clearly shows that this change is concordant for both techniques and, despite the higher detection of patency with 3DCEMRA, their concordance is good. Most important the data on aneurysms recanalization (AR) showed that all the retreated cases (15,6 %) were equally depicted both temporally and in score assignment by both techniques. Moreover most of AR (14 out of 17) were equally depicted at both techniques, while only 3 cases out of 17 were underscored as NR at 3DTOF; none of these 3 patencies with differential 3DTOF/CEMRA NR to AR scores was considered suitable for retreatment. Among the 15 patencies considered suitable for retreatment evaluation, only in one case 3DCEMRA anticipated the presence of aneurysm remnant that was nevertheless disclosed at 3DTOF as well, only later in time. As a consequence a clear influence on patient management of CEMRA better depiction of aneurysms patencies over 3DTOF does not emerge from our data, even if endovascular therapists may feel sometime more confident in the evaluation of aneurysm recanalization on the basis of CEMRA images. The higher detection by CEMRA of aneurysms patencies can be a sum of less sensitivity to slow flow and to susceptibility artifacts related to coils presence, artifacts known to affect 3DTOF evaluation [11]. Due to the higher sensitivity to slow flow of 3DTOF MRA, it is possible that residual flow at the neck of the treated aneurysm is not evident with this technique, as in the presence of a residual aneurysm with slow or turbolent flow where 3DTOF can underestimate the entity of the patency.

Another important result that came out from our study was the stability in time of most cases rated as NR by CEMRA, rated as TO by 3DTOF. The higher

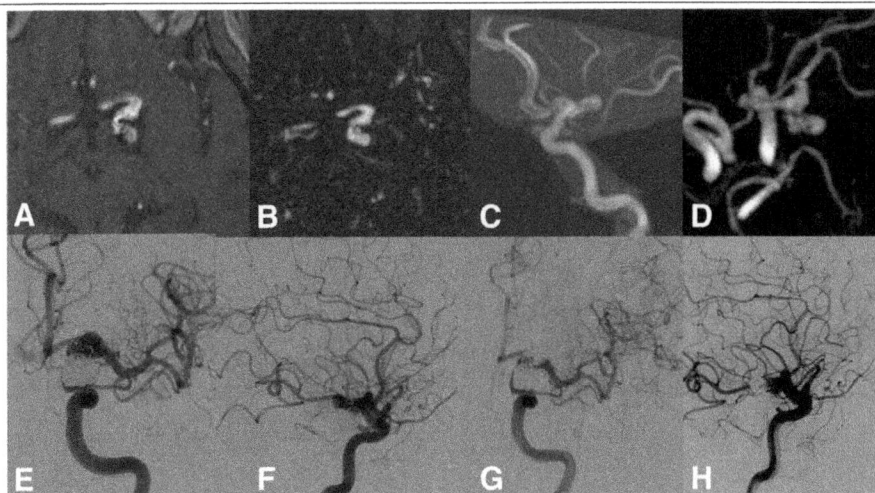

Fig. 2 Internal carotid artery retreated aneurysm. The AR was equally demonstrated at early and late follow up by both 3DTOF (**a**, **c**) and 3DCEMRA (**b**, **d**). DSA confirmed the entity of the patency (**e**, **f**) and the aneurysm was retreated with subtotal occlusion at post procedural DSA (**g**, **h**)

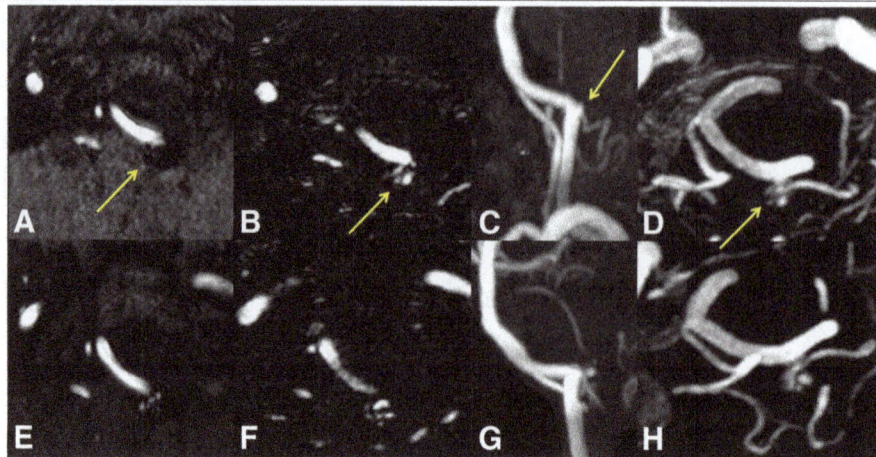

Fig. 3 Left vertebral artery treated aneurysm at 1 year (above) and 4 year (below) FU. At early follow up 3DTOF MRA (**a**, **c**, arrows) scored the aneurysm as NR, while 3DCEMRA (**b**, **d**, arrows) as AR. At late FU the larger remnant was evident also at 3DTOF (**e**, **g**) equally to 3DCEMRA (**f**, **h**)

sensitivity of 3DCEMRA in showing small remnants has been already reported but no data were previously available about the predictive role for further aneurysm recanalization. Our data showed that most of the cases scored as small patencies remained stable and no one enlarged to a higher score.

Another relevant data regard TO rate at one year that in most of the cases (22/28) was equally depicted at both techniques and remained stable (19/22) at following FU. This observation confirms data reported in the literature on large series of treated aneurysms [15].

Sprengers et al. [7] and Pierot et al. [8] had already reported the similar performance of 3DTOF and 3DCEMRA at 3T in the evaluation of aneurysm occlusion, both concluding that the latter is unnecessary in this condition. Our data show that in the presence of aneurysm occlusion at 3DTOF, 3DCEMRA can either show TO or NR, either one avoid of any tendency to further relevant growth in following FU. In this context it seems therefore possible to avoid CEMRA.

Pierot et al. [8] underlie the advantage of 3DTOF in showing coils; indeed the lesser sensitivity to susceptibility artifacts of 3DCEMRA, that allows better evidence of aneurysm enhancing remnant, obscures the images of the aneurysm shape filled of coils that can help in understanding the relationship between the coils and the remnant. On the other hand, if appropriately acquired and timed to the arterial phase, 3DCEMRA acquisitions are less disturbed by movements related artifacts than unenhanced acquisitions.

In our institution we do not regularly perform DSA to follow up coiled aneurysm and arteriography is planned only when a possible aneurysm retreatment is considered. We have a long experience in MRA follow up of coiled aneurysms and from previous published data we have reported a high diagnostic accuracy of both MRA techniques at either 1,5 T and 3T [5, 12]. Moreover as well known, DSA may not always be the ideal technique to disclose aneurysm remnant, due to the frequent possible superimposition of vessels and the consequent

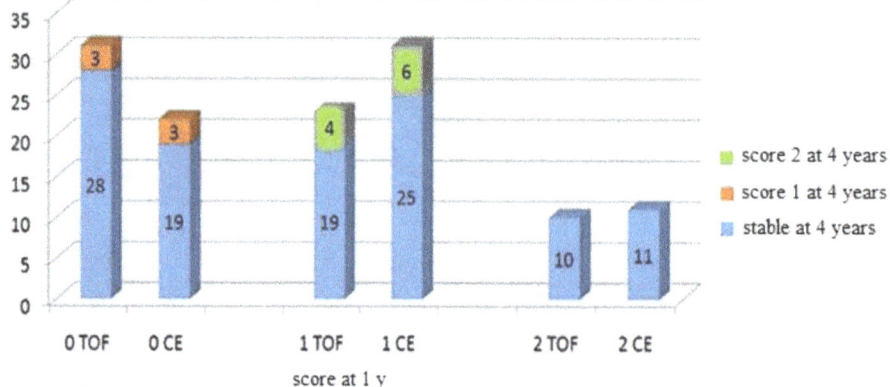

Fig. 4 Treated aneurysms status modifications at 4 years FU compared to 1 year FU

"helmet effect" due to the presence of coils that obscure aneurysm or neck patency. We strongly support the utilization of MRA for coiled aneurysms FU evaluation considering it mature enough to substitute DSA even as gold standard for large series data reporting.

A limitation of this study is the relative small number of cases that does not allow to draw definite conclusions on the possible beneficial impact on outcome of the superiority of CEMRA in the higher demonstration of residual patency in the treated aneurysms.

Nevertheless the data of this first longitudinal follow up evaluation of 3DTOF and 3DCEMRA at 3T in coiled aneurysms show that, despite a higher prevalence of aneurysm and neck remnants demonstrated at 3DCEMRA, no modification in patients management emerged. In front of 3DTOF MRA test negative for residual patency in early FU stages, eventual patencies disclosed by CEMRA proved to be stable at later FU stages.

As opposite, in case of patencies detected at 3DTOF MRA, CEMRA may allow better depiction of the remnant and possibly disclose a larger patency.

Conclusions

Even if from our data CEMRA superiority in the depiction of intracranial aneurysms recanalization is confirmed, a clear impact in patient management is apparently not evident. As a consequence the adjunct of CEMRA to 3DTOF MRA in front of aneurysm patency may be planned on a case to case rather than on a routinary basis, following diagnostic or interventional neuroradiologists judgement. However awareness about a possible underestimation of patencies should be bared in mind.

Evidence of occlusion at 3DTOF FU may not need the addition of a CEMRA study.

Competing interests
The authors declare that they have no competing interest.

Authors' contributions
NANA: project and protocol development, data management, manuscript editing. CDF: data collection and management. FS: data collection, manuscript writing. CG: Statistical analysis. AI: data collection and management. FS: data collection. CR: data collection, protocol design. All authors read and approved the final manuscript.

References

1. Kwee TC, Kwee RM. MR angiography in the follow-up of intracranial aneurysms treated with Guglielmi detachable coils: systematic review and meta-analysis. Neuroradiology. 2007;49:703–13.
2. Urbach H, Dorenbeck U, von Falken hausen M, Wilhelm K, Willinek W, Schaller C, et al. Three dimensional time-of-flight MR angiography at 3T compared to digital subtraction angiography in the follow-up of ruptured and coiled aneurysms. Neuroradiology. 2008;50:383–9.
3. Kaufmann TJ, Huston J, Cloft HJ, Mandrekar J, Gray L, Bernstein MA, et al. A prospective trial of 3T and 1.5T time-of-flight and contrast-enhanced MR angiography in the follow-up of coiled intracranial aneurysms. AJNR Am J Neuroradiol. 2010;31:912–8.
4. Pierot L, Delcourt C, Bouquigny F, Breidt D, Feuillet B, Lanoix O, et al. Follow-up of intracranial aneurysms selectively treated with coils: prospective evaluation of contrast-enhanced MR angiography. AJNR Am J Neuroradiol. 2006;27:744–9.
5. Anzalone N, Scomazzoni F, Cirillo M, Righi C, Simonato F, Cadioli M, et al. Follow-up of coiled aneurysms at 3T: comparison of 3D time-of-flight MR angiography and contrast-enhanced MR angiography. AJNR Am J Neuroradiol. 2008;29:1530–6.
6. Ramgren B, Siemund R, Cronqvist M, Undrén P, Nilsson OG, Holtås S, et al. Follow-up of intracranial aneurysms treated with detachable coils: comparison of 3D inflow MRA at 3T and 1.5T and contrast-enhanced MRA at 3 T with DSA. Neuroradiology. 2008;50:947–54.
7. Sprengers ME, Schaafsma JD, van Rooij WJ, van den Berg R, Rinkel GJ, Akkerman EM, et al. Evaluations of the occlusion status of coiled aneurysms with MR angiography at 3T: is contrast enhancement necessary? AJNR Am J Neuroradiol. 2009;30:1665–71.
8. Pierot L, Portefaix C, Boulin A, Gauvrit JY. Follow-up of coiled intracranial aneurysms: comparison of 3D time-of-flight and contrast-enhanced magnetic resonance angiography at 3T in a large, prospective series. Eur Radiol. 2012;22:2255–63.
9. Gauvrit JY, Leclerc X, Pernodet M, Lubicz B, Lejeune JP, et al. Intracranial aneurysms treated with Guglielmi detachable coils: usefulness of 6-month imaging follow-up with contrast-enhanced MR angiography. AJNR Am J Neuroradiol. 2005 Mar;26(3):515-21.
10. Cirillo M, Scomazzoni F, Cirillo L, Cadioli M, Simonato F, Iadanza A, et al. Comparison of 3D TOF-MRA and 3D CE-MRA at 3T for imaging of intracranial aneurysms. Eur J Radiol. 2013 Dec;82(12):e853-9.
11. Anzalone N, Scomazzoni F, Cirillo M, Cadioli M, Iadanza A, Kirchin MA, et al. Follow-up of coiled cerebral aneurysms: comparison of three-dimensional time-of-flight magnetic resonance angiography at 3 tesla with three-dimensional time-of-flight magnetic resonance angiography and contrast-enhanced magnetic resonance angiography at 1.5 Tesla. Invest Radiol. 2008 Aug;43(8):559-67.
12. Agid R, Willinsky RA, Lee SK, Terbrugge KG, Farb RI. Characterization of aneurysm remnants after endovascular treatment: contrast-enhanced MRA versus catheter digital subtraction angiography. AJNR Am J Neuroradiol. 2008 Sep;29(8):1570-4.
13. Raymond J, Guilbert F, Weill A, Georganos SA, Juravsky L, Lambert A, et al. Long-term angiographic recurrences after selective endovascular treatment of aneurysms with detachable coils. Stroke 2003; 34: 1398-403.
14. Raymond J, Guilbert F, Weill A, Georganos SA, Juravsky L, Lambert A, et al. Long-term angiographic recurrences after selective endovascular treatment of aneurysms with detachable coils. Stroke. 2003;34:1398–403.
15. Roy D, Milot G, Raymond J. Endovascular treatment of unruptured aneurysms. Stroke. 2001;32:1998–2004.
16. Landis JR, Koch GG. The measurement of observer agreement for categorical data. Biometrics. 1977;33:159–74.

17

Cerebral perfusion measurement in brain death with intravoxel incoherent motion imaging

Christian Federau[1,2*], Audrey Nguyen[4], Soren Christensen[5], Luca Saba[3] and Max Wintermark[1]

Abstract

Background: The assessment of brain death can be challenging in critically ill patients, and cerebral perfusion quantification might give information on the brain tissue viability. Intravoxel incoherent motion perfusion imaging is a magnetic resonance imaging technique, which extracts perfusion information from a diffusion-weighted sequence, and provides local, microvascular perfusion assessment without contrast media injection.

Methods: Diffusion weighted images were acquired with 16 b-values (0–900 s/mm^2) in the brain in two patients with cerebral death, confirmed by clinical assessment and evolution, as well as in two age-matched healthy subjects. The intravoxel incoherent motion perfusion fraction maps were obtained by fitting the bi-exponential signal equation model. 8 regions of interest were drawn blindly in the brain neocortex (in the frontal, temporal, parietal, and occipital lobes on both sides) and perfusion fractions were compared between patients with cerebral death and healthy control. Statistical significance was assessed using two-sided Wilcoxon signed rank test, and set to $\alpha < 0.05$.

Results: Intravoxel incoherent motion (IVIM) perfusion fraction was vanishing in the brain of the two patients with cerebral brain death compared to the healthy controls. Mean ($\pm$ standard deviation) cortex perfusion fraction was 0.016 ± 0.005 respectively 0.005 ± 0.008 in the cerebral death patients, compared to respectively 0.052 ± 0.021 ($p = 0.02$) and 0.071 ± 0.042 ($p = 0.008$) in the age-matched controls.

Conclusion: Intravoxel incoherent motion perfusion imaging is a promising tool to assess local brain tissue viability in critically ill patients.

Keywords: Perfusion, IVIM, Brain, Cerebral death

Background

The diagnosis of brain death, as adopted by most countries, is based on clinical criteria that include coma, absence of brain-stem reflexes, and apnea [1]. Nevertheless, additional non-invasive quantitative methods to assess brain tissue viability are of interest, in particular in critically ill patients under anesthesia, in whom clinical assessment is difficult. In this context, perfusion imaging is of particular interest [2].

Intravoxel Incoherent Motion (IVIM) MR perfusion imaging [3] is a method that extracts perfusion information (using a bi-exponential signal equation model)

from diffusion-weighted images acquired at multiple b-values, including low b-values < 200 s/mm^2 (which is the threshold under which perfusion effects are the most prominent). The percentage of "diffusion signal" arising from the microvascular compartment is called the perfusion fraction f, and should be understood as an "effective" cerebral blood volume (in the sense of participating to the "diffusion signal"). While the method can be seen as technically challenging, improvements in hardware and pulse sequences have caused a regain in interest in IVIM perfusion imaging in recent years [4], in particular in the brain [5], mainly because it permits to obtain local cerebral perfusion information without intravenous contrast injection. We applied the IVIM perfusion method in two cases of cerebral brain death, and compared the

* Correspondence: cfederau@stanford.edu
[1]Department of Radiology, Division of Neuroradiology, Stanford University, 300 Pasteur Drive, Stanford 94305-5105, CA, USA
[2]University Hospital Center and University of Lausanne (CHUV-UNIL), Lausanne, Switzerland
Full list of author information is available at the end of the article

results to two healthy age-matched controls, as well as to the conventional Dynamic Susceptibility Contrast (DSC) perfusion imaging.

Methods
IVIM and DSC sequence parameters
A monopolar diffusion-weighted spin-echo EPI sequence was acquired with 16 b-values (0, 10, 20, 40, 80, 110, 140, 170, 200, 300, 400, 500, 600, 700, 800, 900 s/mm^2) in 3 orthogonal directions, from which the trace was calculated. Further acquisition parameters were TR 4000 ms, TE 99 ms, in-plane resolution 1.2x1.2 mm^2, slice thickness 4 mm, parallel imaging acceleration factor 2, 75 % partial Fourier encoding, receiver bandwidth 1086 Hz/pixel. Total acquisition time was 3 min 7 s. IVIM perfusion fraction maps were obtained as previously described [6]. DSC acquisition parameters were: TR/TE = 1950/43 ms; voxel size 1.8 x 1.8 x 6 mm^3); injection dose 0.2 mL/kg; injection rate 3 mL/s.

Quantitative perfusion fraction assessment in cortical regions
Standardized regions of interest of 1 cm^3 were placed blindly by an experienced neuroradiologist on the b0 images, in frontal, temporal, partial, occipital cortex, bilaterally, in the patients and aged matched healthy controls. Statistical significance was assessed using two-sided Wilcoxon signed rank test, and set to $\alpha < 0.05$. Ethic committee approval of the Canton de Vaud, Switzerland, has been obtained for this study.

Patient 1
This 52-year-old patient was transferred from an outside hospital to our emergency department after swallowing 10 g of aconite root extract in suicidal attempt. Starting during the transfer and for 12 h following hospitalization, the patient had multiple episodes of tachycardia and ventricular fibrillation that were treated with multiple electric cardioversions and cardiac massages. A treatment with an intravenous fat emulsion was attempted, with the rational that the structure of aconitine resembles local anesthetics. On hospital day 2, the patient returned to sinus rhythm, but developed acute renal failure, probably on tubular necrosis following the multiple cardiac arrests. The neurologic evolution was unfavorable. The patient never regained consciousness and developed progressively bilateral mydriasis. On hospital day 5, an MRI with IVIM was obtained. On hospital day 7, a clinical examination confirmed cerebral death. External support was withdrawn and his viable organs donated to other patients.

Patient 2
This 7 month-old patient, without history of any known disease, was found with a blue skin tone on the back without spontaneous respiration, 20 min after being seen sleeping normally. Cardiac massage was started immediately and the patient was transferred to our institution. The patient received a total of 600 μg adrenaline intraosseously, and normal cardiac rhythm was re-established 45 min after the start of the reanimation. On neurological examination, the patient presented with a nonreactive bilateral mydriasis, no spontaneous movements and no brain stem reflexes. Images were obtained the day of the admission. The patient presented with multiorgan failure the day after admission, and died.

Results
Patient 1
The MRI obtained demonstrated a diffuse brain edema, bilateral necrotic pallidi and severe swelling of the brain stem and cerebellum, with compression of the mesencephalon and tonsillar herniation through the foramen magnum (Fig. 1a and b). DSC imaging demonstrated a lack of brain perfusion, but preserved perfusion of the scalp, which belongs to the external carotid artery territory (Fig. 1c). Similarly, IVIM perfusion imaging demonstrates no brain perfusion, and similarly to dynamic susceptibility contrast, preserved perfusion of the scalp (Fig. 2). There is some limited residual IVIM signal visible in some posterolateral sulci, which arise probably from incoherent motion of cerebrospinal fluid induced by scanner vibration. Mean (± standard deviation) cortex perfusion fraction in the 8 cortical regions of interest was 0.016 ± 0.005, compared to 0.052 ± 0.021 in the aged-matched healthy ($p = 0.02$).

Patient 2
The MRI showed a diffusely edematous brain, with compression of the brain stem, and herniation through the foramen magnum, with no brain perfusion visible with DSC (Fig. 3). The absence of brain perfusion is well seem on IVIM as well (Fig. 4), and interestingly in this patient, the conserved scalp perfusion is better visible on IVIM compared to DSC, which might be due to slow flow. Mean (± standard deviation) cortex perfusion fraction was 0.005 ± 0.008, compared to 0.071 ± 0.042 in the aged-matched healthy ($p = 0.008$).

Discussion
In these two patients with cerebral brain death, we showed that IVIM could demonstrate lack of cerebral perfusion similarly to DSC. The demonstration of a lack of cerebral circulation can be used as a marker of cerebral death, in addition to neurologic examination. Although cerebral angiography is considered the standard method, CT-angiography [7] and CT perfusion [2] have

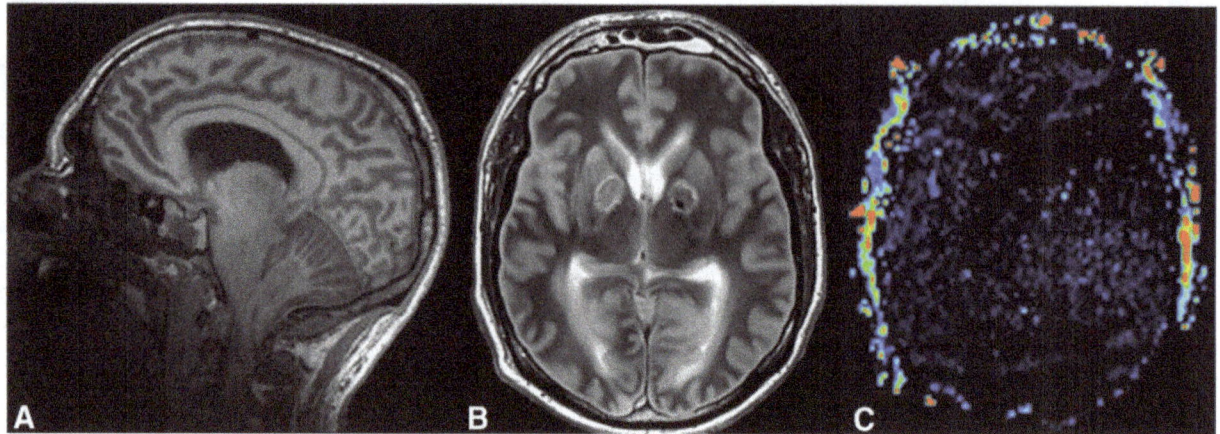

Fig. 1 Patient 1. **a** Sagittal T1-weigthed images demonstrating severe cerebellar edema with brainstem compression and foramen magnum herniation. **b** The T2-weighted axial brain slice shows bilateral basal ganglia necrosis. **c** The dynamic susceptibility contrast MRI cerebral blood volume map shows a lack of brain perfusion, but preserved perfusion of the scalp, which belongs to the perfusion territory of the external carotid artery

also been proposed. IVIM might be of additional interest, because it generates essentially local perfusion maps of microvascular origin, (i.e. from the incoherent motion of blood due to it passage through the microvasculature), therefore using a different paradigm than inflow techniques such as arterial spin labeling or DSC MRI. In other words, IVIM might add complementary perfusion information to currently used perfusion technics. IVIM might add perfusion information of particular interest in the context of slow flow, which may be particularly relevant in cases of brain death, but also, importantly, in the assessment of acute stroke [8, 9].

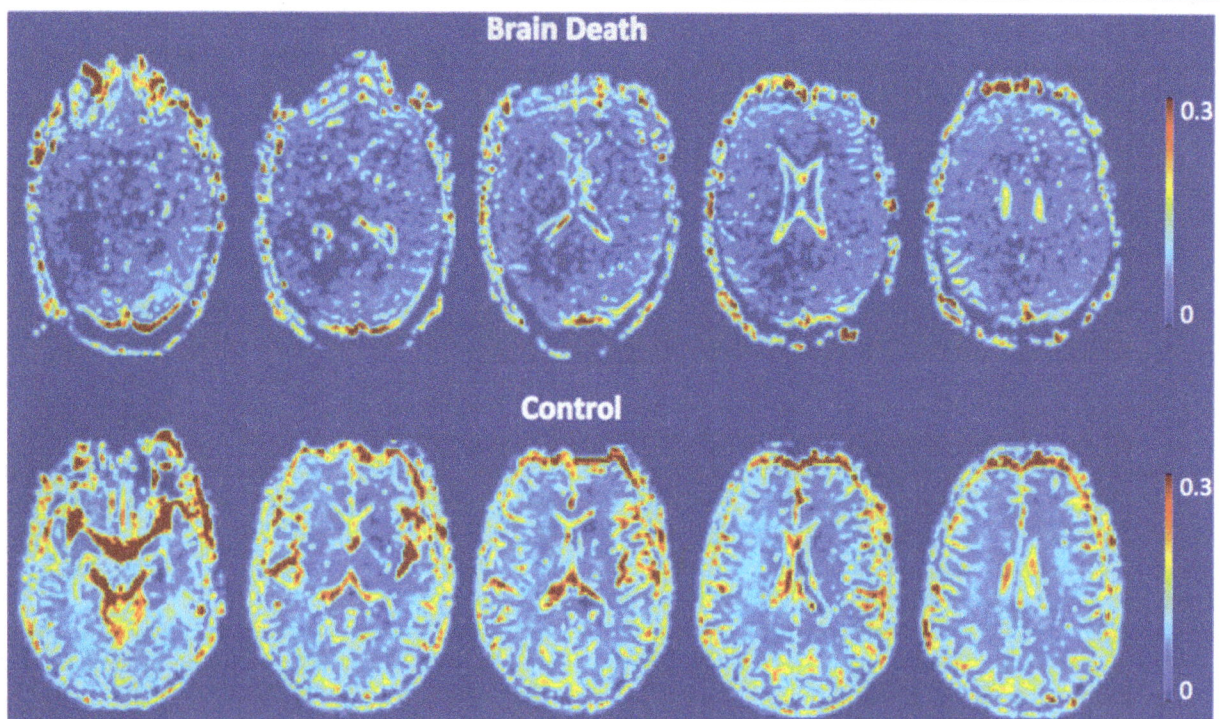

Fig. 2 Patient 1. IVIM perfusion fraction color maps (colorbar unitless), showing a lack of brain perfusion, but preserved perfusion of the scalp, which belongs to the perfusion territory of the external carotid artery. The lower row shows the normal IVIM perfusion fraction in a 25-year-old healthy control

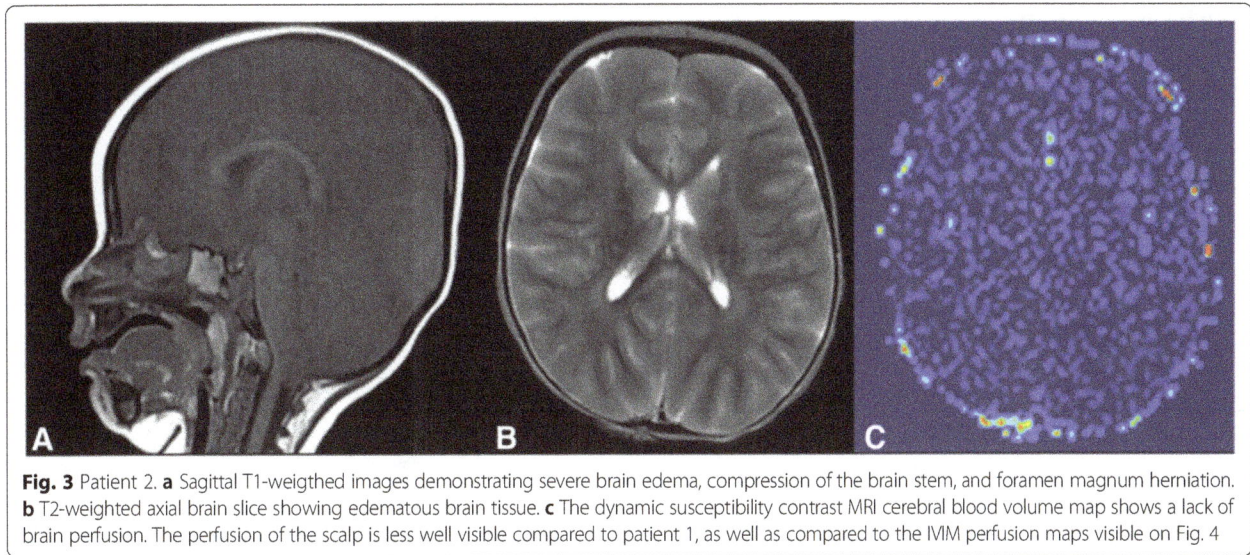

Fig. 3 Patient 2. **a** Sagittal T1-weigthed images demonstrating severe brain edema, compression of the brain stem, and foramen magnum herniation. **b** T2-weighted axial brain slice showing edematous brain tissue. **c** The dynamic susceptibility contrast MRI cerebral blood volume map shows a lack of brain perfusion. The perfusion of the scalp is less well visible compared to patient 1, as well as compared to the IVIM perfusion maps visible on Fig. 4

In addition, no exogenous contrast agent is required with IVIM, and can therefore be used without concerns in critically ill patients, who often have impaired renal function. Nevertheless, the production of high quality IVIM brain perfusion images remains challenging, because the relatively low cerebral perfusion fraction in the brain requires high signal-to-noise-ratio of the raw diffusion-weighted images. In addition, images can be degraded by cerebrospinal fluid pulsations [10], susceptibility artefacts, or the dependence of the IVIM parameters on the cardiac cycle [11].

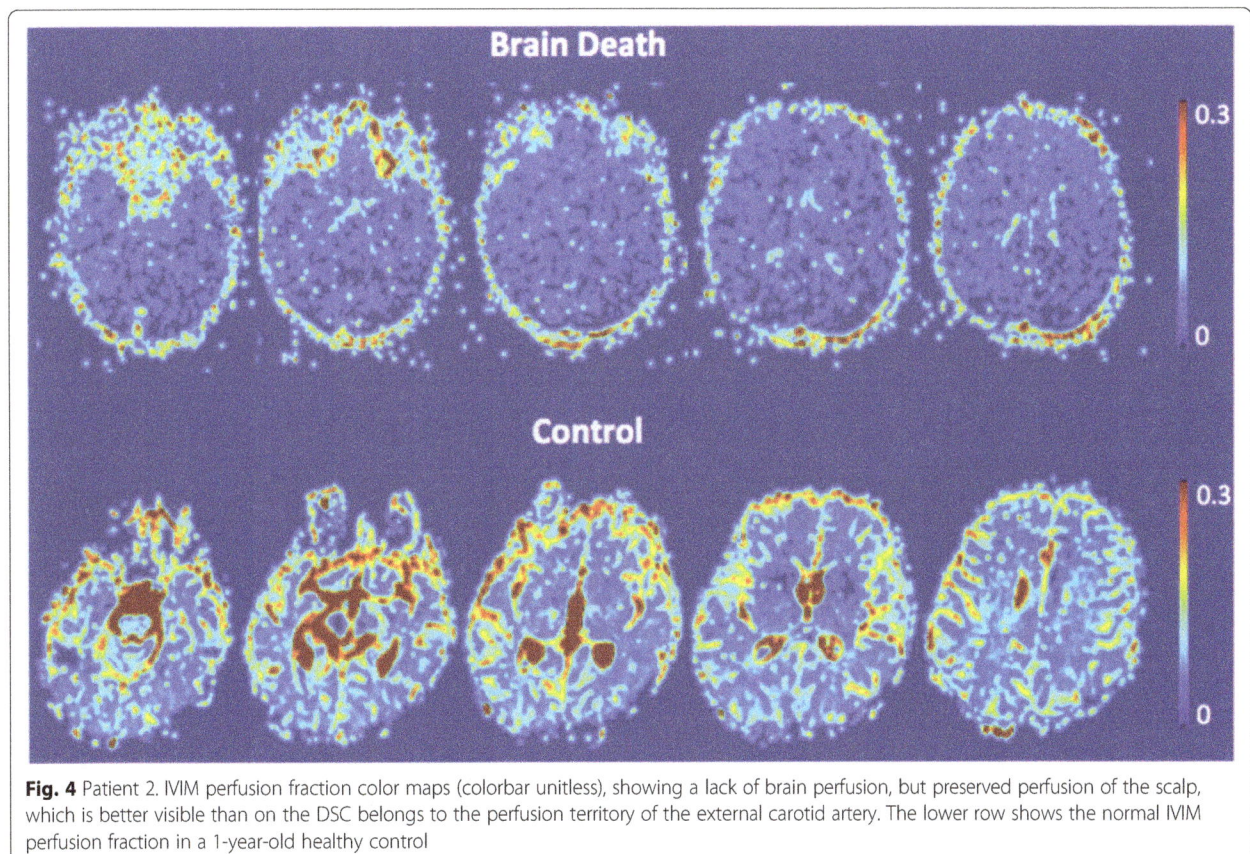

Fig. 4 Patient 2. IVIM perfusion fraction color maps (colorbar unitless), showing a lack of brain perfusion, but preserved perfusion of the scalp, which is better visible than on the DSC belongs to the perfusion territory of the external carotid artery. The lower row shows the normal IVIM perfusion fraction in a 1-year-old healthy control

Conclusion

This report demonstrates that global brain viability can be probed using IVIM perfusion MRI.

Consent

Patient consent was waived by the ethical committee.

Competing interests

The authors declare that they have no competing interests.

Authors' contributions

CF acquired the data, reconstructed the images, analyzed the data, and wrote the manuscript. AN participated in images reconstruction and edited the manuscript. SC participated in data analysis and edited the manuscript. LS and MW participated in the design and coordination of the study. All authors read and approved the final manuscript.

Acknowledgement

Christian Federau was supported by the Swiss National Science Foundation.

Author details

[1]Department of Radiology, Division of Neuroradiology, Stanford University, 300 Pasteur Drive, Stanford 94305-5105, CA, USA. [2]University Hospital Center and University of Lausanne (CHUV-UNIL), Lausanne, Switzerland. [3]Department of Radiology, Azienda Ospedaliero Universitaria di Cagliari, Cagliari, Italy. [4]University of Lausanne, Faculty of Biology and Medicine, Rue du Bugnon 21, Lausanne 1011, Switzerland. [5]Stanford Stroke Center, Stanford University School of Medicine, Stanford, CA, USA.

References

1. Wijdicks EF. The diagnosis of brain death. N Engl J Med. 2001;344(16):1215–21. doi: 10.1056/NEJM200104193441606. [published Online First: Epub Date]|.
2. Shankar JJ, Vandorpe R. CT perfusion for confirmation of brain death. AJNR Am J Neuroradiol. 2013;34(6):1175–9. doi: 10.3174/ajnr.A3376. [published Online First: Epub Date]|.
3. Le Bihan D, Breton E, Lallemand D, et al. Separation of diffusion and perfusion in intravoxel incoherent motion MR imaging. Radiology. 1988; 168(2):497–505. doi: 10.1148/radiology.168.2.3393671. [published Online First: Epub Date]|.
4. Iima M, Le Bihan D. Clinical Intravoxel Incoherent Motion and Diffusion MR Imaging: Past, Present, and Future. Radiology. 2016;278(1):13–32. doi: 10.1148/radiol.2015150244. [published Online First: Epub Date]|.
5. Federau C, O'Brien K, Meuli R, et al. Measuring brain perfusion with intravoxel incoherent motion (IVIM): initial clinical experience. J Magnetic Resonance Imaging. 2014;39(3):624–32. doi: 10.1002/jmri.24195. [published Online First: Epub Date]|.
6. Federau C, Maeder P, O'Brien K, et al. Quantitative measurement of brain perfusion with intravoxel incoherent motion MR imaging. Radiology. 2012; 265(3):874–81. doi: 10.1148/radiol.12120584. [published Online First: Epub Date]|.
7. Frampas E, Videcoq M, de Kerviler E, et al. CT angiography for brain death diagnosis. AJNR Am J Neuroradiol. 2009;30(8):1566–70. doi: 10.3174/ajnr. A1614. [published Online First: Epub Date]|.
8. Federau C, Sumer S, Becce F, et al. Intravoxel incoherent motion perfusion imaging in acute stroke: initial clinical experience. Neuroradiology. 2014;56(8): 629–35. doi: 10.1007/s00234-014-1370-y. [published Online First: Epub Date]|.
9. Suo S, Cao M, Zhu W, et al. Stroke assessment with intravoxel incoherent motion diffusion-weighted MRI. NMR Biomed. 2016;29(3):320–8. doi: 10. 1002/nbm.3467. [published Online First: Epub Date].
10. Federau C, O'Brien K. Increased brain perfusion contrast with T(2)-prepared intravoxel incoherent motion (T2prep IVIM) MRI. NMR Biomed. 2015;28(1):9–16. doi: 10.1002/nbm.3223. [published Online First: Epub Date]|.
11. Federau C, Hagmann P, Maeder P, et al. Dependence of brain intravoxel incoherent motion perfusion parameters on the cardiac cycle. PLoS One. 2013;8(8):e72856. doi: 10.1371/journal.pone.0072856. [published Online First: Epub Date]|.

18

Multimodality CT based imaging to determine clot characteristics and recanalization with intravenous tPA in patients with acute ischemic stroke

Fahad S. Al-Ajlan[1,2,3*], Emmad Qazi[1,2], Chi Kyung Kim[1,4], E. Prasanna Venkatesan[1], Lexi Wilson[1]
and Bijoy K. Menon[1,2,5,6]

Abstract

Acute ischemic stroke (AIS) is a common neurovascular emergency causing significant burden to society. Currently the main focus of AIS treatment is to restore blood flow to at risk brain tissue. For the last twenty years, intravenous tissue plasminogen activator (tPA) was the only proven therapy for patients with AIS. More recently, five randomized clinical trials established the efficacy of endovascular therapy with or without intravenous tPA in selected patient populations with AIS.

Not all stroke patients benefit from intravenous tPA or endovascular treatment. Nonetheless, the concept of early recanalization of occluded arteries resulting in better clinical outcomes is well established. In this focused review, we will discuss how imaging modalities such as Non-Contrast CT, CT-Angiography, and CT-Perfusion can potentially help physicians determine which patients are likely to recanalize early with intravenous tPA and therefore benefit from this therapy.

Keywords: CT, Stroke, Clot, Imaging, Thrombolysis, Angiography, Perfusion

Background

Stroke is the second leading cause of mortality worldwide [http://www.who.int/mediacentre/factsheets/fs310/en/]. In acute ischemic stroke (AIS), clot lysis and early restoration of blood flow to ischemic brain tissue is the ultimate goal of all reperfusion therapies. Recent data from the ESCAPE trial demonstrated that regardless of treatment modality, early effective restoration of blood supply was associated with smaller infarct volumes and better clinical outcome [1].

The recent endovascular clinical trials established the superiority of endovascular therapy (EVT) over intravenous tissue plasminogen activator (IVT) in patients presenting with large vessel anterior circulation occlusions [2–6]. However, in these trials, 5–12% of patients

successfully achieved recanalization (TICI 2b/3) early during first angiography run before EVT (Table 1). An ability to predict which clots will recanalize early with IVT is crucial in the new endovascular era. Identification of this population can lead to better utilization of resources and avoid unnecessary endovascular procedures. This focused review article presents current research on clot characteristics identified using multi-modality CT that can predict early recanalization with IVT alone.

Main text

Theory of clot formation within intracranial arteries

The pathophysiology of clot formation in myocardial infarction is secondary to plaque rupture and thrombosis in situ in 95% [7], while in ischemic stroke it is more diverse and multifactorial (cardio-embolic, arterio-embolic, thrombosis in situ, lacunar, and cryptogenic). The composition of intracranial clots may vary, depending on specific endothelial and blood flow conditions at the source of clot formation (Fig. 1). Old, platelet rich and well-organized clots formed

---
* Correspondence: dr.f-alajlan@hotmail.com
[1]Calgary Stroke Program, Department of Clinical Neurosciences, University of Calgary, Calgary, Canada
[2]Department of Radiology, University of Calgary, Calgary, Canada
Full list of author information is available at the end of the article

Table 1 Percentage of patients achieving successful early recanalization "TICI 2b/3" with IV tPA alone in the recent endovascular trials, evaluated during the first angiography run

Trial	Percentage of patients received IV tPA in control arm	Percentage of patients received IV tPA in EVT arm	Percentage of TICI 2b/3 in first angiography run
MR CLEAN	87.1%	90.6%	no data available
ESCAPE	78.7%	72.7%	5%
EXTEND-IA	100%	100%	12%
SWIFT-PRIM	100%	100%	7%
REVASCAT	77.7%	68%	5%

under flow conditions are likely more resistant to thrombolysis than fresh, fibrin- and red blood cell-rich clots formed under conditions of stasis. Time can also affect clot composition: as time passes, extensive fibrin deposition and cross-linking results in complex organized clots that are more resistant to lysis with IVT. The concept of "Time is Brain" is now being qualified

by another statement "Time is Clot". Clot formation within the intracranial tree is therefore a dynamic time-dependent process. The efficacy of IVT potentially depends on the age of the clot. As time passes, extensive fibrin deposition and cross-linking results in complex and organized clots makes them more resistant to lysis with IVT. Muchada et al. [8] found that the effect of IVT on early recanalization decreases over time. Another recent study revealed that clot volume reduction was independently related to time from stroke symptom onset to IVT [9].

To better explain clot formation and organization over time within the intracranial tree in patients with acute ischemic stroke, we recently suggested a theoretical framework wherein intracranial clots have two components [10]. The first is the "original clot" that comes from a proximal source or is formed in-situ due to endo-luminal factors, and the second is new clot that forms over time from stasis of blood flow around the original clot (Figs. 2 and 3). The extent of new clot formation due to stasis around the original clot is dependent on the patient's collateral status and

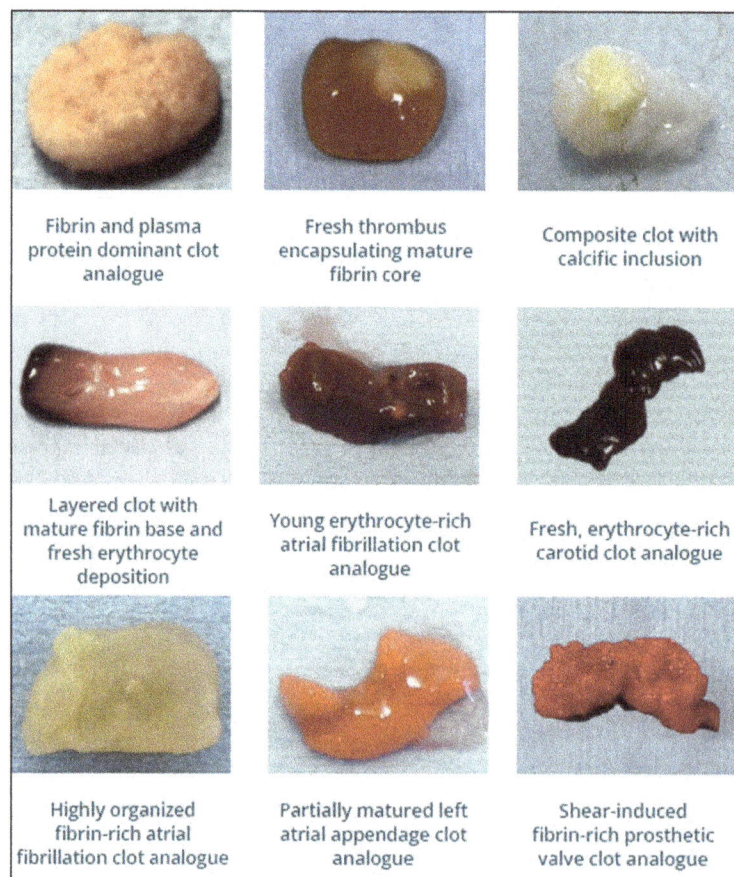

Fig. 1 Clot analogues showing that the composition of the clot material and clot structure may differ, based on endothelial factors and flow dynamic of the source [46]

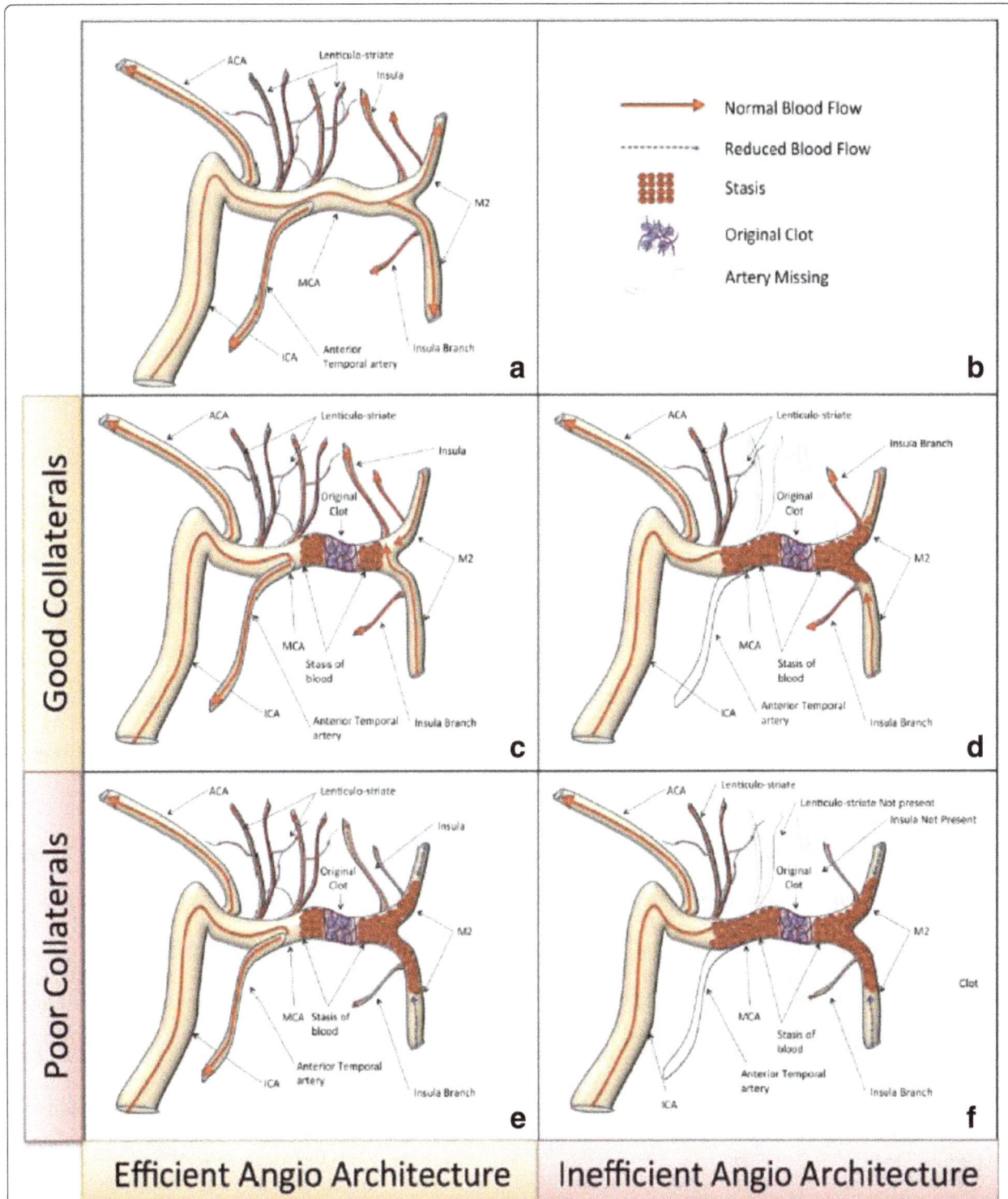

Fig. 2 The length of a clot depends on pial collateral status, and the branching pattern of arteries (angio-architecture) around the original clot. Panel (**a**) shows normal internal carotid artery and its branching vessels. (**b**) is the explanation of the sympoles. We think it is a self-explanatory. Panels (**c-f**) show varying clot lengths depending on pial collateral status and angio-architecture around the original clot. Panel **c** shows small clot with minimal stasis due to good collaterals and efficient angio-architecture. Panel (**d**) shows longer overall clot with good collaterals but inefficient angio-architecture. Panel (**e**) shows long clot due to poor collaterals. Panel (**f**) shows a very long clot because of poor collaterals and inefficient angio-architecture. Adapted from Qazi et al. 2015 [10]

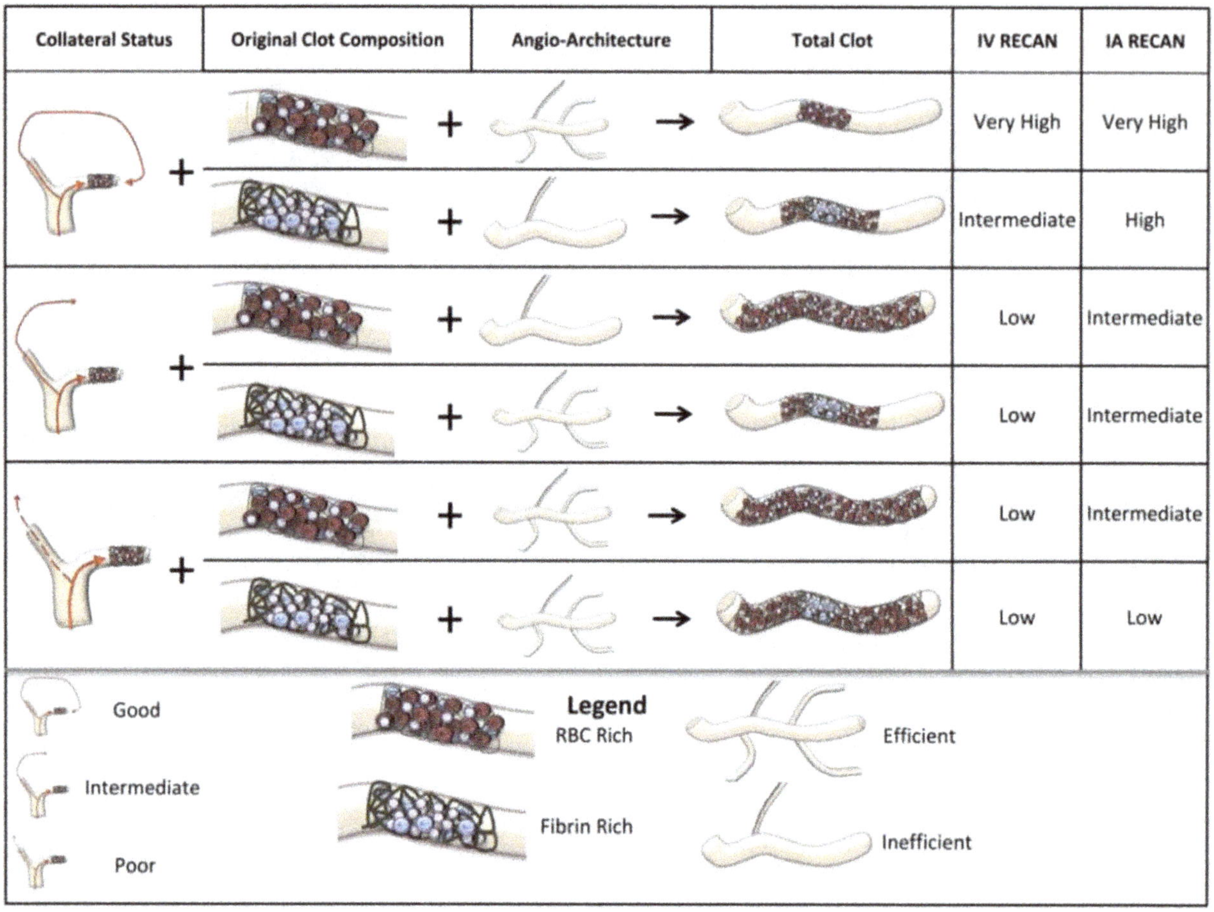

Collateral Status	Original Clot Composition	Angio-Architecture	Total Clot	IV RECAN	IA RECAN
				Very High	Very High
				Intermediate	High
				Low	Intermediate
				Low	Intermediate
				Low	Intermediate
				Low	Low

Legend

Good — Intermediate — Poor

RBC Rich — Fibrin Rich

Efficient — Inefficient

Fig. 3 A theoretical explanation of recanalization response to IV tPA and intra-arterial therapy based on collateral status, original composition of clot, and efficiency of angio-architecture. All possible combinations are not included. Adapted from Qazi et al. 2015 [10]

branching pattern of vessels around the clot (angio-architecture) (Figs. 1 and 2). The original clot can be either RBC- or platelet-rich depending on where it is formed, but the new clot that is formed around the original clot is RBC rich to begin with. Over time, this new clot becomes organized and undergoes changes. In this review, we use this theoretical model to explain how CT-based clot imaging can predict clot lysis with IVT.

Non-contrast computed tomography

NCCT is quick, safe, non-invasive, widely accessible, and well tolerated by critically ill patients. Given these advantages, NCCT has become the primary neuroimaging modality for the assessment of patients with acute neurological emergencies. In evaluating patients with AIS, NCCT is used to rule out intra-cranial hemorrhage and to assess early ischemic changes (EIC) (Fig. 4) [11]. NCCT can also be used to evaluate clot characteristics.

Clot density

The hyperdense artery sign on NCCT has been shown to predict recanalization. This sign is a marker of clot on NCCT within the cerebral arterial network and normally measures 45–80 Hounsfield units (HU). Post-mortem studies have demonstrated that ischemic stroke can be caused by white, red, or mixed blood cell clots [12]. In in vitro experiments, platelet-enriched plasma and whole blood were mixed to produce samples with varying hematocrit levels ranging from 0 to 0·35. These artificial clots were then evaluated by NCCT at various time points from 6 to 144 h. 'Red clots', with the highest hematocrit content, showed densities around 70 HU. 'White clots', with the highest platelet content, were about 20 HU [13]. Interestingly, clots with lower HU were less likely to recanalize compared to clots with higher HU [14, 15]

Problems with detection of the hyperdense artery sign include false positives and false negatives. The average width of the middle cerebral artery (MCA; the most common site of occlusion in AIS) is 3–4 mm [16]. Scans that

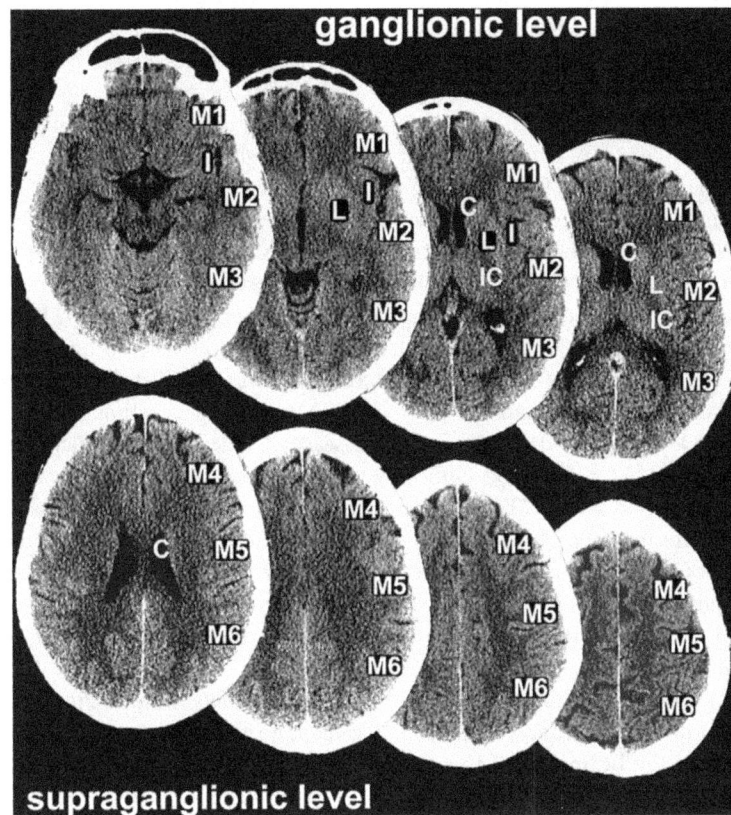

Fig. 4 ASPECTS scoring scheme. The *upper row* demonstrates axial CT cuts of the ganglionic ASPECTS level (M1–M3, insula [I], lentiform nucleus [L], caudate nucleus [C], posterior limb of the internal capsule [IC]). The *lower row* demonstrates CT cuts of the supraganglionic ASPECTS level (M4–M6). As illustrated in the figure, the authors prefer to use cuts in the inferior orbitomeatal line (rather than superior orbitomeatal line). All axial cuts are reviewed for ASPECTS scoring. EIC in the caudate nucleus are scored in the ganglionic level (head of caudate) and supraganglionic level (body and tail of caudate). Adapted from Puetz et al. 2009 [47]

exceed this width and are of average signal may potentially miss detecting the hyperdense sign because of the phenomenon of partial volume averaging. Thin slice NCCT (≤2.5 mm) minimizes volume averaging, significantly improving the signal to noise ratio and producing higher object contrast. [17, 18] Thin slice widths (≤2.5 mm) allow for more sensitive and reliable detection of clots occluding the proximal MCA [19]. The clot detectability is slightly reduced in cases with very small clots or if the site of occlusion is superimposed with imaging artifacts [20]. Recent data from the Third International Stroke Trial (IST-3) showed that the sensitivity, but not specificity, of detecting the hyperdense vessel sign improved with thinner NCCT slices. Slice thickness ≤3 mm had a sensitivity 62%, specificity 98%; versus >3 mm slices, sensitivity 41%, specificity 92%, ($p = 0.031$, $p = 0.089$, respectively) [21]. A major question to be addressed by future studies involves whether a patient specific threshold, taking the hematocrit level and other patient factors for detecting clot length into consideration, is superior to a priori fixed thresholds.

Clot length on NCCT

The length of the hyperdense sign on NCCT is believed to represent the length of the clot. In a 138-patient study, Reidel et al. showed that clots measuring greater than 8 mm on NCCT had less than 1% chance of recanalization with IVT alone and were associated with worse outcome [22]. Recanalization was assessed on follow up TCD, magnetic resonance angiography (MRA), or CT-angiography (CTA). However, clot length in this study was measured on thin slice NCCT (≤2.5 mm) using a three dimensional semi-automated method, which is very time intensive and currently not used in the clinical world. Nevertheless, a more recent study using CTA and 4D-CTA to calculate the clot length challenges the idea that clot length of 8 mm is the longest clot IV tPA can recanalize, indicating that 11 mm may be a more optimal cut-off value [23].

Computed tomography angiography (CTA)

Although conventionally NCCT is the only requisite before IVT administration, additional information provided by CTA is useful in decision-making. CTA is obtained from aortic arch to vertex and it provides information on presence of clot, characteristics of thrombus, tissue ischemia and collaterals.

Assessment of Clot

The location and extent of clot on CTA is an important predictor of clinical outcome in AIS. EVT is only performed for those with target clots in CTA [24, 25]. Successful recanalization by IVT is dependent on clot length [22, 26] or clot burden as measured by CT angiography [27]. In analyses of predictors of early reperfusion using baseline imaging, where early reperfusion was defined as TICI 2a/2b/3, and median clot length in the early reperfusers was 19 mm (IQR 12.9 mm) compared with the non-reperfusers (34.9 mm, IQR 30.7 mm, P .001) [26]. Early recanalization is an independent factor for good clinical outcome [28]. In 80 patients treated with IVT for acute M1 occlusion, Rohan et al. determined clot length using CTA and temporal maximum intensity projection. They found that length of less than 12 mm was an independent predictor for recanalization and good outcome [23]. Another approach for measuring the clot length on CTA used the distance from the carotid T (origin of MCA) to the proximal end of the clot; this study found that a long distance from the carotid T to the beginning of the clot measure on coronal maximum intensity projection images (i.e. more distal clot) was significantly correlated with a good clinical outcome, defined as mRS ≤2 at 90 days [29].

Measuring clot length is challenging. Another method of quantifying clot characteristics is the clot burden score (CBS), a scoring system to define the extent of thrombus in proximal anterior circulation (Fig. 5). It assigns a score of 0–10, determined by subtracting 2 if thrombus is found in each of the supraclinoid ICAs, the proximal half of the MCA trunk, and the distal half of MCA trunk. A score of 1 is subtracted if thrombus is found in the infraclinoid ICA,

anterior cerebral artery (ACA), and for each affected M2 branch. A score of 10 is normal, implying no clot, while a lower score implies greater clot burden. Among 85 patients, those with higher CBS >6 demonstrated smaller final infarct volume and better clinical outcome. A CBS >6 also predicted good recanalization rate with IVT [30]. Analysis of 306 patients with baseline CTA in the Interventional Management of Stroke III (IMS III) Trial was followed by a CTA or MRA after 24 h. It was found that 4.4% of terminal ICA occlusions and 75 –80% of distal M1 and M2 occlusions recanalized with IV tPA [31]. A study of 388 patients with proximal arterial occlusion found that the rates of recanalization were: distal internal carotid artery (ICA) 4.4%; M1-MCA (with or without ICA neck occlusion or stenotic disease) 32.3%; M2-MCA 30.8%; and basilar artery 4% [32].

Multiphase CT angiography (mCTA) is a time-resolved imaging technique that allows assessment of the pial arterial filling by acquiring temporal information at three data points. Hence, it can give a better estimation of clot length and greater insight into the likelihood of arterial recanalization with IVT (Fig. 6) [33].

Clot permeability using multiphase CTA/value of CTA in evaluating the clot

Thrombolysis in any vascular bed depends on the ability of blood and thrombolytic agents to permeate clot [34, 35] Permeation of blood flow through the clot or part of it is defined as residual blood flow; this allows the IVT to reach beyond the proximal part of the clot, leading to higher chance of recanalization. Residual blood flow can be observed in CTA source images by clearly visibly increased contrast attenuation through the clot compared with surrounding brain parenchyma [26]. In the TCD studies, this concept was applied to occluded brain arteries [36, 37]. Using CTA, residual flow within clot was graded – grade 0: clot with no

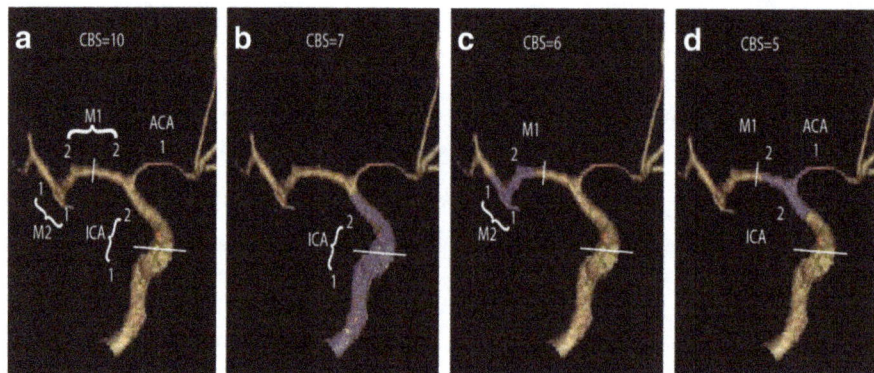

Fig. 5 Illustration of CBS. a, A 10-point score is normal, implying absence of thrombus. Two points (as indicated) are subtracted for thrombus found on CTA in the supraclinoid ICA and each of the proximal and distal halves of the MCA trunk. One point is subtracted for thrombus found in the infraclinoid ICA and A1 segment and for each affected M2 branch. b, Occlusion of infra- and supraclinoid ICAs with a CBS of 7. c, Distal M1 and 2 M2 branch occlusions produce a CBS of 6. d, Occlusion of the terminal ICA, proximal M1, and A1, with a resultant CBS of 5. Adapted from Tan et al. 2009 [30]

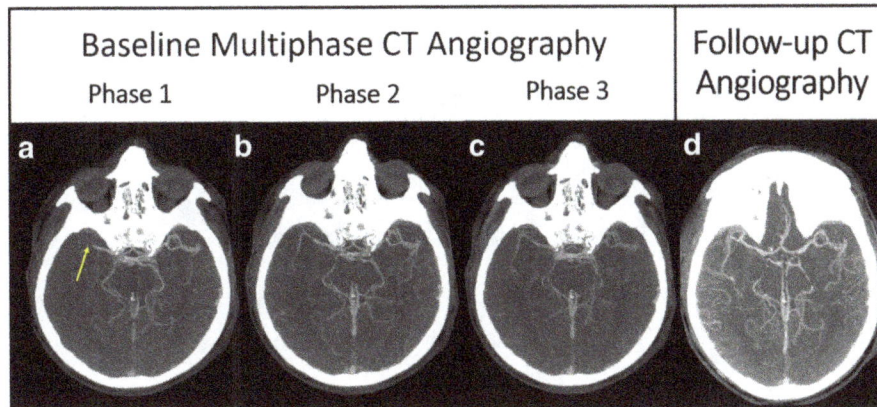

Fig. 6 Multiphase CT angiography image, with each phase and follow-up CT angiography. **a** Peak-arterial Phase 1 image showed right M1 MCA occlusion (*arrow*). **b, (c)** Peak venous Phase 2 and late venous Phase 3 images demonstrate excellent arterial filling beyond the M1 MCA thrombus and no proximal M2 occlusion which was very short in this example (2 mm). **d** Follow-up CT angiography after intravenous thrombolysis administration showed complete recanalization of the arterial occlusion

contrast permeation and attenuation similar to that in surrounding brain parenchyma; grade I: clot appearing denser than surrounding brain parenchyma, with contrast potentially permeating through the clot; grade II: hairline or streak of well-defined contrast across the partial or complete length of clot (Fig. 7). Patients with residual flow within the clot were 5 times more likely to reperfuse than those without (Fig. 8). Residual flow within the clot may not always be visible to the naked eye due to partial volume effects on CTA. If, however, contrast signals at the proximal and distal clot interfaces (in an appropriate venous-weighted scan) are similar, the similarity is a potential marker of residual flow through the clot or of good collateral status. Accordingly, the authors suggested another indirect marker for residual blood flow on CTA: clot interface ratio in Hounsfield units (cirHU). (Figure 9) This is defined as the ratio of proximal thrombus interface HU to distal clot interface

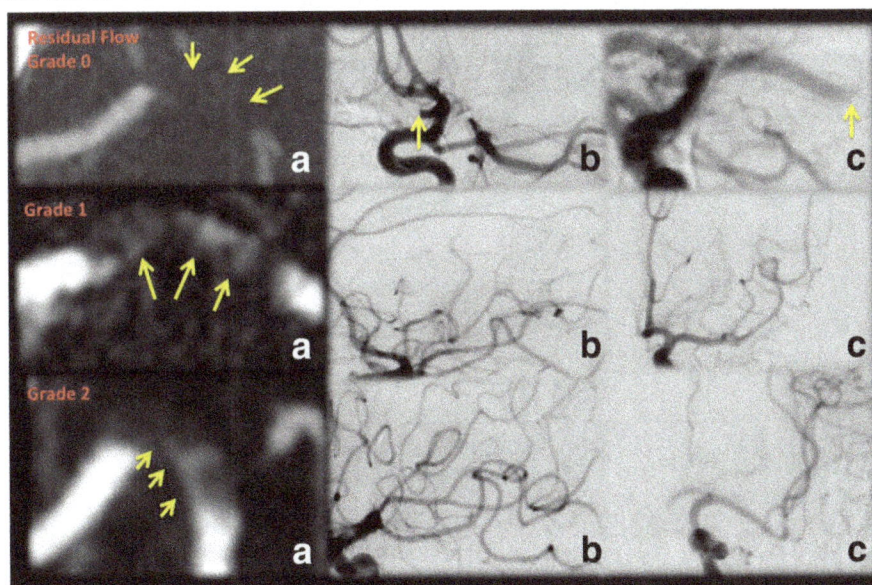

Fig. 7 Residual flow on baseline CT angiography along with early reperfusion with IV tPA assessed on the first angiogram of the ipsilesional arterial tree. The *top panel* shows a patient with a left M1 MCA clot and no residual flow ((**a**), grade 0 residual flow, *yellow arrows*, density similar to that of surrounding brain parenchyma). The first angiogram shows no recanalization (**b** and **c**). The *middle panel* shows a left M1 MCA clot with grade 1 residual flow (A, *yellow arrows*, denser than surrounding brain parenchyma). The first angiogram shows excellent reperfusion (**b** and **c**). The *bottom panel* shows a left M1 MCA clot with grade 2 residual flow (A, *yellow arrows*, hairline or streak of well-defined contrast across the partial or complete length of the clot). The first angiogram shows excellent reperfusion (**b** and **c**). Adapted from Mishra et al. AJNR 2014 [26]

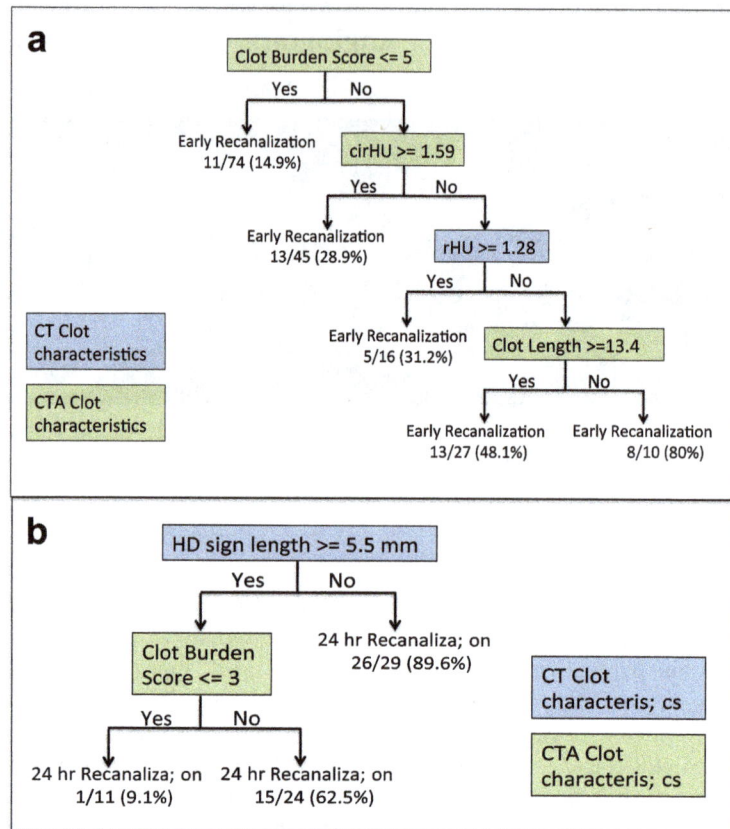

Fig. 8 Panel **a**, CART model determining early recanalization with IV tPA. Panel **b**, CART model determining 24-h recanalization with IV tPA

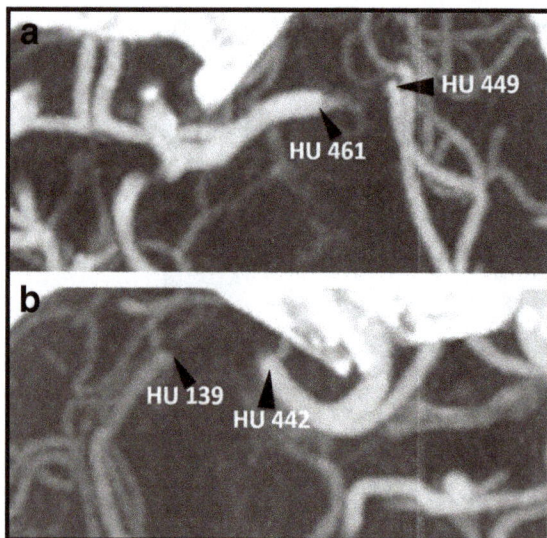

Fig. 9 Clot interface Hounsfield unit ratio calculated by measuring the Hounsfield units in a region of interest selected at the proximal and distal clot interface only in scans that are mid- to late arterial- or appropriate venous-weighted. cirHU is calculated by dividing the proximal clot interface Hounsfield unit by the distal clot interface Hounsfield unit. In (**a**), a patient with a left M1 MCA clot has a cirHU of 1.05 while in (**b**), a patient with a left M1 MCA clot has a cirHU of 3.21 Adapted from Mishra et al. AJNR 2014 [26]

HU. Clot interface ratio >2 implies reduced residual blood flow through the thrombus and is associated with poor recanalization [26].

With these two markers (visible residual flow and cirHU ≥ 2) related to permeability of clots, the researchers suggested a predictive model for early recanalization of occluded arteries after intravenous thrombolysis, incorporating other characteristics of clots (length, location, and distance from the M1 MCA origin to the proximal clot interface) [26].

In most cases, distinguishing between permeable and non-permeable clot requires time-resolved images; because of this, mCTA and CTP have a clear advantage over single-phase CTA for detecting anterograde blood flow through the clot. In a post-hoc analysis of MR CLEAN trial, using quantitative methods on baseline single-phase CTA and NCCT (seen in 44%), Santos et al. showed that permeable clots were associated with improved functional outcome, smaller final infarct volume, higher recanalization rate, and may be associated with improved response to EVT [38]. Although one research group observed that discrepancy of clot length according to phases of CTA in dual-phase CT was associated with collateral status, anterograde flow on DSA, and poor clinical outcomes, they could not find the meaning of this discrepancy of clot length with respect to permeability of clots [39].

Putting it All together: NCCT + CTA

More recent studies on imaging in stroke have endeavoured to assess early and late recanalization by incorporating information from both NCCT and CTA. Menon et al. at presented an abstract at the Radiological Society of North America meeting in 2014 that used data from the interventional management of stroke trial III (IMS III) and utilized clot characteristics from both NCCT and CTA to develop a Classification And Regression Tree (CART) model to predict early and late recanalization success. The clot characteristics derived from NCCT that were included were hyperdense sign (HDS) location, length, and ratio of maximal HDS Hounsfield Unit (HU) to maximal contralateral MCA HU (rHU). CTA clot characteristics included clot burden score, length, residual flow through clot, and ratio of contrast HU at the proximal and distal clot interfaces (cirHU). Early recanalization was assessed on first run digital subtraction angiography on patients given IV-tPA who also underwent endovascular treatment, while late recanalization was assessed on 24 h CTA in patients only treated with IV-tPa. The results show that patients with a clot burden of >5, cirHU <1.59, rHU < 1.28 and clot length of <13.4 still have an 80% chance of early recanalization with IV-tPA alone (Fig. 8). They also show that 62.5% of patients with clots that are >5.5 mm on NCCT but with a clot burden of >3 recanalize within 24 h (Figs. 9 and 10) [26]. Major limitations to this approach are mainly due to the subjectivity of quantifying the residual blood flow. Another point of critique is that calculating the clot interface ratio is not practical in the acute care setting [40].

Computed tomography perfusion

Although CTP is mainly used to evaluate the perfusion status of brain parenchyma in acute stroke patients, some researchers describe the benefits of 4-dimensional (4-D) CTA from CTP source images using multidetector CT scanners. Recent studies have been able to use 4-D CTA to evaluate collateral status more precisely [41, 42] and demarcate thrombus burden better than was possible using conventional CTA [43]. In addition, anterograde flow across occlusion sites of cerebral arteries could be distinguished from retrograde collateral

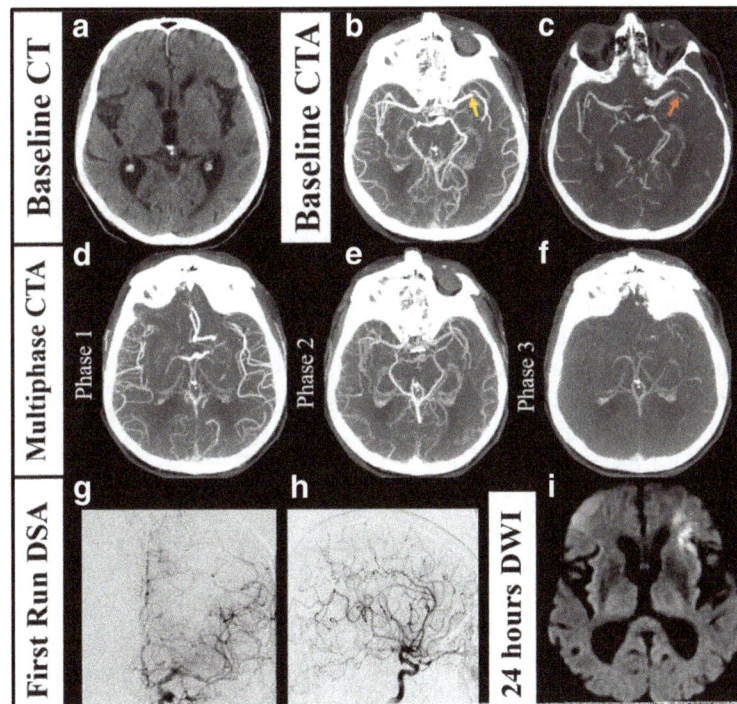

Fig. 10 68-year-old lady presented with acute left MCA syndrome with NIHSS score of 12 treated with IVT 103 min after symptoms onset after reviewing the NCCT. **a.** Axial NCCT at ganglionic level with ASPECTS of 10. **b.** Axial CTA, the *yellow arrow* points to distal M1-MCA occlusion. **c.** Axial CTA, the *red arrow* points to well-defined contrast permeation within the clot. **d – f.** Multiphase CTA MIP images, showing good collaterals with best arterial backfilling seen in phase 1. **g – h.** Conventional cerebral angiogram performed immediately after IVT, the first intracranial run demonstrates a successful reperfusion (TICI 3) with IVT. **i.** Follow-up diffusion-weighted MRI (DWI), obtained 2 days later, shows shows small areas of restricted diffusion in the territory of the MCA. The patient 90 day mRS was zero

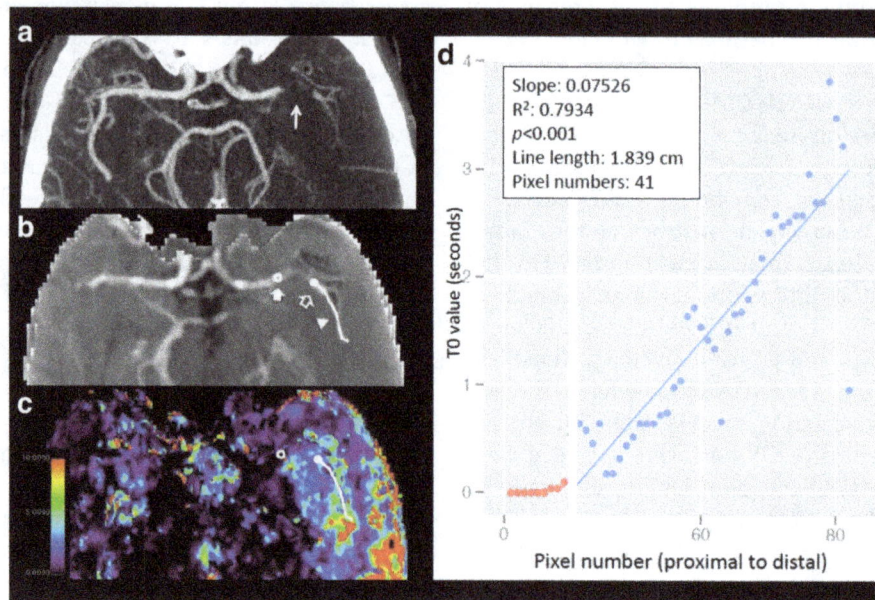

Fig. 11 After identifying a complete occlusion on computed tomographic angiography (CTA; **a**; *white arrow*), regions of interest are drawn at the proximal (**b**), *solid white arrow*) and distal thrombus interface (B, *hollow white arrow*) of the thrombus on the CT perfusion (CTP) average map (**b**). A line profile (*white arrow head*) is drawn along the silhouette of the artery distal to the thrombus on the CTP-average map. The CTP-average map is then coregistered with the CTP T0 map (**c**). T0 values vs distance (pixel number) along the line profile are then plotted and the line of best-fit determined (**d**); T0 values at proximal and distal thrombus interface are also measured. **d**, In this patient, the presence of a positive artery profile slope suggests the presence of anterograde flow distal to thrombus. Adapted from Ahn et al. Stroke 2015 [45]

filling noninvasively by 4-D CTA [44]. In addition to this indirect contribution of CTP to imaging of occluded vessels, a recent study shows a direct parameter of CTP that can be used to evaluate the occult anterograde flow of cerebral artery occlusion in acute stroke patients [45]. Using perfusion maps that measure delay in arrival time of contrast within the intracranial artery tree (T0 maps), a positive sloped regression line of T0 values measured along artery silhouette distal to clot was observed as a marker of occult anterograde flow (permeable clot). This marker was associated with early recanalization of occluded arteries after intravenous thrombolysis (67% for anterograde flow versus 30% for retrograde flow). Moreover, the difference in median T0 value between proximal and distal interface of clot was also related to early recanalization (71% for ≤ 2 s versus 26% > 2 s) – lower difference between two T0 values indicated occult anterograde flow on clots in occluded vessels (Fig. 11). The use of CTP to quantify the occult anterograde flow has limitations, however. It is technically challenging and can only be measured using experts' input. CTP is also susceptible to motion artifacts.

Conclusion

Multimodality CT has become an essential tool to evaluate patients with AIS and facilitate treatment decisions. It can provide more details about clot

characteristics and can be used to tailor the treatment decision of whether further recanalization with EVT should be attempted. More research effort is needed to help aid the clinical decision about proceeding with EVT or treating with IVT only. Furthermore, neuroimaging of the clot is an important topic in modern stroke management and should be pursued to a greater extent.

Abbreviations
AIS: Acute ischemic stroke; CTA: Computed tomography angiography; CTP: Computed tomography perfusion; EVT: Endovascular therapy; IVT: Intravenous tissue plasminogen activator

Acknowledgements
None.

Funding
No funding to report.

Authors' contributions
FSA, BKM review concept and design, drafting the manuscript, critical revision of the manuscript content. EQ, CKK, EPV, LW drafting the manuscript, critical revision of the manuscript content. All authors read and approved the final manuscript.

Competing interests
All authors declare that they have no competing interests.

Declarations

Our current manuscript does not report any studies involving human participants, human data or human tissue.

Author details

[1]Calgary Stroke Program, Department of Clinical Neurosciences, University of Calgary, Calgary, Canada. [2]Department of Radiology, University of Calgary, Calgary, Canada. [3]Department of Neurosciences, King Faisal Specialist Hospital & Research Centre, PO Box 3354 Riyadh11211, MBC 76, Riyadh, Saudi Arabia. [4]Department of Neurology, Korea University Guro Hospital, Seoul, South Korea. [5]Department of Community Health Sciences, University of Calgary, Calgary, Canada. [6]Hotchkiss Brain Institute, Calgary, Canada.

References

1. Al-Ajlan FS, Goyal M, Demchuk AM, et al. Intra-arterial therapy and post-treatment infarct volumes: insights from the ESCAPE randomized controlled trial. Stroke. 2016;47(3):777–81.
2. Berkhemer OA, Fransen PS, Beumer D, et al. A randomized trial of intraarterial treatment for acute ischemic stroke. N Engl J Med. 2015;372(1):11–20.
3. Campbell BC, Mitchell PJ, Kleinig TJ, et al. Endovascular therapy for ischemic stroke with perfusion-imaging selection. N Engl J Med. 2015;372(11):1009–18.
4. Goyal M, Demchuk AM, Menon BK, et al. Randomized assessment of rapid endovascular treatment of ischemic stroke. N Engl J Med. 2015;372(11):1019–30.
5. Saver JL, Goyal M, Bonafe A, et al. Stent-retriever thrombectomy after intravenous t-PA vs. t-PA alone in stroke. N Engl J Med. 2015;372(24):2285–95.
6. Jovin TG, Chamorro A, Cobo E, et al. Thrombectomy within 8 h after symptom onset in ischemic stroke. N Engl J Med. 2015;372(24):2296–306.
7. Arbustini E, Dal Bello B, Morbini P, et al. Plaque erosion is a major substrate for coronary thrombosis in acute myocardial infarction. Heart. 1999;82(3):269–72.
8. Muchada M, Rodriguez-Luna D, Pagola J, et al. Impact of time to treatment on tissue-type plasminogen activator-induced recanalization in acute ischemic stroke. Stroke. 2014;45(9):2734–8.
9. Kim YD, Nam HS, Kim SH, et al. Time-Dependent Thrombus Resolution After Tissue-Type Plasminogen Activator in Patients With Stroke and Mice. Stroke. 2015;46(7):1877–82.
10. Qazi EM, Sohn SI, Mishra S, et al. Thrombus Characteristics Are Related to Collaterals and Angioarchitecture in Acute Stroke. Can J Neurol Sci. 2015;42(6):381–8.
11. Barber PA, Demchuk AM, Zhang J, Buchan AM. Validity and reliability of a quantitative computed tomography score in predicting outcome of hyperacute stroke before thrombolytic therapy. ASPECTS Study Group. Alberta Stroke Programme Early CT Score. Lancet. 2000;355(9216):1670–4.
12. Castaigne P, Lhermitte F, Gautier JC, Escourolle R, Derouesne C. Internal carotid artery occlusion. A study of 61 instances in 50 patients with post-mortem data. Brain. 1970;93(2):231–58.
13. Kirchhof K, Welzel T, Mecke C, Zoubaa S, Sartor K. Differentiation of white, mixed, and red thrombi: value of CT in estimation of the prognosis of thrombolysis phantom study. Radiology. 2003;228(1):126–30.
14. Puig J, Pedraza S, Demchuk A, et al. Quantification of thrombus hounsfield units on noncontrast CT predicts stroke subtype and early recanalization after intravenous recombinant tissue plasminogen activator. AJNR Am J Neuroradiol. 2012;33(1):90–6.
15. Moftakhar P, English JD, Cooke DL, et al. Density of thrombus on admission CT predicts revascularization efficacy in large vessel occlusion acute ischemic stroke. Stroke. 2013;44(1):243–5.
16. Rai AT, Hogg JP, Cline B, Hobbs G. Cerebrovascular geometry in the anterior circulation: an analysis of diameter, length and the vessel taper. J Neurointerv Surg. 2013;5(4):371–5.
17. Barber PA, Demchuk AM, Hudon ME, Pexman JH, Hill MD, Buchan AM. Hyperdense sylvian fissure MCA "dot" sign: A CT marker of acute ischemia. Stroke. 2001;32(1):84–8.
18. Koo CK, Teasdale E, Muir KW. What constitutes a true hyperdense middle cerebral artery sign? Cerebrovasc Dis. 2000;10(6):419–23.
19. Riedel CH, Jensen U, Rohr A, et al. Assessment of thrombus in acute middle cerebral artery occlusion using thin-slice nonenhanced Computed Tomography reconstructions. Stroke. 2010;41(8):1659–64.
20. Riedel CH, Zoubie J, Ulmer S, Gierthmuehlen J, Jansen O. Thin-slice reconstructions of nonenhanced CT images allow for detection of thrombus in acute stroke. Stroke. 2012;43(9):2319–23.
21. Mair G, Boyd EV, Chappell FM, et al. Sensitivity and specificity of the hyperdense artery sign for arterial obstruction in acute ischemic stroke. Stroke. 2015;46(1):102–7.
22. Riedel CH, Zimmermann P, Jensen-Kondering U, Stingele R, Deuschl G, Jansen O. The importance of size: successful recanalization by intravenous thrombolysis in acute anterior stroke depends on thrombus length. Stroke. 2011;42(6):1775–7.
23. Rohan V, Baxa J, Tupy R, et al. Length of occlusion predicts recanalization and outcome after intravenous thrombolysis in middle cerebral artery stroke. Stroke. 2014;45(7):2010–7.
24. Menon BK, Demchuk AM. Computed Tomography Angiography in the Assessment of Patients With Stroke/TIA. Neurohospitalist. 2011;1(4):187–99.
25. Menon BK, Campbell BC, Levi C, Goyal M. Role of imaging in current acute ischemic stroke workflow for endovascular therapy. Stroke. 2015;46(6):1453–61.
26. Mishra SM, Dykeman J, Sajobi TT, et al. Early reperfusion rates with IV tPA are determined by CTA clot characteristics. AJNR Am J Neuroradiol. 2014;35(12):2265–72.
27. Puetz V, Dzialowski I, Hill MD, et al. Intracranial thrombus extent predicts clinical outcome, final infarct size and hemorrhagic transformation in ischemic stroke: the clot burden score. Int J Stroke. 2008;3(4):230–6.
28. Bhatia R, Hill MD, Shobha N, et al. Low rates of acute recanalization with intravenous recombinant tissue plasminogen activator in ischemic stroke: real-world experience and a call for action. Stroke. 2010;41(10):2254–8.
29. Friedrich B, Gawlitza M, Schob S, et al. Distance to thrombus in acute middle cerebral artery occlusion: a predictor of outcome after intravenous thrombolysis for acute ischemic stroke. Stroke. 2015;46(3):692–6.
30. Tan IY, Demchuk AM, Hopyan J, et al. CT angiography clot burden score and collateral score: correlation with clinical and radiologic outcomes in acute middle cerebral artery infarct. AJNR Am J Neuroradiol. 2009;30(3):525–31.
31. Demchuk AM, Goyal M, Yeatts SD, et al. Recanalization and clinical outcome of occlusion sites at baseline CT angiography in the Interventional Management of Stroke III trial. Radiology. 2014;273(1):202–10.
32. Bhatia R, Bal SS, Shobha N, et al. CT angiographic source images predict outcome and final infarct volume better than noncontrast CT in proximal vascular occlusions. Stroke. 2011;42(6):1575–80.
33. Menon BK, d'Esterre CD, Qazi EM, et al. Multiphase CT Angiography: A New Tool for the Imaging Triage of Patients with Acute Ischemic Stroke. Radiology. 2015;275(2):510–20.
34. Blinc A, Francis CW. Transport processes in fibrinolysis and fibrinolytic therapy. Thromb Haemost. 1996;76(4):481–91.
35. Diamond SL, Anand S. Inner clot diffusion and permeation during fibrinolysis. Biophys J. 1993;65(6):2622–43.
36. Saqqur M, Tsivgoulis G, Molina CA, et al. Residual flow at the site of intracranial occlusion on transcranial Doppler predicts response to intravenous thrombolysis: a multi-center study. Cerebrovasc Dis. 2009;27(1):5–12.
37. Ma M, Berger J. A novel TCD grading system for residual flow in stroke patients. Stroke. 2001;32(10):2446.
38. Santos EM, Marquering HA, den Blanken MD, et al. Thrombus Permeability Is Associated With Improved Functional Outcome and Recanalization in Patients With Ischemic Stroke. Stroke. 2016;47(3):732–41.
39. Park M, Kim KE, Shin NY, et al. Thrombus length discrepancy on dual-phase CT can predict clinical outcome in acute ischemic stroke. Eur Radiol. 2015.
40. Menon BK, Goyal M. Clots, Collaterals, and the Intracranial Arterial Tree. Stroke. 2016;47(8):1972–3.
41. Smit EJ, Vonken EJ, van Seeters T, et al. Timing-invariant imaging of collateral vessels in acute ischemic stroke. Stroke; a journal of cerebral circulation. 2013;44(8):2194–9.
42. Frolich AM, Wolff SL, Psychogios MN, et al. Time-resolved assessment of collateral flow using 4D CT angiography in large-vessel occlusion stroke. Eur Radiol. 2014;24(2):390–6.
43. Frolich AM, Schrader D, Klotz E, et al. 4D CT angiography more closely defines intracranial thrombus burden than single-phase CT angiography. AJNR Am J Neuroradiol. 2013;34(10):1908–13.
44. Frolich AM, Psychogios MN, Klotz E, Schramm R, Knauth M, Schramm P. Antegrade flow across incomplete vessel occlusions can be distinguished from retrograde collateral flow using 4-dimensional computed tomographic angiography. Stroke; a journal of cerebral circulation. 2012;43(11):2974–9.
45. Ahn SH, d'Esterre CD, Qazi EM, et al. Occult anterograde flow is an under-recognized but crucial predictor of early recanalization with intravenous tissue-type plasminogen activator. Stroke. 2015;46(4):968–75.

19

Occurrence of intracranial large vessel occlusion in consecutive, non-referred patients with acute ischemic stroke

Debbie Beumer[1,2†], Maxim J. H. L. Mulder[2,4*†], Ghesrouw Saiedie[2,4], Susanne Fonville[2], Robert J. van Oostenbrugge[1], Wim H. van Zwam[3], Philip J. Homburg[5], Aad van der Lugt[4] and Diederik W. J. Dippel[2]

Abstract

Background: The relative frequency of acute intracranial large vessel occlusion (LVO) in patients with acute ischemic stroke (AIS) who could be candidate for intra-arterial treatment (IAT) is not well known. In this study, we determined clinical variables associated with LVO and the proportion of patients with LVO among patients presenting with AIS within 6 h of symptom onset.

Methods: Data of consecutive patients with AIS presenting at the emergency department (ED) of the Erasmus University Medical Center, in the Netherlands, was used. Referrals from other hospitals were excluded.

Results: From 2006 January 1st to 2012 April 30th, 1063 non-referred patients presented at our ED with AIS. 445 (42 %) arrived within 6 h of onset of symptoms. Computed tomography angiography was not performed or was of insufficient quality in 50 patients (11 %) and performed late (≥1 day) in 57 patients (13 %). The remaining 338 with AIS were included in the final analysis. 106 patients (31 %) had LVO, mostly in the anterior circulation (72 %). National Institutes of Health Stroke Scale score was the only variable associated with the presence of LVO (adjusted OR 1.23 per point [95 % Confidence interval: 1.17–1.29]).

Conclusion: Of all patients with acute ischemic stroke who arrive within 6 h of symptom onset at the emergency department, almost one out of three have a intracranial large vessel occlusion and may be candidate for intra-arterial treatment.

Keywords: Large vessel occlusion, Acute ischemic stroke, Thrombectomy candidates, Endovascular procedures, Intra-arterial treatment

Abbreviations: A1, Proximal anterior cerebral artery; AF, Atrial fibrillation; AIS, Acute ischemic stroke; aOR, Adjusted odds ratio; BA, Basilar artery; CI, Confidence interval; ED, Emergency department; ICA, Intracranial internal carotid artery; IAT, Intra-arterial treatment; IVA, Intracranial vertebral artery; IVT, Intravenous alteplase treatment; LVO, Large vessel occlusion; M1, Proximal middle cerebral artery; M2, Distal middle cerebral artery; NIHSS, National Institutes of Health Stroke Scale; P1, Proximal posterior cerebral artery; P2, Distal posterior cerebral artery

* Correspondence: m.mulder@erasmusmc.nl
†Equal contributors
2Department of Neurology, Erasmus MC University Medical Center, Rotterdam, The Netherlands
4Department of Radiology, Erasmus MC University Medical Center, Rotterdam, The Netherlands
Full list of author information is available at the end of the article

Background

Recently published randomized clinical trials showed that intra-arterial treatment (IAT) with retrievable stents for acute ischemic stroke (AIS) was safe and effective in patients with acute intracranial large vessel occlusion (LVO) if they were treated within 6 h of symptom onset [1–6]. Updated guidelines indicate that IAT is now standard of care for AIS patients with LVO [7, 8]. This has great impact on stroke care providers, as the number of performed procedures increases rapidly and resources are limited. To estimate the number of candidates for IAT, it is important to know how many patients with AIS present with LVO.

Observational studies report that 10–61 % of the patients who present at the emergency department (ED) with presumed AIS have LVO. However, these studies did not include unselected, consecutive patients [9], did not use appropriate neuro-imaging in all patients [10], included patients who were transferred from other hospitals [11, 12], or used a restricted time window [13].

Knowledge of the occurrence of LVO is important clinically, for manpower planning and for resource allocation. In this study we describe the occurrence of LVO cases in a consecutive population of all AIS patients admitted to emergency department (ED) within 6 h after onset of symptoms. Moreover, we evaluate clinical predictors of LVO.

Methods

Patients

This retrospective single center study of a consecutive patient cohort was executed by the Erasmus University Medical Center, Rotterdam, the Netherlands. The patient population represents an urban population in a large city, where stroke patients are referred from general practitioners and other centers. Patients with AIS were identified from our Erasmus Stroke Registry, which is operational since 1990. All patients admitted to the ED with a presumed diagnosis of acute stroke are seen by a neurologist or a resident in neurology as part of clinical routine. Patients with AIS were entered into the registry after review and confirmation of the diagnosis by a vascular neurologist. For the present study electronic medical charts and imaging were used. No additional data collection was performed and institutional review board was not needed. All non-referral patients with AIS in the period of From 2006 January 1st to 2012 April 30th who were admitted to the ED were included. Patients had to be 18 years or older. Patients arriving later than 6 h after onset of symptoms at the emergency department were excluded. Patients who did not receive a Computed Tomography Angiography (CTA) or in whom the CTA was of insufficient quality, and patients in whom a CTA was made more than 24 h after intravenous alteplase treatment (IVT) or more than 48 h after

stroke onset were also excluded from the present study. Magnetic resonance imaging was never used instead of CTA.

Clinical variables

We determined the clinical location of the occlusion by categorizing symptoms, described by the attending neurologist or resident in neurology in the medical chart, as belonging to occlusion in the territory of the right or left carotid artery or the vertebrobasilar arteries. Furthermore, the National Institutes of Health Stroke Scale (NIHSS) on admission and time from onset of symptoms to arrival at the ED were assessed. Data on medical history were collected from medical records of the patients. The diagnosis of atrial fibrillation (AF) could be based on pre-existing AF, identified through medical history and de novo AF during hospitalization. All patients were monitored during the first 24 h after AIS and the diagnosis of de novo AF was confirmed by 12-lead ECG. The diagnosis of previous stroke was based on history, transient ischemic attack was not included.

CTA acquisition and analysis

CTA was performed with a 16-slice multidetector CT (MDCT) scanner (Siemens, Sensation 16, Erlangen, Germany), a 64-slice MDCT scanner (Siemens, Sensation 64, Erlangen, Germany) or a 128 slice MDCT scanner (Siemens, Definition AS, Erlangen, Germany) with a standardized optimized contrast-enhanced protocol (100–120 kVp, collimation 16×0.75 mm, 64×0.6 mm, or 128×0.6 mm, pitch ≤1) [14, 15]. The CTA scan ranged from the ascending aorta to the intracranial circulation. Contrast material was given in a bolus of 80 ml (Iodixanol 320 mg/ml, Visipaque, Amersham Health, Little Chalfont, UK), followed by a 40 ml saline bolus chaser. The injection rate was 4 ml/s for both Iodixanol and saline. At the level of the ascending aorta contrast material passage was detected by real time bolus tracking followed by data acquisition. The images were reconstructed by a 100 mm field of view, matrix size 512×512 (real in-plane resolution 0.6x0.6 mm), slice thickness ≤1.0 mm, increment ≤0.6 mm and with an intermediate reconstruction algorithm.

CTA images were sent to a stand-alone workstation (Leonardo, Siemens Medical Solutions, Forchheim, Germany) with dedicated 3D analysis software, and were assessed by experts (GS, PH, AL) who had no clinical information other than a clinical diagnosis of AIS. Of all CTAs the extracranial and intracranial circulation were evaluated blinded without knowledge of the clinical data with multiplanar reformatting software, which allows also reconstruction of sagittal, coronal, and oblique maximum intensity projections from axial sections.

The location of LVO was categorized as: intracranial internal carotid artery (ICA), anterior cerebral artery (A1 segment), proximal middle cerebral artery (M1 segment), distal middle cerebral artery (M2 segment), intracranial vertebral artery (IVA), basilar artery (BA), proximal posterior cerebral artery (P1 segment), distal posterior cerebral artery (P2 segment). Patients suffering from occlusions in multiple segments were categorized by their most proximal intracranial occlusion at the level of the circle of Willis. In addition, occlusions in the extracranial carotid artery and vertebral artery were assessed.

Outcome
LVO was defined as an occlusion in one of the intracranial arteries (ICA, A1, M1, M2, IVA, BA, P1 and P2), accompanied by clinical symptoms that could be attributed to ischemia in the territory of the occluded artery.

Statistical analysis
We used cross tabulation, univariable and multivariable logistic regression analysis. We expressed associations as odds ratios with 95 % confidence intervals (CIs). Statistical analyses were performed with Stata/SE 14.1 (StataCorp. Texas. USA). We considered NIHSS, previous ischemic stroke and AF as possible predictors of occlusion, and we adjusted for age, gender and time to ED.

Results
Over a 6-year period 1063 patients with AIS were admitted to our ED. Of these 1063 patients, 618 (53 %) were excluded because they arrived more than 6 h after onset of symptoms at the emergency department (Fig. 1).

Of the 445 patients who presented within 6 h after onset of symptoms CTA was not performed or of insufficient quality in 50 patients (11 %), and CTA was performed $\geq$ 24 h after IVT or $\geq$48 h after stroke onset in 57 patients (13 %) (Fig. 1). Most of these 107 patients with no or late CTA were admitted in the early phase after implementation of acute CTA in AIS patients (2006–2008). Clinical characteristics, including NIHSS at baseline in these 107 patients (median = 5; IQR:2–12) were similar to the total 338 patients (median = 5; IQR:2–11) with CTA in the acute phase (p = 0.67). Of the remaining 338 patients with clinical symptoms of AIS, 106 patients (31 %) had LVO. These patients had a mean age of 64 ± 15 years and 53 patients (50 %) were male (Table 1). The median NIHSS on admission was 13 (6–18). Of these, 77 patients (73 %) had an occlusion in the anterior circulation and 29 patients (27 %) had an occlusion in the posterior circulation (Table 2).

Clinical predictors of LVO
Only admission NIHSS was associated with LVO (adjusted Odds Ratio (aOR) = 1.23 per NIHSS point increase [95 % CI: 1.17–1.29]) (Table 1). Patients with NIHSS of 1 or 2 had a 10 % likelihood of LVO (Fig. 2). A score of exactly 12 points on NIHSS indicates a likelihood of 50 % for LVO. When NIHSS $\geq$ 12, likelihood of LVO is 75 %. NIHSS of 7 and above corresponds with a > 50 % likelihood of LVO. When NIHSS $\geq$ 20, 21 (91 %) of 23 patients had LVO. Of the two patients with NIHSS $\geq$ 20 without LVO, one had had a previous stroke, with consequently a pre-stroke modified Rankin Scale score of 3 with a spastic hemiparesis; new stroke symptoms

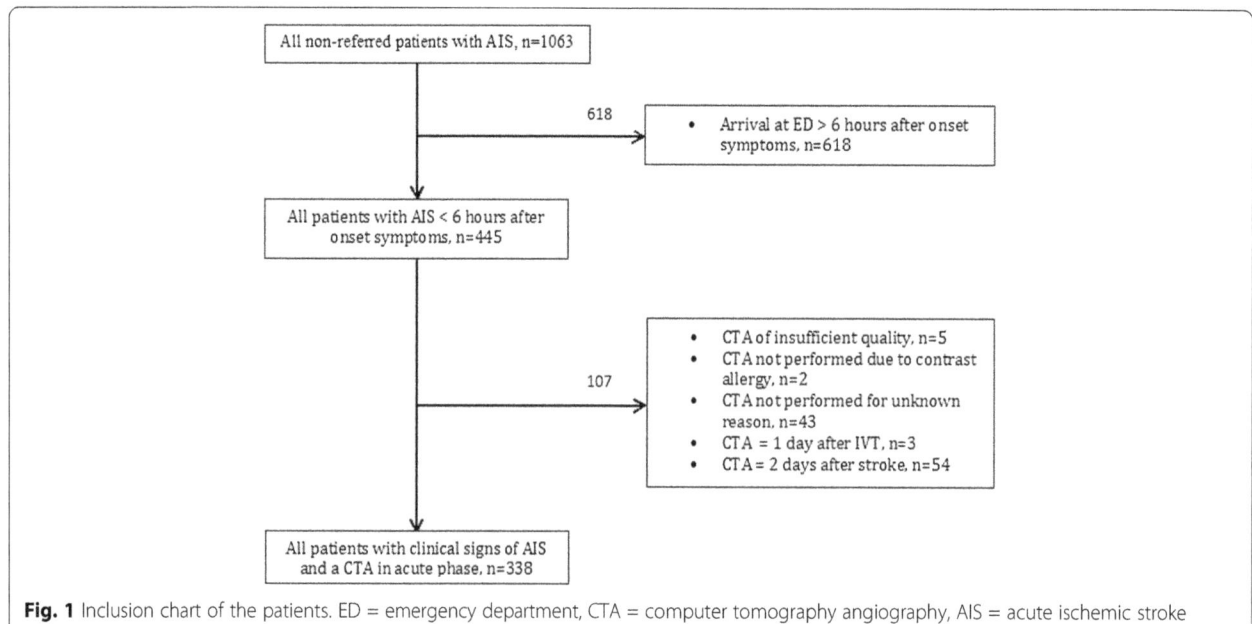

Fig. 1 Inclusion chart of the patients. ED = emergency department, CTA = computer tomography angiography, AIS = acute ischemic stroke

Table 1 Baseline characteristics of the study population with and without acute intracranial large vessel occlusion (LVO)

	LVO (n = 106)	No LVO (n = 232)	P-value
Age (years), mean (SD)	64 (15)	62 (16)	0.26
Male sex, n (%)	53 (50 %)	116 (50 %)	1.00
Caucasian ethnicity, n (%)	81 (76 %)	184 (79 %)	0.55
Systolic blood pressure, mean (SD)	161 (38)	167 (33)	0.16
Diastolic blood pressure, mean (SD)	85 (21)	89 (19)	0.11
BMI (kg/m^2), mean (SD)	28 (3.8)	27 (5.1)	0.50
Glucose (mmol/L), mean (SD)	7.6 (2.4)	7.3 (2.8)	0.33
Previous ischemic stroke, n (%)	18 (17 %)	52 (23 %)	0.22
Previous heart disease, n (%)	14 (13 %)	41 (18 %)	0.28
Atrial fibrillation, n (%)	14 (13 %)	19 (8 %)	0.16
NIHSS on admission, median (IQR)	13 (6-18)	3 (2–7)	<0.01

All patients arrived at the emergency department within 6 h after onset of symptoms and received a CT-angiography of the intracranial circle of Willis in the acute phase. NIHSS on admission significantly differed between both groups

BMI body mass index, *NIHSS* National Institutes of Health Stroke Scale. NIHSS on admission significantly differed between both groups

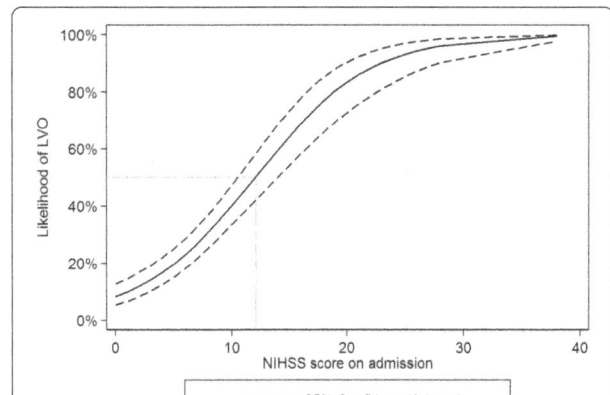

Fig. 2 The association between National Institutes of Health Stroke Scale (NIHSS) and the likelihood of the presence of acute intracranial large vessel occlusion (LVO) confirmed by CTA, in 338 patients with acute ischemic stroke, admitted within 6 h of symptom onset. For each point increase in NIHSS, aOR is 1.23 (95 % CI: 1.17-1.29) for having LVO. At NIHSS 12 the chance of having LVO is 0.5 (50 %)

were aphasia and facial palsy. The other patient who had a NIHSS score of 22, experienced rapid recovery without IVT. No association was found between the presence of LVO and AF (aOR = 1.10 [95 % CI: 0.43–2.79]) or previous ischemic stroke (aOR = 0.69 [95 % CI: 0.34–1.44]) (Table 1).

Table 2 Distribution and location of acute intracranial large vessel occlusion (LVO)

Anatomical location LVO	Number and percentage of total LVO (n = 106)
Anterior circulation (n = 77)	
Anterior cerebral artery, A1 segment, n (%)	0
Intracranial carotid artery, n (%)	23 (22 %)
Middle cerebral artery, M1 segment, n (%)	38 (36 %)
Middle cerebral artery, M2 segment, n (%)	16 (15 %)
Posterior circulation (n = 29)	
Intracranial vertebral artery, n (%)	9 (9 %)
Posterior cerebral artery, P1 segment, n (%)	8 (8 %)
Posterior cerebral artery, P2 segment, n (%)	3 (2 %)
Basilar artery, n (%)	9 (9 %)

A1 first segment of anterior cerebral artery, *M1* first segment of middle cerebral artery, *M2* second segment of middle cerebral artery, *P1* first segment of posterior cerebral artery, *P2* second segment of the posterior cerebral artery

Discussion

This study of an unselected non-referred consecutive cohort of AIS patients arriving at the ED within 6 h of symptom onset, showed that almost one out of three have LVO and may be IAT candidate.

Clinical practice

Our study suggests that almost one third of all patients with AIS may be candidates for IAT, since they had LVO in the proximal anterior or posterior circulation and these LVO locations are currently treated in clinical practice in the Netherlands and registered in the MR CLEAN Registry (www.mrclean-trial.org). This is in concordance with data from Copenhagen where 29 % had LVO. The population in the latter study was different from ours, since only IVT candidates were studied, which implies a restricted time window and extra criteria for candidates in comparison to IAT candidates [13]. However, both these estimates are based on a consecutive AIS population presenting at EDs. In two large and well documented studies from Bern, using an overlapping population, 40–61 % of patients had LVO [12]. However, these studies included patients who were referred from other centers, which implies selection and at least partly explains the higher proportion of patients with LVO. This makes it difficult to extrapolate these estimates to other settings.

Our results confirm that NIHSS score at baseline is the most important predictor of LVO, as reported previously [12, 13, 16]. We found that a vast majority (91 %) of patients with NIHSS ≥ 20 had LVO. This high percentage of occlusion in patients with severe clinical symptoms is in concordance with other studies, where more than 95 % of patients with NIHSS ≥ 20 had an occlusion [12, 13]. However, our study also emphasizes that patients with low NIHSS could have LVO.

Limitations

Several limitations may influence the generalizability of our study results. First, our study was a single center study in an academic hospital. However, our center is a centrally located comprehensive stroke center and it has no restrictions on access to the ED. We present a consecutive series of non-referred patients, which we believe is representative for any urban population in a large city like Rotterdam. Second, 107 patients (24 %) who presented at the ED within 6 h after symptom onset did not get a CTA in the acute phase. Most of these patients were admitted to our hospital in the first years after implementation of acute CTA in AIS patients, in 2006. In that early period CTA was sometimes performed later or not at all, despite being part of standard protocol. Most importantly there was no selection bias based on stroke severity as there was no difference in baseline NIHSS between the patients with and without CTA. Since NIHSS at baseline is the most important predictor of LVO, there is no reason to assume that the rate of LVO in these patients differs from in those who had CTA in the acute phase and were included in our analysis.

Conclusion

Of all patients with acute ischemic stroke who arrive within 6 h of symptom onset at the emergency department, almost one out of three will have an intracranial large vessel occlusion and may be eligible for intra-arterial treatment.

Acknowledgements
None.

Funding
None.

Authors' contributions
DB & MM contributed equally to this paper: literature search, figures, study design, data analysis, data interpretation, writing. GS: data collection, data analysis & writing of first draft. SF & PH: data analysis & writing. RVO & WZ: study conception & critical review of the manuscript. DD & AL: study conception, data analysis & critical review of the manuscript. All authors read and approved the final manuscript.

Competing interests
DD was PI of the MR CLEAN trial, which was partly funded by the Dutch Heart Foundation and by unrestricted grants from AngioCare BV, Medtronic/Covidien/EV3®, MEDAC Gmbh/LAMEPRO, Penumbra Inc., Stryker®, and Top Medical/Concentric.
Erasmus MC received funds from Stryker® and Bracco Imaging® for consultations by DD.
MUMC received funds from Stryker® and dePuySynthes® for consultations by WZ.

Author details
[1]Department of Neurology, Cardiovascular Research Institute Maastricht (CARIM), Maastricht University Medical Center, Maastricht, The Netherlands. [2]Department of Neurology, Erasmus MC University Medical Center, Rotterdam, The Netherlands. [3]Department of Radiology, Cardiovascular Research Institute Maastricht (CARIM), Maastricht University Medical Center, Maastricht, The Netherlands. [4]Department of Radiology, Erasmus MC University Medical Center, Rotterdam, The Netherlands. [5]Department of Rehabilitation, Erasmus MC University Medical Center, Rotterdam, The Netherlands.

References

1. Berkhemer OA, Fransen PS, Beumer D, et al. A randomized trial of intraarterial treatment for acute ischemic stroke. N Engl J Med. 2015;372:11–20.
2. Campbell BC, Mitchell PJ, Kleinig TJ, et al. Endovascular therapy for ischemic stroke with perfusion-imaging selection. N Engl J Med. 2015;372:1009–18.
3. Goyal M, Demchuk AM, Menon BK, et al. Randomized assessment of rapid endovascular treatment of ischemic stroke. N Engl J Med. 2015;372:1019–30.
4. Goyal M, Menon BK, van Zwam WH, et al. Endovascular thrombectomy after large-vessel ischaemic stroke: a meta-analysis of individual patient data from five randomised trials. Lancet. 2016.
5. Jovin TG, Chamorro A, Cobo E, et al. Thrombectomy within 8 h after symptom onset in ischemic stroke. N Engl J Med. 2015;372:2296–306.
6. Saver JL, Goyal M, Bonafe A, et al. Stent-retriever thrombectomy after intravenous t-PA vs. t-PA alone in stroke. N Engl J Med. 2015;372:2285–95.
7. Casaubon LK, Boulanger JM, Blacquiere D, et al. Canadian Stroke Best Practice Recommendations: Hyperacute Stroke Care Guidelines, Update 2015. Int J Stroke. 2015;10:924–40.
8. Powers WJ, Derdeyn CP, Biller J, et al. 2015 American Heart Association/American Stroke Association Focused Update of the 2013 Guidelines for the Early Management of Patients With Acute Ischemic Stroke Regarding Endovascular Treatment: A Guideline for Healthcare Professionals From the American Heart Association/American Stroke Association. Stroke. 2015;46:3020–35.
9. Smith WS, Lev MH, English JD, et al. Significance of large vessel intracranial occlusion causing acute ischemic stroke and TIA. Stroke. 2009;40:3834–40.
10. Weimar C, Goertler M, Harms L, Diener HC. Distribution and outcome of symptomatic stenoses and occlusions in patients with acute cerebral ischemia. Arch Neurol. 2006;63:1287–91.
11. Heldner MR, Hsieh K, Broeg-Morvay A, et al. Clinical prediction of large vessel occlusion in anterior circulation stroke: mission impossible? J Neurol. 2016;26:1633-40.
12. Heldner MR, Zubler C, Mattle HP, et al. National Institutes of Health stroke scale score and vessel occlusion in 2152 patients with acute ischemic stroke. Stroke. 2013;44:1153–7.
13. Hansen CK, Christensen A, Ovesen C, Havsteen I, Christensen H. Stroke severity and incidence of acute large vessel occlusions in patients with hyper-acute cerebral ischemia: results from a prospective cohort study based on CT-angiography (CTA). Int J Stroke. 2015;10:336–42.
14. de Monye C, Cademartiri F, de Weert TT, Siepman DA, Dippel DW, van Der Lugt A. Sixteen-detector row CT angiography of carotid arteries: comparison of different volumes of contrast material with and without a bolus chaser. Radiology. 2005;237:555–62.
15. de Monye C, de Weert TT, Zaalberg W, et al. Optimization of CT angiography of the carotid artery with a 16-MDCT scanner: craniocaudal scan direction reduces contrast material-related perivenous artifacts. AJR Am J Roentgenol. 2006;186:1737–45.
16. Fischer U, Arnold M, Nedeltchev K, et al. NIHSS score and arteriographic findings in acute ischemic stroke. Stroke. 2005;36:2121–5.

20

Carotid artery intra-plaque attenuation variability using computed tomography

Luca Saba[1*] [iD], Michele Anzidei[2], Carlo Nicola de Cecco[3], Michele Porcu[1], Antonella Balestrieri[1], Roberto Sanfilippo[4], Marco Francone[2], Alessio Mereu[1], Pierleone Lucatelli[2], Roberto Montisci[4], Jasjit S. Suri[5] and Max Wintermark[6]

Abstract

Background: In the CT assessment of the carotid plaque, the analysis of the attenuation value is a fundamental parameter in order to classify the type of the tissue that composes the plaque. The purpose of this paper is to assess the intra-plaque attenuation variability in order to verify the potential reproducibility of HU measurements.

Methods: In this retrospective study, 68 consecutive patients (males 42; average age 64 ± 11 years) that underwent CT of carotid arteries were included. Exams were performed before and after administration of contrast medium and in each slice 4 different circular or elliptical ROIs (≥ 1 and ≤ 2 mm^2) were traced and attenuation values were recorded. Wilcoxon and Mann-Whitney test were used to test the differences between the ROI.

Results: A total of 192 slices were analysed. The average value of attenuation before contrast medium was 41. 591(SD 8.1) HU and 54.159 (SD 15.7) in post-contrast scan. Mann-Whitney test did not find statistically significant difference among the ROI in the pre-contrast scan whereas a statistically significant differences was found in post-contrast scan. Wilcoxon analysis showed a statistically significant difference (p value = 0.001) between pre and post-contrast attenuation.

Conclusion: In conclusion, results of our study suggest that ROI sampling performed in the CT dataset acquired after administration of contrast medium show significant degree of heterogeneity and a statistically significant differences compared to the baseline measurement. This effect may be driven by a different amount of contrast acquisition in some areas of the carotid artery plaque.

Background

Cerebrovascular ischemic events are the third leading cause of death after acute myocardial infarction and cancer and represent the second cause of disability in the Western world [1, 2]. A significant portion of the ischemic events have their cause in the embolization occurred from the carotid artery [3, 4].

In the past years it was thought that the stenosis degree was the leading parameter related to the patient's risk to develop cerebrovascular events [5] but in the last decade several researches have demonstrated that the plaque morphology and characteristics play a fundamental role in the development of embolic cascade [6, 7]. Therefore identification of carotid artery features that are associated with plaque vulnerability is extremely important in order to correctly stratify the risk of occurrence of cerebrovascular events [8, 9] that's why several imaging techniques are trying to identify those characteristics [10, 11].

Ultrasonography (US) is nowadays considered the first-line exam [12] but in most of centres Magnetic Resonance Imaging (MRI) or Computed Tomography (CT) are required to confirm or to rule out the presence of pathological stenosis and\or plaque's characteristics related to the vulnerability [13, 14]. MRI offers, other than the potentiality of quantify the degree of stenosis, the opportunity to identify the presence of intra-plaque-hemorrhage (IPH), lipid-rich necrotic core (LRNC) as well as the status of the fibrous cap [15, 16].

In the assessment of the carotid arteries, CT is a frequently used technique because of the wide availability, the rapid time execution and its potentiality to identify some features related to the plaque vulnerability [17–19]. In the CT assessment of the carotid plaque the analysis

---

* Correspondence: lucasaba@tiscali.it
[1]Department of Radiology, Azienda Ospedaliero Universitaria (A.O.U.), di Cagliari – Polo di Monserrato, s.s. 554 Monserrato, Cagliari 09045, Italy
Full list of author information is available at the end of the article

of the attenuation value is a fundamental parameter in order to classify the type of the tissue that composes the plaque [20].

The purpose of this paper is to assess the intra-plaque attenuation variability in order to verify the potential reproducibility of HU measurements.

Methods
Study design and patient population
In this retrospective study, 68 consecutive patients (males 42, females 16; median age 64 ± 11 years, age range 44–82 years) that underwent CTA between January 2012 and May 2012 were included. The IRB approval was obtained and because of the retrospective nature of the analysis patient's consent was waived.

In our Hospital CTA is performed after ultrasonography that is used as exam to rule-out significant atherosclerotic disease of the supra-aortic vessels. In particular CTA is performed when a) carotid sonography shows a pathological stenosis (>50% according to the NASCET criteria [21]) or plaque's features related to plaque vulnerability (such as ulcers of irregular luminal morphology) b) sonography cannot adequately assess degree of stenosis and plaque's characteristics because of anatomical conditions.

CTA technique
None of the patients included in this research had any contraindications to iodinated contrast media. CTA was performed using a 16-multi-detector row CT system (Philips Brilliance, Eindhoven, Netherlands). Acquisitions were performed from the aortic arch to the circle of Willis before and after administration of contrast medium. Bolus tracking technique was used in all cases. The ROI trigger threshold was placed into the aortic arch and six seconds after the beginning of the i.v. administration of 80 ml of pre-warmed contrast medium (Ultravist 370; Schering, Berlin, Germany) into median cubital vein (flow rate of 5 ml/s) the monitor scanning began. The trigger threshold was set at + 80 HU above the baseline. Four seconds after having reached the threshold the angiographic phase began. CT technical parameters were: matrix 512×512, field of view 14–19 cm; slice thickness 0.6 mm, interval 0.3 mm, 180–220 mAs; 120–140 kV. C-filter algorithm of reconstruction was applied.

Plaque analysis
The window parameters (center/level) was set at W850:L300 according to *Saba et al* [21] and in the first phase the observer (XX, 12 years of experience in vascular imaging) analysed the dataset acquired after administration of contrast material. The carotid artery plaque was identified and for each slice 4 different circular or elliptical ROIs were traced. The 4 ROI were exactly the same in each slice and their dimension was variable ≥ 1 and ≤ 2 mm^2 in the different slices. When small cluster of calcium were identified, these are avoided in the ROI tracings. We considered 2 main exclusion criteria 1) calcified plaques 2) presence of artefacts (movement or dental artefacts). In the second phase the basal scan were assessed. The observers identified the same slice correspondent to the angiographic phase and the same ROIs (for locations and dimension) used in the angiographic phase were applied in the slices (Fig. 1).

At the end of the analysis the ROI were grouped according to their HU value from the lower to the higher values and ROI 1 represents the lower HU values whereas ROI 4 the higher.

Statistical analysis
In this study the normality of each continuous variable group was tested using the Kolmogorov-Smirnov Z test and appropriate tests for Gaussian or non-Gaussian values were selected. For Gaussian values, continuous data were described as the mean value $\pm$ SD whereas for non-gaussian values median values were given. Wilcoxon test was applied to test the difference of attenuation of the ROIs traced before and after administration of contrast material whereas the Mann-Whitney test was used to test the differences between the ROI. A p value < 0.05 was regarded to indicate statistical significance association and all values were calculated using a two-tailed significance level. R software (www.r-project.org) was employed for statistical analyses.

Results
Of the 136 carotid arteries that were imaged with CTA, sixteen carotid arteries were excluded because no evidence of plaque was found. Other 41 carotid arteries were excluded because their plaque was heavily calcified and other 12 because of the presence of artefacts (movements $n = 6$ and dental artefacts $n = 6$). The remaining 67 carotid artery plaques were analysed and 192 slices were found where it was possible to trace 4 ROIs with area between 1 and 2 mm^2.

In the Table 1 are summarized the results of the attenuation values of the four ROIs in the basal and post-contrast phase. The average value of attenuation before contrast medium was 41.591 HU (SD 8.1) and 54.159 (SD 15.7) after its administration. The average value of the ROI used was 1.532 mm^2 (SD 0.163).

By comparing the attenuation values among the four different ROIs (summarized in the Table 2) we found that in the basal scan no statistic differences among the four ROIs was found whereas in the scan performed after contrast material in most of cases there were difference among the ROI values. Standard deviation analysis was also performed (summarized in the Table 3). In the Fig. 2 is given a box-plot that shows the attenuation

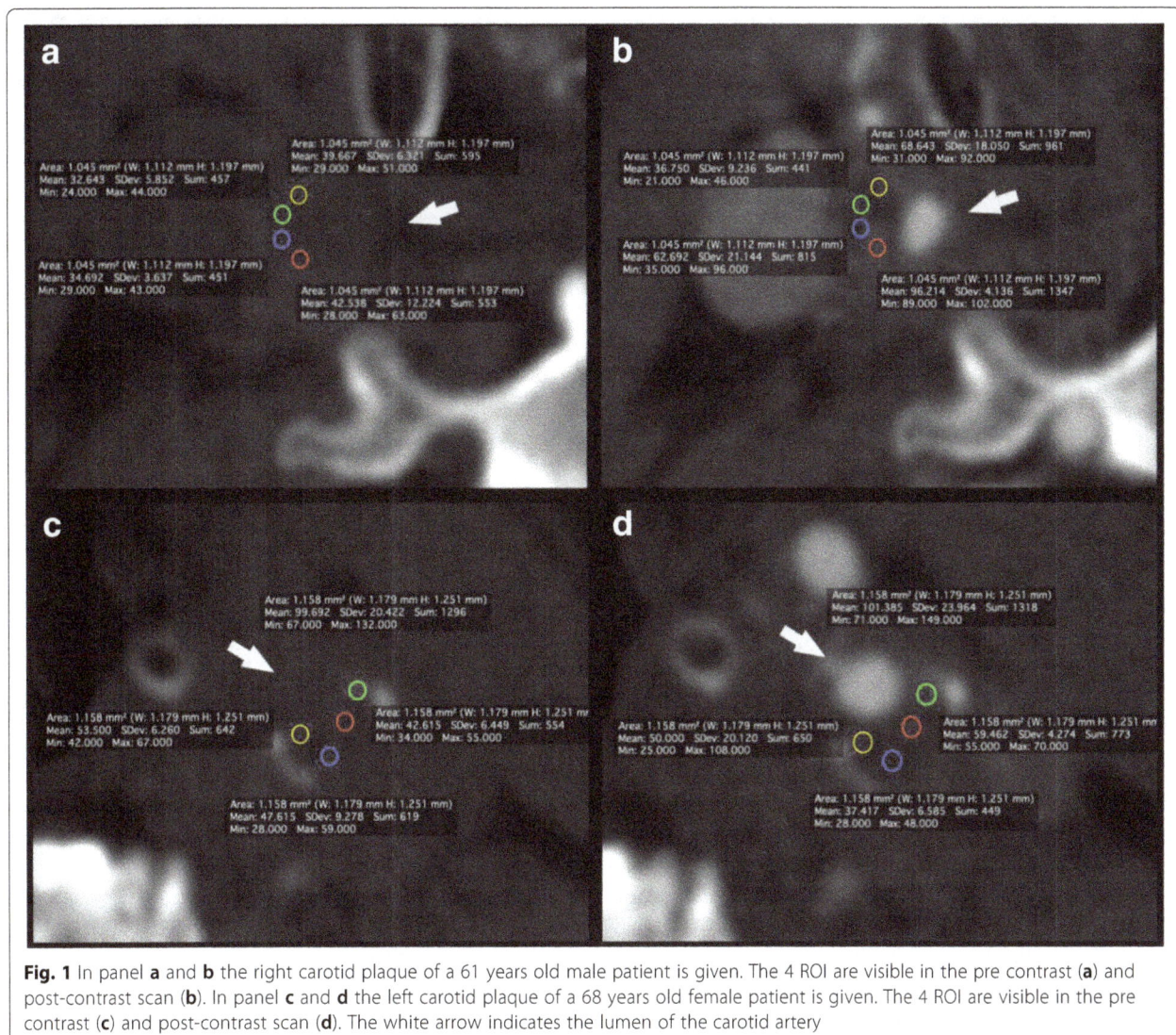

Fig. 1 In panel **a** and **b** the right carotid plaque of a 61 years old male patient is given. The 4 ROI are visible in the pre contrast (**a**) and post-contrast scan (**b**). In panel **c** and **d** the left carotid plaque of a 68 years old female patient is given. The 4 ROI are visible in the pre contrast (**c**) and post-contrast scan (**d**). The white arrow indicates the lumen of the carotid artery

values of the ROI and the Standard Deviations before and after administration of contrast material.

Wilcoxon analysis was used to assess the difference of attenuation before and after administration of contrast material. By comparing the overall attenuation of the ROI of the plaques before and after administration of contrast medium we found a statistically significant difference (p value = 0.001).

Discussion

Attenuation analysis of carotid artery plaque represents an important criterion for the identification of plaque's vulnerability because some types of tissue (fatty ones) are associated with an increased risk [22] of cerebrovascular events whereas others (calcified tissues) are associated with a reduced risk [23]. In this study our purpose was to assess the intra-plaque attenuation variability in order to verify the potential reproducibility of

HU measurements and to assess the polymorphism of the plaque.

Our analysis relies to previous histopathological studies that have been demonstrated that multiple type of tissues are present in the carotid artery plaques [24, 25] and that this features can be visible also in the CT images.

We excluded from the ROI tracings those areas where small calcium deposits or cluster of calcium were visible and we considered as exclusion criteria for a slice the presence of heavily calcified plaques (that determines HU values usually very high up to 800–1000). Nowadays it is extremely important to obtain information that allows to identify and distinguish the fatty plaque (components) from the mixed plaques (components).

Moreover the structure of the carotid artery plaque, when big calcification are present, is characterized by the peripheral location of the calcium components with the

Table 1 Summary values of attenuation (measured in HU) of the ROIs before and after administration of contrast medium (with the Standard Deviation)

	Mean	SD	Minimum	Maximum	2.5–97.5 P	Normal Distr.
ROI 1 basal	33.818	11.0074	14	49	14.000–49.000	0.3899
ROI 1 contrast	40.273	9.1879	24	51	24.000–51.000	0.6966
ROI 2 basal	41.364	7.5534	28	52	28.000–52.000	0.5753
ROI 2 contrast	51.273	10.2868	31	62	31.000–62.000	0.0512
ROI 3 basal	41.909	11.5884	27	57	27.000–57.000	0.0872
ROI 3 contrast	56.273	13.8859	31	72	31.000–72.000	0.3031
ROI 4 basal	49.273	20.7079	28	99	28.000–99.000	0.0254
ROI 4 contrast	68.818	19.0778	43	101	43.00–101.000	0.8457
SD ROI 1 basal	7.545	2.1616	5	11	5.000–11.000	0.5274
SD ROI 1 contrast	10.364	4.081	5	20	5.000–20.000	0.0547
SD ROI 2 basal	11.818	4.3547	4	17	4.000–17.000	0.6073
SD ROI 2 contrast	17.091	9.7719	5	34	5.000–34.000	0.6494
SD ROI 3 basal	7.909	2.0226	5	11	5.000–11.000	0.3265
SD ROI 3 contrast	10.091	4.6574	4	18	4.000–18.000	0.6571
SD ROI 4 basal	10.455	4.5905	5	20	5.000–20.000	0.5176
SD ROI 4 contrast	15.545	6.1703	9	25	9.000–25.000	0.157

lipid components close to the intima layer and it is this part of the plaque that may evolve to rupture and embolization.

By comparing the attenuation values among the four different ROIs the Mann-Whitney test did not show statistical differences among the four ROIs in the basal scan, whereas in the scan performed after contrast material administration in most cases there were difference among ROI values. This is an interesting point because shows 2 different types of information: 1) in the basal scan there are some differences (Table 1) but these are not statistically significant 2) After contrast material the differences between the ROI are statistically significant.

These results indicate that ROI sampling for the HU assessment of the carotid artery plaque in the scan acquired after administration of contrast material can produce heterogeneous results according to the position of the ROI in the plaque and that the values are statistically different in the different part of the plaque. Moreover this heterogeneity is mainly due to the effect of the contrast material, as demonstrated by the fact that in the basal scan these differences are not significant whereas after contrast medium become statistically significant. Therefore, the difference of attenuation identified in the ROI may represent a difference of contrast material

Table 2 Mann-Whitney analysis of the ROI attenuation values (*p* values are given)

Basal Attenuation values

	ROI 1	ROI 2	ROI 3	ROI 4
ROI 1	x	0,1006	0,2122	0,078
ROI 2		x	0,695	0,524
ROI 3			x	0,722
ROI 4				x

Post contrast Attenuation values

	ROI 1	ROI 2	ROI 3	ROI 4
ROI 1	x	0,0086*	0,0053*	0,0008*
ROI 2		x	0,1311	0,0488*
ROI 3			x	0,0115*
ROI 4				x

*statistically significant difference

Table 3 Mann-Whitney analysis of the Standard Deviation of ROI attenuation values (*p* values are given)

Basal Attenuation values

	ROI 1	ROI 2	ROI 3	ROI 4
ROI 1	x	0,0196	0,691	0,1062
ROI 2		x	0,0351	0,3579
ROI 3			x	0,1779
ROI 4				x

Post contrast Attenuation values

	ROI 1	ROI 2	ROI 3	ROI 4
ROI 1	x	0,1306	0,818	0,0562
ROI 2		x	0,071*	0,9215
ROI 3			x	0,0417
ROI 4				x

*statistically significant difference

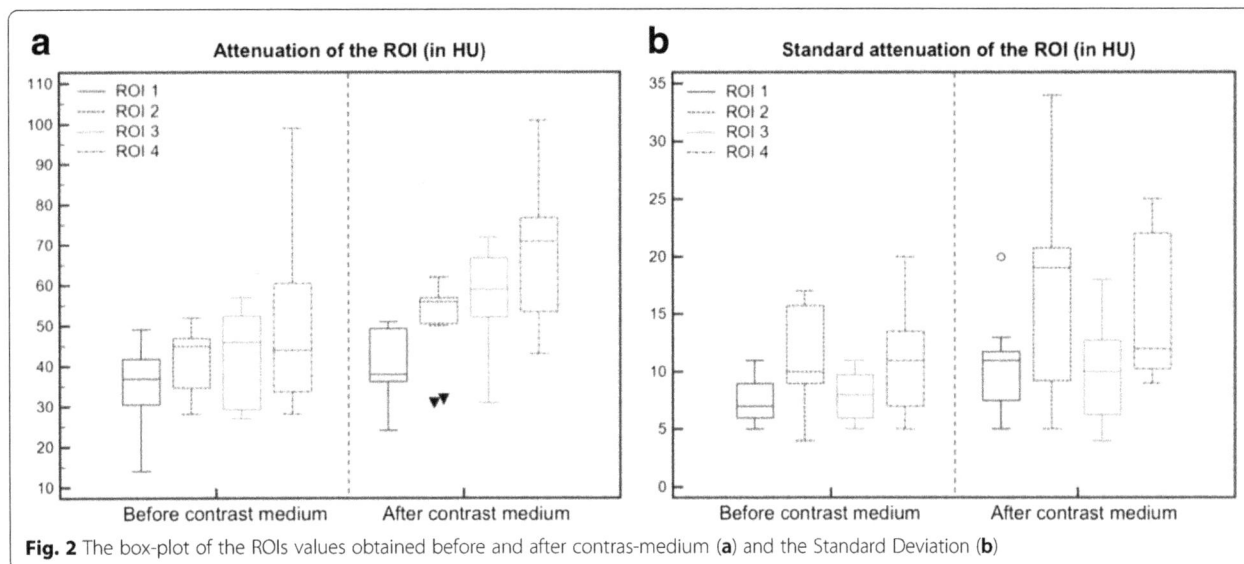

Fig. 2 The box-plot of the ROIs values obtained before and after contras-medium (**a**) and the Standard Deviation (**b**)

acquisition in different areas of the plaque. These results are in line with previously published papers that have demonstrated how carotid artery plaques shows enhancement after administration of contrast material [26–29]. Therefore, the attenuation value of the carotid artery plaque after administration of contrast material seems to represent not only the plaque type but also the amount of contrast material that enters in some areas of the plaques that is mainly due to the neovascularization or to the rupture of the fibrous cap [9, 30]. This approach suggests that for the HU quantification of the tissue type the only pre-contrast CT should be performed and not the one after contrast material. This finding is concordant with a the study results of a paper published by *Park et al* [12] in 2012 where the authors demonstrated in a small cohort of carotid arteries ($n = 43$) that is the attenuation value obtained in he pre-contrast scan that is associated with the cerebrovascular symptoms whereas the attenuation values obtained after contrast medium do not show statistically significant association with the cerebrovascular symptoms. Further analysis are needed to assess if the basal scan may be helpful to stratify the risk to develop cerebrovascular events.

We also assessed, using the Wilcoxon analysis, the global variation of attenuation of the plaque's ROI before and after contrast medium (basal value = 41.591 HU; contrast value = 54.159) and we found a statistically significant difference (p value = 0.001).

Conclusion

In conclusion, results of our study suggest that the ROI sampling performed in the CT dataset acquired after administration of contrast medium show significant degree of heterogeneity and that the ROI have a statistically significant differences. This effect may be driven by a different amount of contrast acquisition in some areas of the carotid artery plaque.

Abbreviations
CT: Computed tomography; CTA: Computed tomography angiography; HU: Hounsfield units; MRI: Magnetic resonance imaging; ROI: Region of interest; US: Ultrasound

Acknowledgements
None.

Funding
None.

Authors' contributions
LS Manuscript ideation; data analysis; data collection; manuscript contribution and revision. MA Data analysis; manuscript contribution and revision. CDC Manuscript ideation; manuscript contribution and revision. MP Data analysis; data collection; manuscript contribution and revision. AB Data analysis; data collection; manuscript contribution and revision. RS Manuscript ideation; manuscript contribution and revision. MF Manuscript ideation; data analysis. AM Manuscript ideation; manuscript contribution and revision. PL Manuscript ideation; manuscript contribution and revision. RM Manuscript ideation; manuscript contribution and revision. JSS data analysis; manuscript contribution and revision. MW data analysis; manuscript contribution and revision. All authors read and approved the final manuscript.

Competing interests
The authors declare that they have no competing interests.

Author details
[1]Department of Radiology, Azienda Ospedaliero Universitaria (A.O.U.), di Cagliari – Polo di Monserrato, s.s. 554 Monserrato, Cagliari 09045, Italy. [2]Department of Radiological, Oncological and Pathological Sciences, Sapienza University of Rome, Rome, Italy. [3]Department of Radiological

Sciences, Oncology and Pathology, University of Rome Sapienza-Polo Pontino, Latina, Italy. [4]Department of Vascular Surgery, Azienda Ospedaliero Universitaria (A.O.U.), di Cagliari – Polo di Monserrato, s.s. 554 Monserrato, Cagliari 09045, Italy. [5]Stroke and Monitoring Division, AtheroPoint, Roseville, CA, USA. [6]Department of Radiology, Neuroradiology Section, Stanford University, Stanford, California, USA.

References

1. Go AS, Mozaffarian D, Roger VL, Benjamin EJ, Berry JD, Borden WB, Bravata DM, Dai S, Ford ES, Fox CS, Franco S, Fullerton HJ, Gillespie C, Hailpern SM, Heit JA, Howard VJ, Huffman MD, Kissela BM, Kittner SJ, Lackland DT, Lichtman JH, Lisabeth LD, Magid D, Marcus GM, Marelli A, Matchar DB, McGuire DK, Mohler ER, Moy CS, Mussolino ME, Nichol G, Paynter NP, Schreiner PJ, Sorlie PD, Stein J, Turan TN, Virani SS, Wong ND, Woo D, Turner MB, American Heart Association Statistics Committee and Stroke Statistics Subcommittee. Heart disease and stroke statistics–2013 update: a report from the American Heart Association. Circulation. 2013;127(1):e6–245.
2. Roger VL, Go AS, Lloyd-Jones DM, Benjamin EJ, Berry JD, Borden WB, Bravata DM, Dai S, Ford ES, Fox CS, Fullerton HJ, Gillespie C, Hailpern SM, Heit JA, Howard VJ, Kissela BM, Kittner SJ, Lackland DT, Lichtman JH, Lisabeth LD, Makuc DM, Marcus GM, Marelli A, Matchar DB, Moy CS, Mozaffarian D, Mussolino ME, Nichol G, Paynter NP, Soliman EZ, Sorlie PD, Sotoodehnia N, Turan TN, Virani SS, Wong ND, Woo D, Turner MB, American Heart Association Statistics Committee and Stroke Statistics Subcommittee. Executive summary: heart disease and stroke statistics–2012 update: a report from the American Heart Association. Circulation. 2012;125(1):188–97.
3. Imray CH, Tiivas CA. Are some strokes preventable? The potential role of transcranial doppler in transient ischaemic attacks of carotid origin. Lancet Neurol. 2005;4(9):580–6.
4. Rothwell PM, Warlow CP. Prediction of benefit from carotid endarterectomy in individual patients: a risk-modelling study. European Carotid Surgery Trialists' Collaborative Group. Lancet. 1999;353(9170):2105–10.
5. Alamowitch S, Eliasziw M, Algra A, Meldrum H, Barnett HJ, North American Symptomatic Carotid Endarterectomy Trial (NASCET) Group. Risk, causes, and prevention of ischaemic stroke in elderly patients with symptomatic internal-carotid-artery stenosis. Lancet. 2001;357(9263):1154–60.
6. Parmar JP, Rogers WJ, Mugler JP 3rd, Baskurt E, Altes TA, Nandalur KR, Stukenborg GJ, Phillips CD, Hagspiel KD, Matsumoto AH, Dake MD, Kramer CM. Magnetic resonance imaging of carotid atherosclerotic plaque in clinically suspected acute transient ischemic attack and acute ischemic stroke. Circulation. 2010;122(20):2031–8.
7. Hellings WE, Peeters W, Moll FL, Piers SR, van Setten J, Van der Spek PJ, de Vries JP, Seldenrijk KA, De Bruin PC, Vink A, Velema E, de Kleijn DP, Pasterkamp G. Composition of carotid atherosclerotic plaque is associated with cardiovascular outcome: a prognostic study. Circulation. 2010;121(17):1941–50.
8. Zainon R, Ronaldson JP, Janmale T, Scott NJ, Buckenham TM, Butler AP, Butler PH, Doesburg RM, Gieseg SP, Roake JA, Anderson NG. Spectral CT of carotid atherosclerotic plaque: comparison with histology. Eur Radiol. 2012;22(12):2581–8.
9. Saba L, Tamponi E, Raz E, Lai L, Montisci R, Piga M, Faa G. Correlation between fissured fibrous cap and contrast enhancement: preliminary results with the use of CTA and histologic validation. AJNR Am J Neuroradiol. 2013; 24 [Epub ahead of print].
10. Park JK, Sung YH, Jeong SY, Lee JH. Higher precontrast CT density of the carotid plaque in the symptomatic patients. Eur J Radiol. 2012;81(9):2386–8.
11. Saba L, Raz E, Grassi R, Di Paolo PL, Iacomino A, Montisci R, Piga M. Association between the volume of carotid artery plaque and its subcomponents and the volume of white matter lesions in patients selected for endarterectomy. AJR Am J Roentgenol. 2013;201(5):W747–52.
12. Dean N, Lari H, Saqqur M, Amir N, Khan K, Mouradian M, Salam A, Romanchuk H, Shuaib A. Reliability of carotid doppler performed in a dedicated stroke prevention clinic. Can J Neurol Sci. 2005;32(3):327–31.
13. Singh N, Moody AR, Rochon-Terry G, Kiss A, Zavodni A. Identifying a high risk cardiovascular phenotype by carotid MRI-depicted intraplaque hemorrhage. Int J Cardiovasc Imaging. 2013;29(7):1477–83.
14. Saba L, Caddeo G, Sanfilippo R, Montisci R, Mallarini G. CT and ultrasound in the study of ulcerated carotid plaque compared with surgical results:

15. potentialities and advantages of multidetector row CT angiography. AJNR Am J Neuroradiol. 2007;28(6):1061–6.
15. Chu B, Yuan C, Takaya N, Shewchuk JR, Clowes AW, Hatsukami TS. Images in cardiovascular medicine. Serial high-spatial-resolution, multisequence magnetic resonance imaging studies identify fibrous cap rupture and penetrating ulcer into carotid atherosclerotic plaque. Circulation. 2006;113(12):e660–1.
16. Kampschulte A, Ferguson MS, Kerwin WS, Polissar NL, Chu B, Saam T, Hatsukami TS, Yuan C. Differentiation of intraplaque versus juxtaluminal hemorrhage/thrombus in advanced human carotid atherosclerotic lesions by in vivo magnetic resonance imaging. Circulation. 2004;110(20):3239–44. E.
17. Saba L, Argiolas GM, Siotto P, Piga M. Carotid artery plaque characterization using CT multienergy imaging. AJNR Am J Neuroradiol. 2013;34(4):855–9.
18. Anzidei M, Napoli A, Zaccagna F, Di Paolo P, Saba L, Cavallo Marincola B, Zini C, Cartocci G, Di Mare L, Catalano C, Passariello R. Diagnostic accuracy of colour Doppler ultrasonography, CT angiography and blood-pool-enhanced MR angiography in assessing carotid stenosis: a comparative study with DSA in 170 patients. Radiol Med. 2012;117(1):54–71.
19. Saba L, Anzidei M, Marincola BC, Piga M, Raz E, Bassareo PP, Napoli A, Mannelli L, Catalano C, Wintermark M. Imaging of the carotid artery vulnerable plaque. Cardiovasc Intervent Radiol. 2013. [Epub ahead of print], PubMed PMID: 23912494.
20. de Weert TT, de Monyé C, Meijering E, Booij R, Niessen WJ, Dippel DW, van der Lugt A. Assessment of atherosclerotic carotid plaque volume with multidetector computed tomography angiography. Int J Cardiovasc Imaging. 2008;24(7):751–9. doi:10.1007/s10554-008-9309-1.
21. Saba L, Mallarin G. Window settings for the study of calcified carotid plaques with multidetector CT angiography. AJNR Am J Neuroradiol. 2009;30(7):1445–50.
22. Nandalur KR, Baskurt E, Hagspiel KD, Phillips CD, Kramer CM. Calcified carotid atherosclerotic plaque is associated less with ischemic symptoms than is noncalcified plaque on MDCT. AJR Am J Roentgenol. 2005;184(1):295–8.
23. Saba L, Montisci R, Sanfilippo R, Mallarini G. Multidetector row CT of the brain and carotid artery: a correlative analysis. Clin Radiol. 2009;64(8):767–78.
24. Redgrave JN, Lovett JK, Gallagher PJ, Rothwell PM. Histological assessment of 526 symptomatic carotid plaques in relation to the nature and timing of ischemic symptoms: the Oxford plaque study. Circulation. 2006;113(19):2320–8.
25. Lovett JK, Redgrave JN, Rothwell PM. A critical appraisal of the performance, reporting, and interpretation of studies comparing carotid plaque imaging with histology. Stroke. 2005;36(5):1091–7.
26. Saba L, Piga M, Raz E, Farina D, Montisci R. Carotid artery plaque classification: does contrast enhancement play a significant role? AJNR Am J Neuroradiol. 2012;33(9):1814–7.
27. Saba L, Mallarini G. Carotid plaque enhancement and symptom correlations: an evaluation by using multidetector row CT angiography. AJNR Am J Neuroradiol. 2011;32(10):1919–25.
28. Horie N, Morikawa M, Ishizaka S, Takeshita T, So G, Hayashi K, Suyama K, Nagata I. Assessment of carotid plaque stability based on the dynamic enhancement pattern in plaque components with multidetector CT angiography. Stroke. 2012;43(2):393–8.
29. Romero JM, Babiarz LS, Forero NP, Murphy EK, Schaefer PW, Gonzalez RG, Lev MH. Arterial wall enhancement overlying carotid plaque on CT angiography correlates with symptoms in patients with high grade stenosis. Stroke. 2009;40(5):1894–6.
30. Saba L, Lai ML, Montisci R, Tamponi E, Sanfilippo R, Faa G, Piga M. Association between carotid plaque enhancement shown by multidetector CT angiography and histologically validated microvessel density. Eur Radiol. 2012;22(10):2237–45.

21

An historical and contemporary review of endovascular therapy for acute ischemic stroke

Karl Boyle[1*], Raed A. Joundi[1] and Richard I. Aviv[2]

Abstract

Long standing, evidence based approved therapies for acute ischemic stroke include intravenous thrombolysis therapy (IVT) with alteplase (recombinant tissue plasminogen activator, rtPA) given within 4.5 h; aspirin therapy within 48 h; management in an acute stroke unit and hemicraniectomy in cases of malignant infarction. Multiple recent positive randomized controlled trials (RCTs) have now also established endovascular therapy with mechanical thrombectomy as the standard of care for acute ischemic stroke involving a large vessel occlusion in the anterior circulation.

This article will review the history of endovascular treatments for acute ischemic stroke and will review the recent positive and negative randomized controlled trial evidence for its efficacy. Current guidelines and dilemmas regarding appropriate patient selection will be discussed.

Keywords: Thrombolysis, Endovascular, Imaging, Stroke, Trials, CT, Perfusion

Background

IVT is the standard of care for acute ischemic stroke [1–3]. Yet IVT must be delivered rapidly within 4.5 h, and has many contraindications. Furthermore, many patients with large or proximal clots may not achieve adequate reperfusion with thrombolysis, and treatment carries the risk of intracranial haemorrhage, which can be fatal.

As a result, there have been a wide variety of dedicated trials over the past 20 years to treat proximal clots not responsive to thrombolysis with interventional and mechanical means. As reviewed below, early trials in endovascular therapy did not demonstrate a benefit in patients with acute ischemic stroke, whereas newer trials have demonstrated substantial efficacy in the treatment of proximal occlusions producing a major breakthrough for treatment options in hyperacute ischemic stroke.

Early experience with endovascular treatment in acute stroke

Intra-arterial thrombolysis (IAT)

The PROACT trials introduced the initial promise of intra-arterial treatment for ischemic stroke [4, 5]. PROACT I demonstrated IAT administration of 6 mg pro-urokinase in patients with M1 or M2 occlusions resulted in higher recanalization rates, although all patients received intravenous heparin, and clinical outcomes were not measured. In PROACT II, patients with angiographically proven proximal MCA occlusions were randomized to receive IAT with 9 mg of pro-urokinase (given proximal to the clot and mechanical clot disruption with the guide wire was not allowed) plus heparin or heparin only in the control arm. Pro-urokinase administration within 6 h resulted in a significantly higher number of patients with modified Rankin scale (mRS) score of 2 or less at 90 days (40% v 25%), with recanalization rates of 66% v 18%. Symptomatic intracranial haemorrhage occurred in 10% versus 2% in controls and mortality was 25% versus 27% in controls. Pro-urokinase was never approved by the FDA for this indication, citing the need for a confirmatory trial that was never performed.

* Correspondence: Karl.Boyle@sunnybrook.ca
[1]Department of Medicine, Division of Neurology, Sunnybrook Health Science Centre and University of Toronto, 2075 Bayview Avenue, Toronto M4N 3M5, Canada
Full list of author information is available at the end of the article

First generation thrombectomy devices

Following the results of the 1999 PROACT II trial, the MERCI retriever device was developed. This was the first generation of mechanical thrombectomy devices approved by the FDA, and propelled an era of interventional stroke trials. MERCI devices were found to achieve recanalization rates (defined as thrombolysis in myocardial infarction score (TIMI) 2 or 3 flow in internal carotid artery (ICA), M1 and M2 (first and second portion of the middle cerebral artery (MCA) branches) of 46% in the first MERCI trial and 55% in the follow up MULTI MERCI trial [6, 7]. Good clinical outcome (modified Ranking Scale, mRS ≤ 2) was 28 and 36% in the two trials but mortality remained high (44 and 34% respectively). However both trials, which treated patients within 8 h, were single arms trials compared to historical controls. Nevertheless, patients with successful recanalization were more likely to achieve good clinical outcome, establishing a clinical rationale for early recanalization after acute stroke.

Second generation thrombectomy devices

The results of a second generation device, the Penumbra aspiration system, were reported in the Penumbra Pivotal Stroke Trial [8]. This trial was not randomized but rather the goal of the trial was to provide substantial equivalence in safety and effectiveness to the MERCI device in opening occluded blood vessels in stroke. High vessel revascularization rates (defined as TIMI 2 or 3 flow at the site of primary occlusion only) of 82% were achieved compared to those reported for the MERCI device. However clinical outcomes remained poor with only 25% achieving a good clinical outcome (mRS ≤ 2) and high all-cause mortality rate of 33%. Complication rates were high with 12.8% of patients experiencing a procedural complication, of which 2.4% were considered serious, and a 24 h intracranial haemorrhage (ICH) rate of 28% with a symptomatic ICH rate of 11.2%. Similar to the MERCI trials, an 8 h time window was used.

Third generation thrombectomy devices

The SOLITAIRE and Trevo devices were both retrievable stents, a technology that continued the evolution of thrombectomy device. Promising recanalization rates and clinical outcomes, as compared to the Merci device, were reported in the SWIFT and TREVO 2 trials, heralding what was to come in later RCTs [9, 10].

2013 – the year of three negative EVT RCTs (Tables 1, 2, 3 and 4)

In March 2013, three randomized controlled trials, SYNTHESIS, MR RESCUE, and IMS III, were presented at the International Stroke Conference in Hawaii and subsequently published in the same issue of the New England Journal of Medicine. Very disappointingly all three trials reported negative results [11–13].

Using the MERCI retriever or PENUMBRA system, MR RESCUE, completed over an 8 year period, compared patients receiving endovascular therapy versus those receiving standard care. Inclusion criteria included demonstration of intracranial ICA or M1 occlusion, NIHSS greater or equal to 6 and once again the eligible time window was within 8 h. Forty-four percent received tPA in the endovascular arm compared to 30% in the standard care arm. There was no outcome difference between groups, irrespective of whether the patient had a favourable penumbral pattern or nonpenumbral pattern based on perfusion imaging. Reperfusion, defined as modified thrombolysis in cerebral infarction score (mTICI) 2a/3 was 67% and defined as mTICI 2b/3 was only 27%. Good clinical outcome (mRS 0–2) was only demonstrated in 14%. Older generation devices were used and the mean time to endovascular procedure was 6 h and 21 min.

IMS III was a large, randomized controlled trial comparing endovascular therapy plus IVT (IVT stopped at 40 min) to IVT alone. Demonstration of intracranial occlusion was not required. In IMS III, National Institutes of Health Stroke Scale, NIHSS ≥10 was used as a marker of stroke severity and risk of proximal occlusion, but as Computed Tomography Angiography, CTA became more widespread, an amendment mid-way through the trial allowed screening for proximal clots with CTA for patients with NIHSS of 8 or 9. MERCI, PENUMBRA, SOLITAIRE, or Microcatheter delivery of intra-arterial tPA was allowed. As a result, the methods were a mix of pharmacological thrombolysis, manipulation of clot with use of a guidewire or microcatheter, mechanical and aspiration thrombectomy, and stent-retriever technology. The procedure was required to begin within 5 h. Disappointingly, there was no difference in outcome between groups with 41% good clinical outcome (mRS 0–2) in the combined IVT/EVT arm versus 39% in the IVT only arm. Recanalization rate (defined as modified arterial occlusion lesion score mAOL 2–3) was 81% for ICA occlusion and 86% for M1 occlusion; the reperfusion rate (mTICI 2b/3) was 38% for ICA occlusion and 44% for M1 occlusion. Retrievable stents were only used in 14 patients.

The SYNTHESIS trial compared endovascular therapy (intra-arterial thrombolysis with rtPA, mechanical clot disruption or retrieval or a combination of these approaches) to treatment with intravenous tPA alone. Demonstration of vessel occlusion prior to endovascular treatment was not required nor was any clinical severity rating on the NIHSS. Reperfusion rates were not reported. There was no difference in good clinical outcome –42% in the endovascular arm versus 46% in the intravenous tPA arm. A mechanical device was only

Table 1 Study design

	Arms	Size	Era	Centres	Age Range	Clinical Criteria	Vessel occlusion	Time Window (onset to groin puncture)	CT Criteria	Advanced Imaging Criteria
MR RESCUE	Rescue EVT v standard	118	2004 - 2011	North America – 22 sites	18-85 yr	NIHSS 6- 29	CTA/MRA showing persistent occlusion post IVT – ICA, M1 or M2	<8 hr	None	Penumbra assessment with multimodal CT or MRI for stratification but not for trial eligibility
IMS III	Bridging v IVT	656	Aug 2006 – Apr 2012	58 Centres (US, Canada, Australia, Europe)	18-82 yr	NIHSS ≥10 Or NIHSS 8-9 with proven vessel occlusion (ICA, M1, BA)	Not required at randomization	<5 hr	None	None
SYNTHESIS	EVT v IVT	362 (181 v 181)	Feb 2008 – Apr 2012	Italy – 24 centres	18-80 yr	NIHSS >25 excluded	Not required at randomization	<4.5 hr	None	None
PISTE	Bridging v IVT	65 (33 v 32)	Apr 2013- Apr 2015	10 Centres (UK)	≥18 yr	NIHSS ≥6	I-ICA, M1, M2 Extra-cranial-ICA excluded	<5.5 hr	Evidence of extensive established infarction excluded	None
THERAPY	Bridging v IVT	108 (55 v 53)	Mar 2012- Oct 2014	36 Centres (US and Germany)	18-85 yr	NIHSS ≥8	I-ICA, M1	eligible for tPA (<4.5 hr)	Any acute ischemic changes >1/3 MCA excluded	clot length ≥8 mm
MR CLEAN	EVT v standard	500 (233 v 267)	Dec 2010- Mar 2014	Netherlands - 16 centres	≥18 yr	NIHSS ≥2	I-ICA,M1,M2,A1,A2 Additional extra-cranial ICA or dissection at discretion of treating physician	<6 hr	None	None
ESCAPE	EVT v standard	315 (165 v 150)	Feb 2013- Oct 2014	22 Centres (Canada, US, Ireland, South Korea, UK)	≥18 yr	NIHSS >5	I-ICA,M1, 2-M2s, A1 Additional extracranial ICA or dissection at discretion of treating physician	<12 hr	ASPECTS >5	CTA filling >50% of MCA pial collaterals, CTP = vlCBF/CBV ASPECTS >5
EXTEND_IA	Bridging v IVT (Solitaire only)	75 (35 v 35)	Aug 2012- Oct 2014	10 centres (9 Aus, 1 NZ)	≥18 yr	No NIHSS cut-off	ICA, M1 or M2 dissection excluded	<6 hr	None	Target mismatch: mismatch >1.2, rCBF core <70 ml, 6 sec Tmax penumbra >10 ml
SWIFT PRIME	Bridging v IVT (Solitaire only)	196 (98 v 98)	Dec 2012- Nov 2014	39 centres (US and Europe)	18-80	NIHSS 8-29	I-ICA, M1 Extra-cranial-ICA excluded (including dissection)	<6 hr	Revised small core (ASPECTS >5)	Initially target mismatch (core <50 ml, 10 sec Tmax lesion <100 ml, penumbra >15 ml and mismatch ≥1.8)

Table 1 Study design (Continued)

REVASCAT	EVT v standard (Solitaire only)	206 (103 v 103)	Nov 2012-Dec 2014	4 centres Spain (Catalonia)	18-80	NIHSS?>?5	I-ICA,M1,	<8 hr	ASPECTS >6 (>5 on DWI)	No recanalization on CTA/MRA after ≥30 min from start of tPA infusion. If CTA/MRA performed >4.5 hr from onset then CBV ASPECTS, CTA-SI ASPECTS or DWI-MR ASPECTS must be performed
THRACE	Bridging v IVT	412 (208 v 204)	June 2010-Feb 2015	26 centres France (Mothership only model)	18-80	NIHSS 10-25	I-ICA, M1, upper 1/3 basilar artery, Ipsilateral E-ICA, stenosis/occlusion excluded	<5 hr	None	None

Table 2 Baseline characteristics

	Age (median)	Male (%)	NIHSS (median)	Vessel occlusion	Tandem lesion (extrancranial ICA occlusion)	ASPECTS (median)	IVT (%)	Retrievable stent (%)
MR RESCUE	66	50	16	71% ICA or M1*	nr	predicted core 36 ml*	47*	0
IMS III	69	50	17	18% of EVT group had no occlusion	nr	nr	100	4
SYNTHESIS	66	59	13	2% no occlusion	nr	nr	0	41
PISTE	67	39	18	90% carotid T/L or M1	3%	9	100	68
THERAPY	67	62	17	89% I-ICA or M1	excluded	7.5	100	13% (majority used aspiration thrombectomy)
MR CLEAN	66	58	17	92% I-ICA, carotid T or M1	32%	9	87 (44% drip & ship)	82
ESCAPE	71	48 (87% white)	16	96% carotid T/L or M1	13%	9	73	73
EXTEND_IA	69	49	17	88% I-ICA or M1	n/r	n/r (median core 12 ml)	100	100
SWIFT PRIME	65	55 (89% white)	17	86% carotid T/L or M1	excluded	9	100 (44% drip & ship)	100
REVASCAT	65	55	17	90% carotid T/L or M1	19	7	70	70
THRACE	66	57	18	98% ICA or M1	excldued	nr	100 (100% mothership)	77

[a]MR RESCUE values reported for penumbral group receiving embolectomy

used in 56/181 patients randomized to endovascular treatment; however, this trial did see the introduction of the third generation of mechanical devices, the retrievable stents, which were used in 23/56 patients in whom a device was deployed.

Overall, these three trials failed to show a benefit for endovascular intervention in ischemic stroke. However, a variety of limitations were identified and addressed in the design of new endovascular therapy RCTs [14, 15]. Firstly, the use of non-invasive angiography was not universal in patient selection. For example, in IMS III, more than 50% of patients did not undergo CTA, as it was not in widespread use during early patient recruitment. In MR RESCUE, patients were eligible only if angiography showed persistent target occlusion after receiving tPA. Secondly, there were long time delays from stroke onset to

Table 3 Process times

	Onset to IVT (median., min)	Onset to randomisation (median., min)	Onset to groin puncture (median., min)	Onset to first reperfusion (median., min)	Groin puncture to reperfusion (median., min)	IVT to groin puncture (median., min)	CT to groin puncture (median., min)	CT to reperfusion (median., min)
MR RESCUE	nr	nr	381	nr	nr	nr	124	nr
IMS III	122	nr	208	nr	nr	nr	nr	nr
SYNTHESIS	165	148	225	nr	nr	nr	nr	nr
PISTE	120	150	209	259	49*	82	58#	nr
THERAPY	108	181	227	nr	nr	nr	123	nr
MR CLEAN	85	204	260	332	nr	nr	nr	nr
ESCAPE	110	169	208	241	30	51	51	84
EXTEND_IA	127	156	210	248	43	74	93	nr
SWIFT PRIME	111	191	224	252	nr	nr	58	87
REVASCAT	118	223	269	355	59	nr	67	nr
THRACE	150	168	250	nr	nr	nr	nr	nr

[a]Groin puncture to device removal
[b]Randomisation to groin puncture

Table 4 Outcomes

	Recanalization (%, EVT v control)	Reperfusion (mTICI 2b/3, %)	Primary outcome	mRS at day 90	mRS 0-2 at day 90	Final infarct volume (mL)	sICH (PH-2, %)	Death at day 90 (%)	New AIS in a different territory (%)	SAE (%)
MR RESCUE	69	27	mRS 3.8 v 3.4	3.8 v 3.4	21 v 26	32 v 32	9 v 6	18 v 21	1.4	62
IMS III	81 ICA; 86 M1; 88 M2	38 ICA; 44 M1; 44 M2	mRS 0-2 41 v 39%	nr	41 v 39	nr	6 v 6	19 v 21	nr	nr
SYNTHESIS	nr	nr	mRS 0-1 30 v 35%	nr	42 v 46	nr	6 v 6	8 v 6	nr	nr
PISTE	69	87	OR 2.12 mRS 0-2 p = 0.2	nr	51 to 40 vo NNT = 9	nr	0 v 0	7 v 4	nr	45 v 34
THERAPY	nr	70	mRS 0-2 38 v 30% p = 0.44	nr	38 v 30 ns	nr	9.3 v. 9.7	12 v 24	nr	42 v 48
MR CLEAN	75 v 33	59	mRS 3v4 day 90	3 v 4	33 v 19 NNT = 7	49 v 79	6 v 5	21 v 22	5.6	47 v 42
ESCAPE	nr v 31 (mAOL 2-3)	72	cOR 2.6	2 v 4	53 v 29 NNT = 4	nr	4 v 3	10 v 19 (significant)	nr	21 v 18
EXTEND_IA	94 v 43 (TIMI 2-3)	86	24 hr reperfusion 100 v 37% Early neurological recovery 82 v 37%	1 v 3	71 v 40 NNT = 3	23 v 53	0 v 6	9 v 20 (p = 0.18)	5.7	nr
SWIFT PRIME	nr	88	Shift analysis p = 0.0002	2 v 3	60 v 36 NNT = 4	nr	1 v 3	9 v 12 (p = 0.5)	nr	36 v 31
REVASCAT	nr	66	cOR 1.7	nr	44 v 28 NNT = 6	16 v 39	5 v 2	18 v 16	5	30 v 25
THRACE	78	69	mRS 0-2 at day 90 53v42%	nr	53 v 42 NNT = 9	nr	2 v 2	12 v 13	6	8 v 7

EVT endovascular thrombectomy, tPA tissue plasminogen activator, Bridging IV tPA + thrombectomy, NIHSS National Institutes of Health Stroke Scale, I-ICA intracranial internal carotid artery, MCA middle cerebral artery, M1 first portion of the middle cerebral artery, from the origin to the bifurcation/trifurcation, M2 s portion of the middle cerebral artery, CTA Computer Tomography Angiography, CTP Computed Tomography Perfusion, vlCBV very low cerebral blood volume, ASPECTS Alberta Stroke Program Early CT Score, nr not recorded, mAOL modified arterial occlusion lesion score, TIMI thrombolysis in myocardial infarction score, mTICI modified thrombolysis in cerebral infarction score, mRS modified Ranking Scale, sICH symptomatic intracranial haemorrhage, PH-2 parenchymal hematoma 2, ie. >30% of the infarcted area with significant space-occupying effect, or clot remote from infarcted area, AIS acute ischemic stroke, SAE serious adverse events

revascularization, in part due to lack of rapid workflow. Lastly, devices were relatively limited in their ability to achieve recanalization and the new generation retrievable stents were used in a small number of patients.

Recent landmark positive RCTs demonstrating efficacy and safety of EVT (Tables 1, 2, 3 and 4)

In 2015 the landscape completely changed with the publication of five randomized controlled trials showing positive results for endovascular treatment in patients with acute ischemic stroke. presenting with large vessel occlusion in the anterior circulation [16–20]. A sixth positive trial has been published in 2016 [21]. These six trials focused on the previous deficiencies in order to maximize work-flow and patient selection, by 1) mandating universal vascular imaging to identify patients with proximal occlusion 2) emphasizing rapid door-to-recanalization times, and 3) use of advanced retrievable stent technology.

The first landmark positive trial was MR CLEAN, presented at the 9th World Stroke Congress in October 2014. The trial recruited patients within 6 h of onset, with proximal occlusion of the anterior circulation (distal ICA, M1 or M2, first or second portion of Anterior cerebral artery, A1 or A2), and NIHSS >2. This was a very pragmatic trial conducted within a single country (the Netherlands) and it is important to note that neither the basic non contrast Computed Tomography, NCCT brain Alberta Stroke Program Early CT Score, (-ASPECTS score) nor advanced clinical imaging (collateral scoring or perfusion imaging) were used to identify and exclude patients with large core infarction. The vast majority of patients received IVT (89%) and 82% of patients were treated with retrievable stents. This trial shifted from using a dichotomized mRS as the primary outcome to using the adjusted common odds ratio for a shift in the direction of a better outcome on the mRS. The adjusted common odds ratio was 1.67 (95% CI 1.21 to 2.30), representing the first positive RCT for endovascular therapy. Statistically significantly more patients achieved functional independence (mRS 0 to 2) at 90 days in the intervention group, 33% compared to 19% (95% CI 5.9 to 21.2) with an adjusted odds ratio of 2.16 (95% CI 1.39 to 3.38).

Following early interim analyses prompted by these positive results, five other ongoing RCTs stopped recruitment early and swiftly produced concordant results. MR CLEAN therefore remains the only fully powered study. Unpowered studies may overestimate effect size but it is reassuring that the same positive result was obtained in five different prematurely terminated RCTs. Those trials will now be discussed.

The ESCAPE trial, conducted February 2013 to October 2014 across 22 sites in Canada, United States,

Ireland and South Korea, allowed recruitment of patients within 12 h, the longest time window of all the trials, with clinical severity requirements for inclusion set at a NIHSS >6. Additional advanced imaging criteria were also required: (i) NCCT ASPECTS >5 aimed at identifying small core infarcts; (ii) proximal intracranial occlusion of M1, M2, or intracranial ICA was required on vascular imaging, with tandem occlusion of the extra-cranial internal carotid artery also allowed; and (iii) moderate to good collaterals, defined as filling of >50% of MCA pial arterial circulation on CTA, preferably acquired with multiphase CTA. Although not obligatory, if CT perfusion was used, a low CBV or very low CBF ASPECTS >5 was needed. This trial also mandated an imaging-to-groin puncture time of <60 min and a target groin puncture to reperfusion time of < 30 min. Wake up strokes and patients ineligible for intravenous tPA were also accepted if the above criteria were fulfilled. Rapid workflow was emphasized, thus achieving the shortest onset-to-reperfusion time among the trials - the median stroke onset to reperfusion was 4 h. Seventy-six percent of patients received IVT. The trial demonstrated an increase in functional independence (mRS 0–2) at 90 days from 29% in the control group to 53% in the intervention group ($p < 0.001$) and the primary outcome favoured the intervention with a common odds ratio of 2.6 (95% CI 1.7 to 3.8; $p < 0.001$). ESCAPE was the only trial to demonstrate a statistically significant reduction in mortality from 19 to 10% ($p = 0.04$).

The Australian and New Zealand EXTEND-IA trial, conducted from August 2012 through October 2014 across ten sites, had the most stringent selection criteria and was the only one to mandate perfusion imaging, requiring evidence of salvageable tissue using the automated RAPID software (ischemic core of less than 70 mL and target mismatch of >1.2 on perfusion imaging). This was also the only trial to report a screening log - 7798 patients were screened, with 1044 (7%) receiving IVT and 70 (1%) receiving endovascular therapy. Four hundred ninety-five of 1044 (47%) of patients treated with IVT were excluded because CTA did not demonstrate a large artery occlusion. It was estimated that 25% of clinically eligible patients for thrombectomy were excluded on the basis of perfusion imaging alone. All randomized patients received IVT and endovascular treatment commenced within 6 h. This highly selected cohort translated into excellent outcomes – the reperfusion rate was impressive (mTICI 2b/3 86%) and this trial had the largest effect size, with 71% of patients in the intervention group achieving functional independence (mRS 0–2) at 90 days, compared to 40% in the control arm ($p = 0.01$, relative risk, RR 1.8). Furthermore, this trial demonstrated a large trend to mortality benefit (20 to 9%), although unlike the ESCAPE trial the difference was not statistically significant (RR 0.4, 95% CI 0.1–1.5), probably due to the small sample size.

In SWIFT-PRIME, conducted in 39 United States and European sites between December 2012 to November 2014, the initial premise was to select a target-mismatch penumbra profile (core <50 ml, ischemic tissue with time to the peak of the residual function, Tmax >10 s <100 ml, mismatch volume >15 ml and mismatch ratio >1.8) using the automated RAPID penumbral imaging software. However, perfusion mismatch was a requirement in only 71 patients before the protocol was changed to one identifying small core infarcts (NCCT ASPECTS >5) in the next 125 patients. All patients received IVT and the endovascular procedure had to start within 6 h. This trial had the highest rate of reperfusion (mTICI 2b/3 88%) and demonstrated improvement in functional independence (mRS 0–2) at 90 days with 60% in the intervention group versus 36% in controls (RR 1.7, 95% CI 1.23–2.33, $p < 0.001$).

REVASCAT was the last of the five key studies published in 2015 and randomized patients from Nov 2012 to December 2014 from four centres in Catalonia, Spain. A longer time window was allowed (endovascular procedure to start within 8 h of stroke onset) and patients were recruited either due to contraindication to IVT (32%), or lack of revascularization 30 min after tPA infusion. The trial was stopped after the first planned interim analysis when only 25% of patients had completed 90 days of follow-up. Although the pre-specified boundaries for stopping were not met the steering committee elected to stop the trial due to lack of equipoise following the results of the other positive RCTs. REVASCAT included patients with an NIHSS ≥6 with proven vessel occlusion of the intracranial ICA, MCA or M1 trunk; tandem proximal ICA/MCA-M1 occlusions were allowed. This trial used the highest cut-off on ASPECTS score for inclusion (ASPECTS >6) but also demonstrated the challenges around using this score to exclude patients – the core lab would have excluded 25% of participants with ASPECTS ≤ 6 and a further 9% who had occlusion of a single M2 only. REVASCAT had the longest door-to-groin puncture time of 269 min. Nevertheless, there were still positive results: the primary outcome demonstrated a common odds ratio of improvement in the distribution of the mRS score of 1.7 (95% CI 1.05–2.8) and the proportion with good outcome (mRS 0–2) increasing from 28 to 44% (adjusted odd ratio 2.1, 96% CI 1.1 to 4.0).

The THRACE (THRombectomie des Artères CErebrales) trial was the most recently published RCT appearing online in August 2016. Patients were recruited from June 2010 to February 2015 from 26 centres in France. This trial compared IVT within 4 h (changed from 3 h after 14 May 2011 and 80 patients enrolled) to IVT within 4 h plus mechanical thrombectomy starting within 5 h, the shortest time window of all trials. Included patients had NIHSS 10–25 and proximal vessel occlusion. The trial included over 400 patients making it the second largest thrombectomy trial behind MR CLEAN ($n = 500$). THRACE resembled IMS with a bridging IV/IA protocol but used the newest stent retrievers and aspiration devices. Importantly imaging assessment of infarct/ischemic extent using ASPECTS or perfusion was not used to exclude patients representing the widest patient selection profile of all RCTs to date. Interestingly, 17/57 (30%) of patients with ASPECTS 0–4 had a good clinical outcome. Unlike the other trials that incorporated a drip and ship model, THRACE only included patients presenting directly to an interventional centre, representing a mothership model of care. This trial used functional independence (mRS 0–2) at 3 months as the primary outcome and was also a positive trial, with a significantly higher proportion in the mechanical thrombectomy arm reaching this good outcome - 53% versus 42%, (OR 1.55 95% CI 1.05–2.3; $p = 0.028$). The lower difference between intervention and control group was thought to reflect the longer randomization to groin puncture time of 82 min which would have adversely affected the intervention arm. The rate of IA reperfusion (TICI 2b-3) was 69%.

Not all recent RCTs have been positive

THERAPY, using the Penumbra aspiration system rather than a retrievable stent, presented in 2015 and published in September 2016 and PISTE, a pragmatic trial conducted in the UK only, have both reported a trend to improved outcome that did not reach statistical significance [22, 23]. In an attempt to identify the poorest prognosis patients the THERAPY trial targeted patients with a thrombus length of 8mm or longer but failed to show any significant difference in the primary outcome of functional independnece (mRS 0-2) at 90 days, 38% IAT v 30% IVT groups (p=0.52).

Efficacy and safety

The evidence is overwhelmingly in favour of endovascular thrombectomy for large vessel occlusion in patients with acute ischemic stroke. All trials aimed for rapid recanalization, mandated advanced imaging, to greater or lesser degrees, for patient selection, and used newer-generation retrievable stents. These improvements likely resulted in positive effect sizes where previous trials failed. In keeping with this, in a sub-analysis of IMS III, patients with documented occlusion who achieved recanalization within 6 h had a significant benefit [24]. All trials showed increased functional independence at 90 days with treatment with only one study, ESCAPE, showing significantly reduced mortality. Variability in effect size likely relate to slightly different selection criteria, devices used, and speed of treatment.

There was no increase in the rate of intracranial haemorrhage in any of the trials despite concurrent use of thrombolysis for the majority of patients. In the MR CLEAN trial, there was a low rate of distal embolization into new territories (8.6%), procedure-related dissections (1.7%), and vessel perforations (0.9%).

Meta-analyses of trials
Multiple meta-analyses, including various combinations of the three negative RCTs published in 2013 (MR RESCUE, IMS III and SYNTHESIS) with the six positive RCTs published or presented in 2015 (MR CLEAN, ESCAPE, SWIFT-PRIME, EXTEND IA, REVASCAT, THRACE) have confirmed the benefit of endovascular thrombectomy in large vessel occlusion [25–30]. The HERMES collaboration analysed individual patient level data from five of the six positive RCTs published in 2015 (MR CLEAN, ESCAPE, REVASCAT, SWIFT-PRIME and EXTEND-IA; THRACE had not yet been published) [25]. For the primary outcome (the degree of disability on the mRS) the adjusted combined odds ratio for reduced disability at 90 days was 2.49, 95% CI 1.76–3.53, $p < 0.0001$. The number needed to treat for one patient to have reduced disability of at least 1 point on the mRS was 2.6. The adjusted odds ratio for patients achieving functional independence (mRS 0–2) at 90 days was 2.71 (95% CI 2.07–3.55; $p < 0.0001$).

In another meta-analysis, including the negative 2013 RCTs with the same five positive new trials as HERMES, the odds ratio summary statistic for reduction of disability at 90 days was 1.56; 95% CI 1.14–2.13; $p = 0.05$ and the odds ratio for functional independence (mRS 0–2) at 90 days was 1.71 (1.18–2.49) [26]. The largest meta-analysis to date included the above eight trials but also preliminary data from THERAPY and THRACE, and showed similar benefit with risk ratio for good functional outcome (mRS 0–2) at 90 days reported as 1.37; 95% CI 1.14–1.64 [27]. A subgroup of the seven trials published or presented in 2015, more reflective of current practice with improved patient selection and use of retrievable stents, yielded a risk ratio of 1.56 (95% CI 1.38–1.75) for a good functional outcome (mRS 0–2) at 90 days. Consistently, all the various meta-analyses showed no significant difference in mortality or intracranial haemorrhage.

Several cost utility and cost effectiveness analyses have suggested that although EVT is a costly procedure it is likely to be cost effective [31–33].

Patient selection - Guidelines and controversies
Based on the recent positive RCTs, multiple guidelines around the world (eg American Heart Association – AHA, Canadian Stroke Best Practice - CSBP and European Stroke Organization - ESO) have been developed to synthesize the patient selection criteria and facilitate decision making [34–36]. All now recommend endovascular therapy as the new standard of care for patients with acute ischemic stroke presenting with a large vessel intracranial occlusion (i.e. occlusion of the distal internal carotid artery or proximal middle cerebral artery) identified on vascular imaging, and provide their highest level of recommendation for various other clinical and radiological criteria:

(1) neurologic deficits (CSBP – disabling stroke; AHA - NIHSS ≥ 6; ESO - not defined)
(2) time (CSBP – within 6 h with a level B recommendation for patients up to 12 h based on ESCAPE criteria; AHA – 6 h; ESO – 6 h)
(3) lack of an established infarct i.e., a small core, (CSBP - ASPECTS ≥6; AHA - ASPECTS ≥6; ESO – Grade B, level 2a for "large infarcts may be excluded" but no ASPECTS cut-off suggested)
(4) advanced imaging - Intracranial vascular imaging is strongly recommended for decision making, but the benefits of additional imaging such as MRI or CT perfusion are unknown.
(5) baseline function – the AHA guideline is the only one to explicitly mandate a certain level of baseline function, i.e., a pre-stroke mRS score 0 to 1
(6) intravenous tPA – all recommend treatment with IVT for eligible patients prior to endovascular therapy. However both the CSBP and ESO guidelines maintain their highest level of recommendation for patients ineligible for IVT whereas the AHA reduce their level of recommendation for this subgroup (class IIa, level C)
(7) type of anesthesia – conscious sedation is preferred over general anesthesia (unless medically indicated) by both AHA and CSBP recommendations, albeit with reduced levels of evidence (class IIb level C and level B respectively) whereas the ESO guideline leaves this as an individual patient decision. Several RCTs are underway to address this issue [37, 38].
(8) age – an upper age limit is not specified by any of the guidelines with the ESO guideline explicitly stating that "high age alone is not a reason to withhold mechanical thrombectomy", assigning this recommendation Grade A, level 1a evidence.
(9) Tandem occlusions (additional extracranial ICA occlusion): both the CSBP and ESO guidelines do not provide an explicit recommendation for this cohort. However, the AHA guideline states that "angioplasty or stenting of proximal cervical atherosclerotic stenosis or complete occlusion at the time of thrombectomy may be considered but its usefulness is unknown" (Class IIb, Level C)

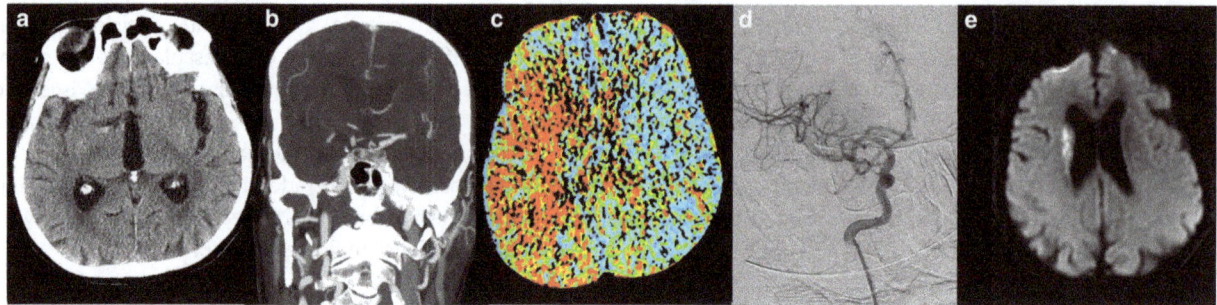

Fig. 1 Illustrative cases of difficult patients pushing boundaries of conventional therapeutic criteria: Advanced age and baseline function. Ninety-five year old male with known dementia – lives at home with his wife, ambulates independently but needs assistance with activities of daily living; pre-stroke mRS 3. Presents with a left MCA syndrome, NIHSS 22. Very early presentation with very favourable imaging – ASPECTS 9 on NCCT (**a**). Note the hyperdense right proximal MCA. CTA (**b**) confirmed a left M1 occlusion with a large clot extending along the M1 trunk into the M2 vessels. Good collaterals were present with a large mismatch on CT perfusion (**c**). The patient was treated with IVT - door to needle (DTN) time 32 min; onset to tPA treatment (OTT) time 74 min. Successful EVT recanalization at 150 min post stroke onset (**d**). A small deep infarct was present on DWI (**e**). Patient was discharged home on day 8 with NIHSS of 5 and was ambulating independently

(10) Type of device – The use of retrievable stents is recommended with the highest level of evidence by all three guidelines, with lower levels of recommendations given to consider other devices based on local protocols. A recent analysis of the MR CLEAN data showed that choice of device did not influence outcomes in that data set. The majority were treated with the Trevo device, 53%, Solitaire device 13% and other device 17% [39].

Conclusions

Endovascular therapy is now the standard of care in patients with large vessel anterior circulation occlusion. This creates challenges in providing care to appropriate patients within a rapid timeframe, since only few highly specialized centres have access to the necessary skills and technology [40, 41]. Peripheral centres may or may not have rapid access to non-invasive angiographic imaging 24/7 in order to screen stroke patients for large vessel occlusion. Therefore currently decisions to transfer patients to tertiary care centre must be made on the basis of patient presentation and non-contrast head CT, which can be challenging. Whether it is best to build the capacity of peripheral centres in providing vascular imaging (providing more accurate diagnosis by screening out clinical false positives but delaying arrival to endovascular centres), or centralizing acute stroke care by transferring all patients who have a possibility of large vessel occlusion (rapid access for selected patients, but many false negatives will place a large burden on tertiary care centres), must be further determined.

The expanded and varying time window used across the trials creates challenges and opportunities in treating patients with proximal occlusion (Fig. 1). "Wake up strokes," typically deemed out of the time window for thrombolysis given the lack of clear time of onset, may be candidates for endovascular therapy if a proximal occlusion is identified (Fig. 2) [42]. Multi-model imaging, including perfusion, and

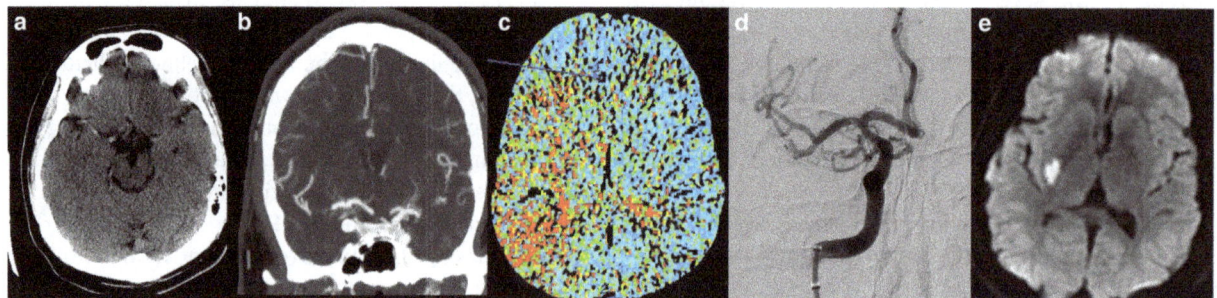

Fig. 2 Illustrative cases of difficult patients pushing boundaries of conventional therapeutic criteria: Unclear time of onset. Twenty-nine year old male last seen normal at 4 am. Found the same day at 1 pm. Presents with right MCA syndrome with severe left sided weakness. NIHSS 8. ASPECTS 10 with hyperdense right MCA (**a**). CTA reveals right intracranial ICA and mid to distal M1 occlusion with good collaterals (**b**). Mismatch demonstrated on CT perfusion (**c**). IVT not given. EVT performed and successful recanalization 13 h 29 min post last seen well time (**d**). DWI confirmed right deep putamen infarct (**e**). Patient was discharged home on day 3 with NIHSS 0

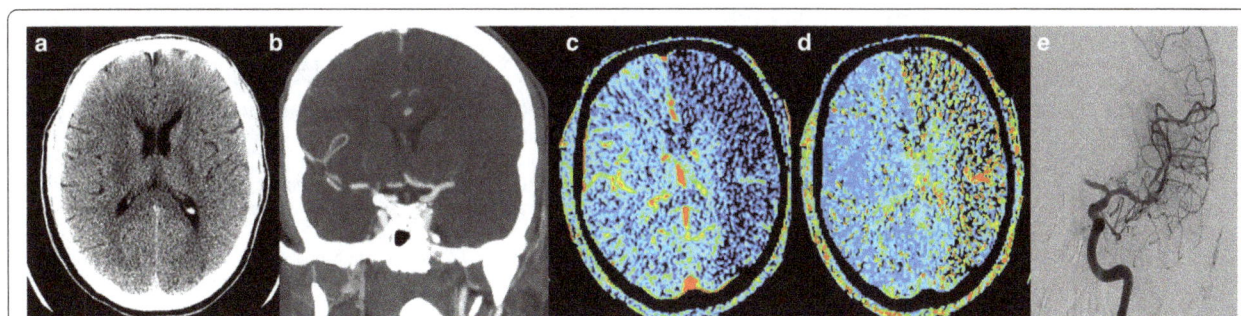

Fig. 3 Illustrative cases of difficult patients pushing boundaries of conventional therapeutic criteria: Poor collaterals but early time to presentation and treatment. Forty-two year old male with witnessed collapse at 19:20. Presents ultra-early, 35 min post collapse, with left MCA syndrome including right sided weakness, forced gaze deviation and mutism with NIHSS 22. Unfavorable imaging including ASPECTS 5 (**a**), hyperdense left MCA vessel, left M1 (CTA **b**), left proximal A2 (not shown) occlusions with poor collaterals and matched CT perfusion defect (CBV, MTT **c**, **d**). Patient was treated with IVT (DTN time 37 min; OTT time 72 min) and EVT (DSA (**e**) with successful recanalization 141 min post stroke onset). No tPA/EVT complications but no neurological improvement with a 24 h NIHSS of 23. Patient developed malignant infarction requiring decompressive hemicraniectomy. Day 90 mRS 2

assessment of collaterals may help identify patients who do not yet have established infarct and who may still benefit from reperfusion despite unknown time of onset [43]. Multimodal imaging has the potential to remove strict time windows on delivering therapy, but rather focus on individualizing therapy to patients with salvageable brain tissue. The role of collaterals in patient selection and outcome remains to be determined (Fig. 3).

The new trials were conducted in patients with occlusion in the ICA, M1, proximal M2, A1, and proximal A2. More distal clots were not adequately assessed in the recent trials and occlusions of the posterior circulation eg basilar artery occlusions, were not even included. Further trials are needed to address the feasibility, efficacy, and safety of extracting clots from the distal M2 or M3 or the posterior circulation. The newer generation retrievable stents, Solitaire and Trevo, have demonstrated superiority in recanalization and clinical outcomes, compared to older generation devices and further technological developments may be geared to reducing complications such as distal embolization.

The future is bright for acute treatment in ischemic stroke but much work remains to be done.

Abbreviations

A1: First portion of anterior cerebral artery; A2: Second portion of anterior cerebral artery; AHA: American Heart Association; AIS: Acute ischemic stroke; ASPECTS: Alberta Stroke Program Early CT Score; Bridging: IV tPA + thrombectomy; CBF: Cerebral blood flow; CSBP: Canadian stroke best practice; CT: Computed tomography; CTA: Computer tomography angiography; CTP: Computed tomography perfusion; ESO: European Stroke Organization; EVT: Endovascular thrombectomy; IAT: Intra-arterial thrombolysis; I-ICA: Intracranial internal carotid artery; IVT: Intravenous thrombolysis; M1: First portion of the middle cerebral artery, from the origin to the bifurcation/trifurcation; M2: Second portion of the middle cerebral artery; mAOL: modified arterial occlusion lesion score; MCA: Middle cerebral artery; mRS: modified Ranking Scale; mTICI: modified thrombolysis in cerebral infarction score; NIHSS: National Institutes of Health Stroke Scale; nr: not recorded; PH-2: Parenchymal hematoma 2, ie. >30% of the infarcted area with significant space-occupying

effect, or clot remote from infarcted area; RCT: Randomized control trial; RR: Relative risk; SAE: Serious adverse events; sICH: symptomatic intracranial haemorrhage; TIMI: Thrombolysis in myocardial infarction score; Tmax: Time to the peak of the residual function; tPA: tissue plasminogen activator; vlCBV: very low cerebral blood volume

Acknowledgements
Not applicable.

Funding
Dr Aviv is funded by CIHR Project Grant 148672. The funding agency played no role in the design of the study and collection, analysis, and interpretation of data or in writing the manuscript.

Authors' contributions
KB was the primary author. All authors (KB,RAJ,RIA) contributed to the literature review, manuscript writing, review and editing. All authors read and approved the final manuscript.

Competing interests
The authors declare that they have no competing interests.

Author details
[1]Department of Medicine, Division of Neurology, Sunnybrook Health Science Centre and University of Toronto, 2075 Bayview Avenue, Toronto M4N 3M5, Canada. [2]Department of Medical Imaging, Division of Neuroradiology, Sunnybrook Health Science Centre and University of Toronto, 2075 Bayview Avenue, Toronto M4N 3M5, Canada.

References
1. The National Institute of Neurological Disorders and Stroke rt-PA Study Group. Tissue plasminogen activator for acute ischemic stroke. N Engl J Med. 1995;333:1581–7. 2.
2. Hacke W, Kaste M, Bluhmki E, et al. Thrombolysis with alteplase 3 to 4.5 hours after acute ischemic stroke. NEJM. 2008;359:1317–29.
3. Emberson J, Lees K, Lyden P, et al. Effect of treatment delay, age and stroke severity on the effects of intravenous thrombolysis with alteplase for acute ischaemic stroke: a meta-analysis of individual patient data from randomised trials. Lancet. 2014;384:1929–35.

4. Del Zoppo G, Higashida R, Furlan A, et al. PROACT: a phase II randomized trial of recombinant Pro-urokinase by direct arterial delivery in acute middle cerebral artery stroke. Stroke. 1998;29:4–11.

5. Furlan A, Higashida R, Wechsler L, et al. Intra-arterial prourokinase for acute ischemic stroke – the PROACT II study: a randomized controlled trial. JAMA. 1999;282:2003–11.

6. Smith W, Sung G, Starkman S, et al. Safety and efficacy of mechanical embolectomy in acute ischemic stroke: results of the MERCI trial. Stroke. 2005;36:1432–8.

7. Smith W, Sunf G, Saver J, et al. Mechanical thrombectomy for acute ischemic stroke: final results of the multi MERCI trial. Stroke. 2008;39:1205–12.

8. The Penumbra Pivotal Stroke Trial Investigators. The penumbra pivotal stroke trial: safety and effectiveness of a New generation of mechanical devices for clot removal in intracranial large vessel occlusive disease. Stroke. 2009;40:2761–8.

9. Saver J, Jahan R, Levy E, et al. Solitaire flow restoration device versus the Meric Retriever in patients with acute ischaemic stroke (SWIFT): a randomized parallel-groip, non-inferiority trial. Lancet. 2012;380:1241–9.

10. Nogueira R, Lutsep H, Gupta R, et al. Trevo versus Merci retrievers for thrombectomy revascularisation of large vessel occlusions in acute ischaemic stroke (TREVO 2): a randomised trial. Lancet. 2012;380:1231–40.

11. Kidwell CS, Jahan R, Gornbein J, et al. MR RESCUE Investigators. A trial of imaging selection and endovascular treatment for ischemic stroke. N Engl J Med. 2013;368:914–23.

12. Broderick JP, Palesch YY, Demchuk AM, et al. Interventional Management of Stroke (IMS) III Investigators. Endovascular therapy after intravenous t-PA versus t-PA alone for stroke. N Engl J Med. 2013;368:893–903.

13. Ciccone A, Valvassori L, Nichelatti M, et al. SYNTHESIS expansion investigators. Endovascular treatment for acute ischemic stroke. N Engl J Med. 2013;368:904–13.

14. Goyal M, Almekhlafi MA, Fan L, et al. Evaluation of interval times from onset to reperfusion in patients undergoing endovascular therapy in the Interventional Management of Stroke III trial. Circulation. 2014;130:265–72.

15. Menon BK, Almekhlafi MA, Pereira VM, et al. Optimal workflow and process-based performance measures for endovascular therapy in acute ischemic stroke: analysis of the Solitaire FR Thrombectomy for Acute Revascularization study. Stroke. 2014;45:2024–9.

16. Berkhemer O, Beumer F, van den Berg L, et al. A randomized trial of intraarterial treatment for acute ischemic stroke (MR CLEAN). NEJM. 2015;372:11–20.

17. Goyal M, Demchuk A, Menon B. Randomized assessment of rapid endovascular treatment of ischemic stroke (ESCAPE). NEJM. 2015;372:1019–30.

18. Campbell B, Mitchell P, Kleinig T, et al. Endovascular therapy for ischemic stroke with perfusion-imaging selection (EXTEND-IA). NEJM. 2015;372:1009–18.

19. Saver J, Goyal M, Bonafe A, et al. Stent-retriever thrombectomy after intravenous t-PA vs. t-PA alone in stroke (SWIFT-PRIME). NEJM. 2015;372:2285–95.

20. Jovin T, Chamorro A, Cobo E, et al. Thrombectomy within 8 hours after symptom onset in ischemic stroke (REVASCAT). NEJM. 2015;372:2296–306.

21. Baccard S, Ducrocq X, Mas J, et al. Mechanical thrombectomy after intravenous alteplase versus alteplase alone after stroke (THRACE): a randomized controlled trial. Lancet Neurol. 2016;15:1138–47.

22. Mocco J, Osama O. Zaidat, Rüdiger von Kummer, et al. Aspiration Thrombectomy After Intravenous Alteplase Versus Intravenous Alteplase Alone (THERAPY). Stroke 2016;47(9):2331-8.

23. Muir k, Ford G, Messow C et al. Endovascular therapy for acute ischaemic stroke: the Pragmatic Ischaemic Stroke Thrombectomy Evaluation (PISTE) randomised, controlled trial. JNNP 2016 Oct 18. doi: 10.1136/jnnp-2016-314117 (Epub ahead of print)

24. Demchuk AM, Goyal M, Yeatts SD, et al. Recanalization and clinical outcome of occlusion sites at baseline CT angiography in the Interventional Management of Stroke III trial. Radiology. 2014;273:202–10.

25. Goyal M, Menon B, van Zwam W, et al. Endovascular thrombectomy after large-vessel ischaemic stroke: a meta-analysis of individual patient data from five randomized controlled trials, (HERMES collaboration). Lancet. 2016;387:1723–31.

26. Badhiwala J, Nassiri F, Alhazzani W, et al. Endovascular thrombectomy for acute ischemic stroke – a meta-analysis. JAMA. 2015;314(17):1832–43.

27. Rodrigues F, Neves J, Caldeira D, et al. Endovascular treatment versus medical care alone for ischaemic stroke: systematic review and meta-analysis. BMJ. 2016;353:i1754. doi:10.1136/bmj.i1754.

28. Balami J, Sutherland B, Edmunds L, et al. A systematic review and meta-analysis of randomized controlled trials of endovascular thrombectomy compared with best medical treatment for acute ischemic stroke. Int J Stroke. 2015;10:1168–78.

29. Elgendy I, Kumbhani D, Mahmoud A, et al. Mechanical thrombectomy for acute ischemic stroke – a meta-analysis of randomized trials. J Am Coll Cardiol. 2015;66:2498–505.

30. Sardar P, Chatterjee S, Giri J, et al. Endovascular therapy for acute ischaemic stroke: a systematic review and meta-analysis of randomized trails. Eur Heart J. 2015. doi:10.1093/eurheartj/ehv270.

31. Ganesalingam J, Pizzo E, Morris S, et al. Cost-utility analysis of mechanical thrombectomy using stent retrievers in acute ischemic stroke. Stroke. 2015;46:2591–8.

32. Leppert M, Campbell J, Simpson J, et al. Cost-effectiveness of intra-arterial treatment as an adjunct to intravenous tissue-type plasminogen activator for acute ischemic stroke. Stroke. 2015;46:1870–6.

33. Xie X, Lambrinos A, Chan B, et al. Mechanical thrombectomy in patients with acute ischemic stroke: a cost-utility analysis. CMAJ Open. 2016. doi:10.9778/cmajo.20150088.

34. Powers WJ, Derdeyn CP, Biller J, Ameri- can Heart Association Stroke Council, et al. 2015 AHA/ASA focused update of the 2013 guidelines for the early management of patients with acute ischemic stroke regarding endovascular treat- ment: a guideline for healthcare professionals from the American Heart Association/American Stroke Association. Stroke 2015;46(10): 3020-35.

35. Casaubon LK, Boulanger J-M, Blacquiere D, et al. Heart and Stroke Foundation of Canada Canadian Stroke Best Practices Advisory Committee. Canadian stroke best practice recommendations: hyper- acute stroke care guidelines, update 2015. Int J Stroke. 2015;10:924–40.

36. Wahlgren N, Moreira T, Michel P, et al. Mechanical thrombectomy in acute ischemic stroke: Consensus statement by ESO-Karolinksa Stroke Update 2014/2015, supported by ESO, ESMINT, ESNR and EAN. Int Stroke. 2016;11(1):134–47.

37. Sedation vs. Intubation for Endovascular Stroke Treatment (SIESTA). ClinicalTrials.gov NCT02126085.

38. General Anesthesia Versus Sedation During Intra-arterial Treatment for Stroke (GASS). ClinicalTrials.gov NCT02822144

39. Dippel D, Majoie C, Roos Y, et al. Influence of device choice on the effect of intra-arterial treatment for acute ichemic stroke in MR CLEAN. Stroke. 2016;47:2574–81.

40. Fisher M, Saver JL. Future directions of acute ischaemic stroke therapy. Lancet Neurol. 2015;14(7):758–67.

41. Goyal M, Hill MD, Saver JL, et al. Challenges and opportunities of endovascular stroke therapy. Ann Neurol. 2015;79(1):11–7.

42. Trevo and Medical Management Versus Medical Management Alone in Wake-Up and Late Presenting Strokes (DAWN, ClinicaTrials.gov NCT02142283)

43. Perfusion Imaging Selection of Ischemic Stroke Patients for Endovascular Therapy (POSITIVE, ClinicalTrials.gov NCT01852201)

22

Intracranial vessel wall MRI: a review of current indications and future applications

Adam de Havenon[1*], Lee Chung[1], Min Park[2] and Mahmud Mossa-Basha[3]

Abstract

Background: Intracranial vessel wall MRI (IVWM) is a new diagnostic imaging approach with the goal of evaluating intracranial vascular pathology by directly visualizing arterial vessel wall abnormalities with MR sequences, preferably at 3 Tesla field strength, that suppress blood and have excellent spatial resolution.

Body: The differentiation of intracranial vascular pathology has historically relied on luminal imaging techniques that depict the alteration of flow created by atherosclerotic stenosis or vasospasm. With IVWM, it is possible to identify distinct radiologic findings of the pathology within the intracranial vessel wall itself, ranging from arterial dissection to vasculitis. Futhermore, IVWM imaging characteristics, such as post-contrast enhancement, can elucidate the temporal relationship between imaging findings and clinical pathology; and may predict future behavior of unruptured aneurysms or atherosclerotic plaques.

Conclusion: We present a review of the basic IVWM imaging techniques and the relevant published literature on IVWM, with a focus on evidence-based diagnostic indications for IVWM and discussion of the strengths and weaknesses of each indication. Finally, we discuss how IVWM can be used to differentiate between intracranial pathology and future directions for IVWM research.

Keywords: Vessel wall MRI, Black blood MRI, High-resolution MRI, Intracranial atherosclerosis, Intracranial aneurysm, CNS vasculitis

Background

Intracranial vessel wall MRI (IVWM) is a term for different MRI sequences that share the common goal of achieving sufficient resolution and contrast such that the vessel wall and overlying tissue, such as atherosclerotic plaque, can be accurately assessed; and to differentiate between intracranial vascular pathologies that were previously evaluated with luminal imaging. IVWM, as compared to extracranial vessel wall imaging, is more challenging due to the small caliber and tortuous course of the intracranial arteries. For example, the middle cerebral artery diameter can range from 3 to 5 mm, with a vessel wall thickness from 0.5 to 0.7 mm [1]. While some protocols have used 1.5T scanners, 3T is preferable because of the need for very high resolution and small voxels to accurately depict the normal arterial wall and differentiate between pathological states.

In addition, with decreased in-plane and through-plane resolution, there is increased likelihood of volume averaging and wall blurring [2]. Both 2D and 3D IVWM techniques can be employed depending on the scanning environment and institutional experience [2–13] (Table 1). An important consideration for intracranial vessel wall imaging is blood and cerebrospinal fluid (CSF) suppression for better outer wall boundary evaluation. For 2D vessel wall imaging techniques, spin echo techniques will generate dark blood and are frequently used, but a major limitation is that with slow or in-plane flow, blood suppression will be lost. Multiplanar 2D techniques permit imaging in a plane perpendicular to the axis of the interrogated artery, allowing more complete visualization of the lesion morphology, assessment of its effects on the lumen, minimization of volume averaging effects and accurate estimation of wall thickness. Vessel obliquity, slice thickness and in-plane resolution are all factors that affect wall measurements and the sharpness of the vessel wall borders [14]. Cardiac gating may be performed for 2D IVWM, but its benefit is debatable [2].

* Correspondence: adam.dehavenon@hsc.utah.edu
[1]Department of Neurology, University of Utah, Salt Lake City, USA
Full list of author information is available at the end of the article

Table 1 Common IVWM pulse sequences with advantages/disadvantages

Pulse sequence	Advantages	Disadvantages
3D time of flight (TOF) MRA (non-contrast)	Flow-related enhancement allows identification of luminal abnormality or aneurysm for measurement and placement of IVWM sequences	Luminal imaging alone may not identify non-stenotic vessel abnormalities (outwardly remodeling plaque, non-stenotic dissection, etc.). TOF overestimates stenosis secondary to flow dephasing artifact. It also shows diminished flow in slow flow or in-plane flow states. These are overcome with contrast-enhanced TOF MRA
2D turbo spin echo (TSE) or fast spin echo (FSE)	Wide availability, good in-plane resolution, flexible tissue contrast, reduced sensitivity to magnetic field inhomogeneities, high SNR, can image focused area of interest in rapid acquisition to limit motion artifact	Low spatial resolution in the slice-select direction leading to partial volume effect that can hide subtle findings, poor reproducibility, inability to create multiplanar reformats. Requires multi-planar scanning which is time consuming
3D variable refocusing flip angle (VRFA) sequences (VISTA, Philips; SPACE, Siemens; CUBE, GE)	High SNR with excellent spatial resolution, superior anatomic coverage, T1/T2/PD weightings available, ability to reformat into multiplanar images that allow viewing of vessel wall, plaque, or aneurysm from any aspect. Shorter overall scan time	Requires research preparation prepulse sequence for blood suppression, longer acquisition times for slab can result in motion artifact, more susceptible to magnetic field inhomogeneities
Blood suppression prepulse: • Double inversion-recovery	Available as a commercial pulse, negligible effect on image contrast weighting	Blood-suppression difficult after contrast administration, does not work with 3D techniques
Blood suppression prepulse: • Motion-sensitive driven equilibrium (MSDE)	3D blood suppression technique, robust to large slab size acquisition, in-flow/outflow independent	Can lead to loss of signal with T2 weighting, inability to implement 180° pulse due to high specific absorption rate, B1 inhomogeneity
Blood suppression prepulse: • Delay alternating with nutation for tailored excitation (DANTE)	Best blood suppression, robust to large slab size acquisition, in-flow/outflow independent, no loss of T2 signal, performs well at 7T, available on research sequences from most vendors	Longer imaging time than MSDE may create artifact from vessel wall motion
Gradient-echo 3D T1-weighted without blood suppression (MP-RAGE, FLASH)	Can identify intraplaque hemorrhage in atherosclerosis, intramural hematoma in dissection, and aneurysmal wall hematoma	Lack of blood suppression can hide pathologic findings, unclear significance of intracranial intraplaque hemorrhage. MP-RAGE is preferred sequence

3D acquisitions allow for improved through-plane resolution and permit multi-planar reformations with isotropic acquisitions. 3D variable refocusing flip angle (VRFA) sequences (VISTA, Philips Healthcare, Best, the Netherlands; SPACE, Siemens Healthcare, Erlangen, Germany; CUBE, GE Healthcare, Milwaukee, WI, USA) have been the most extensively studied 3D techniques to date, as these sequences provide excellent image quality, coverage and blood flow suppression in a shorter scan time [3, 4, 15, 16]. VRFA techniques have been used with T1 and proton density (PD) weightings, both before and after gadolinium contrast administration, as the pattern and degree of contrast enhancement can be helpful in differentiating and characterizing vasculopathies [2, 5]. High-resolution 3D T2-weighted imaging has also shown promise for helping further differentiate intracranial vessel wall pathology [17].

The delay alternating with nutation for tailored excitation (DANTE) pulse train, which is a series of low flip angle nonselective pulses interleaved with gradient pulses with short repetition times, results in optimized blood and CSF suppression without effects on tissue contrast [10]. DANTE allows for improved vessel wall assessment with 3D VRFA techniques while also minimizing artifacts from turbulent or slow flow. In addition to VRFA sequences, another 3D technique that successfully suppresses blood flow is motion sensitized driven equilibrium (MSDE),

which employs flow-sensitive dephasing gradients to suppress flow [18]. However, MSDE can result in T2 signal decay and loss of signal.

IVWM protocols can be performed in a time efficient manner. A 3D PD-weighted VRFA sequence (0.4–0.5 mm³ isotropic voxels) with coverage of the major intracranial arteries can be performed on a 3T system in 7 to 11 min [2]. Thus a full protocol, including TOF MRA for localization and PD-weighted VRFA, pre and post contrast, can be performed in under 30 min. As MRI scanners improve in efficiency, field strength, coil element technology and compressed sensing techniques become more efficient, sequences will further shorten with improved coverage [19]. Currently, the majority of research has been conducted using a 12- or 16-channel coil, although data suggests that a 32-channel coil improves the ability to detect pathology in the more peripheral vessels, and may become more prevalent in the future [20].

Intracranial atherosclerosis (Fig. 1)

Compared to time-of-flight (TOF) MRA, which measures degree of stenosis, IVWM is able to characterize multiple imaging features of intracranial plaque [21] and has been more sensitive for the identification of symptomatic atherosclerotic lesions [5]. IVWM is also helpful to identify the morphology of intracranial vessels at [22] or distal [23] to an arterial occlusion, lesions

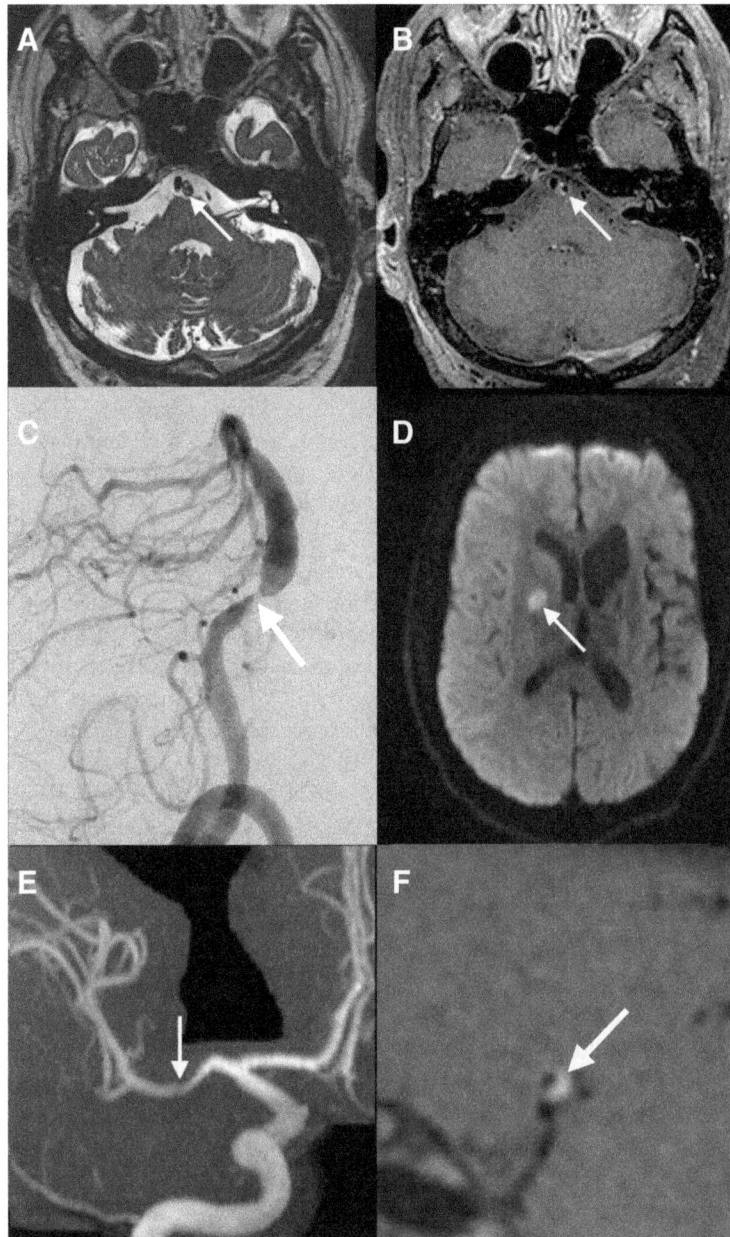

Fig. 1 All images were created with a 3T MRI and 16-channel head coil. **a** 3D axial T2-weighted image of atherosclerotic plaque (*white arrow*) at the vertebrobasilar junction in a patient who presented with a transient ischemic attack. Note the juxtaluminal T2 hyperintensity, depicting the fibrous cap. **b** 3D axial T1-weighted image post-contrast showing eccentric vessel wall enhancement, consistent with a recently symptomatic atherosclerotic plaque, and outward remodeling of the plaque. **c** Digital subtraction angiogram of the same patient in (**a**) and (**b**), showing a lateral view of the atherosclerotic stenosis at the vertebrobasilar junction. **d** Diffusion-weighted image and apparent diffusion coefficient axial images of a second patient who presented with left-sided weakness and was found to have an acute ischemic stroke in the right internal capsule (*white arrows*). **e** TOF MRA shows minimal stenosis in the right M1 segment (*white arrow*) of the middle cerebral artery, at the origin of the lenticulostriate perforators that supplied the distribution of the ischemic stroke. **f** Sagittal reconstruction of the same right M1 segment again demonstrates eccentric wall enhancement, consistent with recently symptomatic atherosclerotic plaque, and outward remodeling at the site of the enhancement

that MRA and CTA do not visualize well. IVWM studies of intracranial stenosis suggest that IVWM is more accurate than MRA at measuring degree of luminal stenosis, [24, 25] and can identify symptomatic non-flow-

limiting intracranial lesions in ischemic stroke that would normally be missed by standard luminal imaging [26].

Compared to asymptomatic MCA atherosclerotic plaques, recently symptomatic plaques are larger and irregularly surfaced with increased ratio of plaque thickening to patent vessel lumen [27–32]. Among MCA plaques with associated deep penetrating artery infarctions, plaque tended to be more superior and less ventral [28, 31]. Symptomatic MCA plaques typically have positive remodeling, characterized by outward remodeling of the stenotic vessel area [26, 28, 29, 33], an association first demonstrated in coronary arterial atherosclerosis [34, 35]. Several studies of pontine ischemic stroke patients have shown that IVWM is more sensitive than TOF MRA to the presence of symptomatic basilar artery (BA) plaque, even in pontine lacunar infarctions, [36] and more predictive of progressive motor deficit during hospitalization [37].

Carotid artery plaque hemorrhage is considered a risk factor of ischemic stroke [38–40]. Histopathological studies of carotid plaque have shown that intraplaque high-intensity signal on vessel wall imaging techniques correlate well with the presence of intraplaque hemorrhage (IPH) [41]. These same principles can be applied to intracranial plaques to both identify the etiology of medium-to-large-vessel stroke and potentially to stratify future risk of ischemic stroke due to intracranial stenosis. For example, T1, T2 and PD weighted IVWM hyperintensity was found to be more common among symptomatic (57.1 %) vs. asymptomatic (22 %) MCA plaques [42], a finding which has been replicated in several studies [43, 44]. In the posterior circulation, a study of 73 patients with >50 % BA stenosis found that IPH, detected on the nonblood suppressed 3D magnetization-prepared rapid gradient-echo (MP-RAGE) sequence, was associated with a 1.64 relative risk of a focal stroke event on DWI ($p < 0.01$), with a sensitivity of 80.0 % and specificity of 46.5 % [45].

Compared to MRA, IVWM permits the evaluation of wall enhancement in intracranial arterial atherosclerosis and the potential identification of sources of acute stroke [12]. This was first demonstrated among 13 ischemic stroke patients who received a 3T IVWM protocol that was compared to CTA, MRA, or catheter angiogram. 12/13 (92.3 %) patients with symptomatic intracranial atherosclerosis had focal areas of eccentric wall enhancement in the relevant major branches of the circle of Willis supplying the area of infarct and 10/12 (83.3 %) had enhancement only in the vessel supplying the infarct [46]. Another study followed acute stroke patients with intracranial atherosclerotic stenosis with IVWM and found strong vessel wall enhancement in all patients imaged within 4 weeks of acute stroke and that the strength and presence of enhancement decreased in the subacute (4–12 weeks) and chronic (>12 weeks) phases [47]. A recent study performed 3T IVWM on 138 patients with symptomatic atherosclerotic plaque of varying degrees

of stenosis (108/138 had plaque enhancement) and followed the patients for a median of 18 months [48] There were 39 stroke recurrences, of which 37/39 were in patients with enhancing plaques, creating a hazard ratio of 7.42 for recurrent stroke among the patients with enhancing plaque.

Given that interobserver reliability for plaque morphology, presence of intracranial IPH and enhancement pattern on contrasted IVWM is excellent [49, 17], it would appear that IVWM could reliably identify symptomatic atherosclerosis. However, it is important to consider that all IVWM findings are also seen in asymptomatic atherosclerosis [4, 33, 45], suggesting that IVWM findings such as plaque enhancement or IPH could be useful for identifying symptomatic atherosclerotic plaque, but only in combination given their individually moderate sensitivity and low specificity. Additional long-term prospective studies with serial radiographic and clinical follow-up, ideally with pathologic correlation, are needed to better understand the clinical significance of these techniques and how they may be combined to optimally characterize intracranial atherosclerosis and predict medical treatment failure, because intracranial atherosclerosis has an annual rate of recurrent stroke that is three times the average of other stroke etiologies (13–18 versus 5 %) and IVWM research suggests it may be even higher in the subgroup of patients with enhancing plaque [48, 50, 51].

Intracranial aneurysm (Fig. 2)

IVWM has been used to identify ruptured intracranial aneurysms (IA). An early study showed that in 5 cases of subarachnoid hemorrhage, the culprit IA consistently demonstrated wall enhancement at the site of rupture [52]. Several of the IAs also demonstrated pre-contrast T1 shortening consistent with intramural hematoma. A larger study of 117 patients, with 61 ruptured and 83 unruptured IAs, used an MSDE 3D pre- and post-contrast protocol that detected "strong/faint enhancement" in 73.8/24.6 % of the ruptured IAs and only 4.8/13.3 % of the unruptured IAs [53]. These results suggest that IA wall enhancement on 3D T1- or PD-weighted post-contrast IVWM could serve as a marker for aneurysm rupture in the 12–20 % of subarachnoid hemorrhage patients found to have multiple IAs, although further investigation is necessary considering that early studies have indicated that unstable unruptured aneurysms may also show wall enhancement [54, 55].

Unruptured intracranial aneurysms (IAs) are a relatively common imaging finding, incidentally found in up to 2 % of luminal imaging studies [56]. Given the historical difficulty in risk stratifying unruptured IAs, IVWM has been used to identify the underlying arterial wall inflammation that is hypothesized to be the driving force

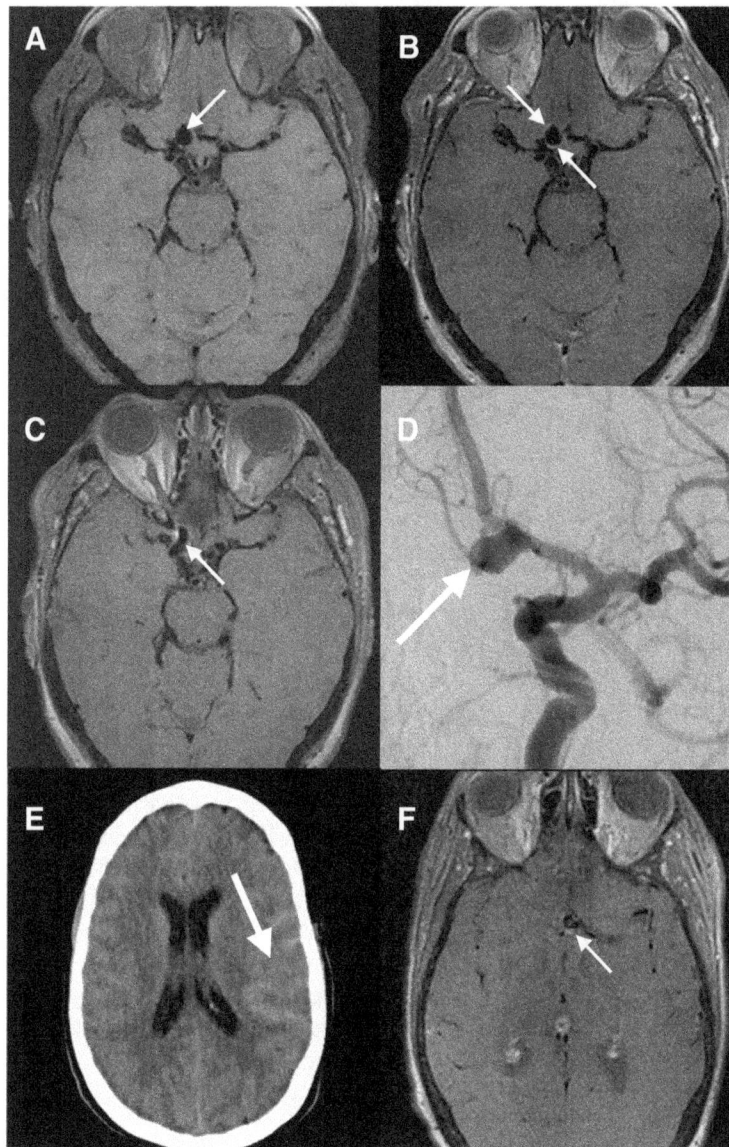

Fig. 2 a 3D axial T1-weighted image showing a large internal carotid artery unruptured aneurysm (*white arrow*). **b** 3D axial T1-weighted post-contrast image showing enhancement of the aneurysm wall, concerning for active inflammation and instability. **c** 3D axial T1-weighted post-contrast image after placement of a flow-diverting stent, which has not yet occluded the aneurysm, but has created a small area of enhancement remote from the aneurysm (*white arrow*), that has been reported after flow-diverting stent placement presumed to be related to local inflammation or thrombosis. **d, e** A second patient who presented with thunderclap headache and was found to have an anterior communicating artery aneurysm (**d**, *white arrow*, digital subtraction angiogram, lateral projection), which had ruptured and caused subarachnoid hemorrhage (**e**, *white arrow*, CT noncontrast, axial). **f** 3D axial T1-weighted post-contrast image showing enhancement of the aneurysm wall, consistent with recent rupture

of IA pathogenesis and, potentially, rupture [57]. The first IVWM study of unruptured IAs imaged 14 patients with saccular IAs using 2D sequences on a 1.5T MRI and found that evaluating IA wall thickness and structure was easier on T1-weighted than T2-weighted sequences [58]. A study of 35 pre-surgical unruptured IAs predicted wall thickness using a combination of a 3D T1 sequence and a 3D steady-state free procession (SSFP) gradient echo sequence, to retain aspects of T2-weighting for contrast generation with spinal fluid [59].

The IVWM prediction agreed with surgical findings in 78 % of cases. The most common reason for an inaccurate pre-surgical IVWM was thrombus within the aneurysm or previous surgical instrumentation [59]. What remains unknown, and of crucial importance, is the ability of IVWM to predict future risk of IA rupture based on imaging characteristics such as wall thickness or enhancement. A retrospective study described IA wall enhancement between 31 "unstable" IAs (ruptured, symptomatic, or undergoing morphological modification) and 77 "stable"

IAs (incidental and nonevolving) [60]. Using a 3T MRI with 3D T1 pre- and post-contrast imaging, wall enhancement was found in 87 % of unstable and only 29 % of the stable IAs.

Several studies have examined IVWM findings after endovascular treatment of IAs. Using standard MRI sequences, it has been identified that IA wall enhancement is common, occurring in 19–66 % of patients treated with endovascular coiling or flow-diversion stents [61–63]. Procedural factors, such as the density of coil packing or coil material and IA-specific characteristics, such as IA size or location, influenced the incidence of wall enhancement, but the MRI findings did not predict IA occlusion success, procedural complications, or post-procedure morbidity such as IA rupture. One case report used IVWM to demonstrate thrombosis of an IA treated with a flow-diversion stent, [64] but otherwise IVWM has not been utilized to study the pathophysiology of IA occlusion following endovascular treatment.

A recently published study examined 11 patients with subarachnoid hemorrhage who had negative catheter angiograms and found that 4/11 had vessel wall enhancement on IVWM near possible sites of IA rupture, raising the possibility of ruptured or thrombosed IAs that may have been missed on luminal imaging modalities [65]. This represents an important future research direction for IVWM studies of patients with non-traumatic subarachnoid hemorrhage who have a negative initial catheter angiogram, which is 10–20 % of patients [66, 67]. The yield of repeat catheter angiography is low in this population and IVWM may allow the identification of the causative pathology and lead to management strategies that reduce future morbidity [68].

Vasculitis (Fig. 3)

Vasculitis, the result of an immune system-mediated attack on the arterial vessel wall, [69, 70] compromises mural integrity and leads to contrast uptake [71]. While there are numerous etiologies for intracranial vasculitis, which have different pathophysiology and temporal courses, the end result of vascular mural inflammation is consistent. Given that IVWM is particularly sensitive to vessel wall enhancement and that other diagnostic tests such as catheter angiogram or cerebrospinal fluid analysis are often inconclusive and lead to invasive brain biopsy, researchers have pursued IVWM in vasculitis. Early research demonstrated the high prevalence of vessel wall enhancement and wall thickening, reported in 23/27 and 25/27 patients in one series [72]. The first 3T study used 2D sequences and identified the concentric pattern of wall enhancement seen in vasculitis, as compared to the eccentric enhancement seen in atherosclerosis [46]. Although reversible cerebral vasospasm syndrome (RCVS) often resembles cerebral vasculitis on luminal imaging modalities such as

MRA or DSA [73], RCVS should exhibit very subtle or no vessel wall enhancement on IVWM as compared to vasculitis [74]. The concentric enhancement pattern of vasculitis has been replicated in subsequent studies [75], but further research is still warranted to verify this finding in a larger cohort with biopsy-proven cerebral vasculitis.

Research has identified more intense enhancement in vasculitis patients than atherosclerosis patients, which has been investigated as a therapeutic efficacy marker [76]. Case reports with longitudinal data have shown improvement of wall enhancement after treatment with immunosuppressive medications [77, 78], but in a study of 4 vasculitis patients there was a decrease in the intensity of enhancement with immunosuppression for 2/4 patients, while in the other 2 the enhancement persisted two months after the index scan despite clinical improvement [76]. Another longitudinal study, using 2D techniques with 3T MRI, showed that on baseline imaging 9/13 vasculitis patients had smooth concentric wall enhancement with wall thickening, 3/13 had eccentric wall enhancement with wall thickening and 1/13 had no identifiable vessel wall abnormality [75]. Follow-up imaging showed variable amounts of improvement in the enhancement after treatment, with some patients continuing to enhance after a year of follow-up despite clinical improvement, highlighting the lack of consistency in follow-up imaging IVWM findings for vasculitis patients. Nonetheless, IVWM's potential role as a marker of treatment response should continue to be investigated given the lack of randomized clinical trials for vasculitis treatment and the heterogeneity of disease activity, patient response, and high rate of adverse effects associated with treatment and uncertain necessary duration of treatment.

Intracranial dissection (Fig. 3)

Arterial vessel wall dissection can be difficult to differentiate from atherosclerotic stenosis/occlusion on conventional luminal imaging modalities [79]. T1-weighted spin echo and gradient echo MRI sequences have long been used to identify the often crescentic intramural hematoma associated with dissection in the aorta, extracranial carotid and extracranial vertebral arteries [80–84]. Similar findings have been described in intracranial vessels [85–88], but inadequate resolution was a significant limitation for the diminutive intracranial vasculature [79]. Sub-millimeter resolution and suppression of intraluminal blood signal on 3T 3D IVWM allows detection of intracranial intramural hematomas and more detailed visualization of secondary features of dissection such as intimal flaps in the vessel lumen, the morphology of the false lumen, or the contours of a dissecting pseudoaneurysm [89].

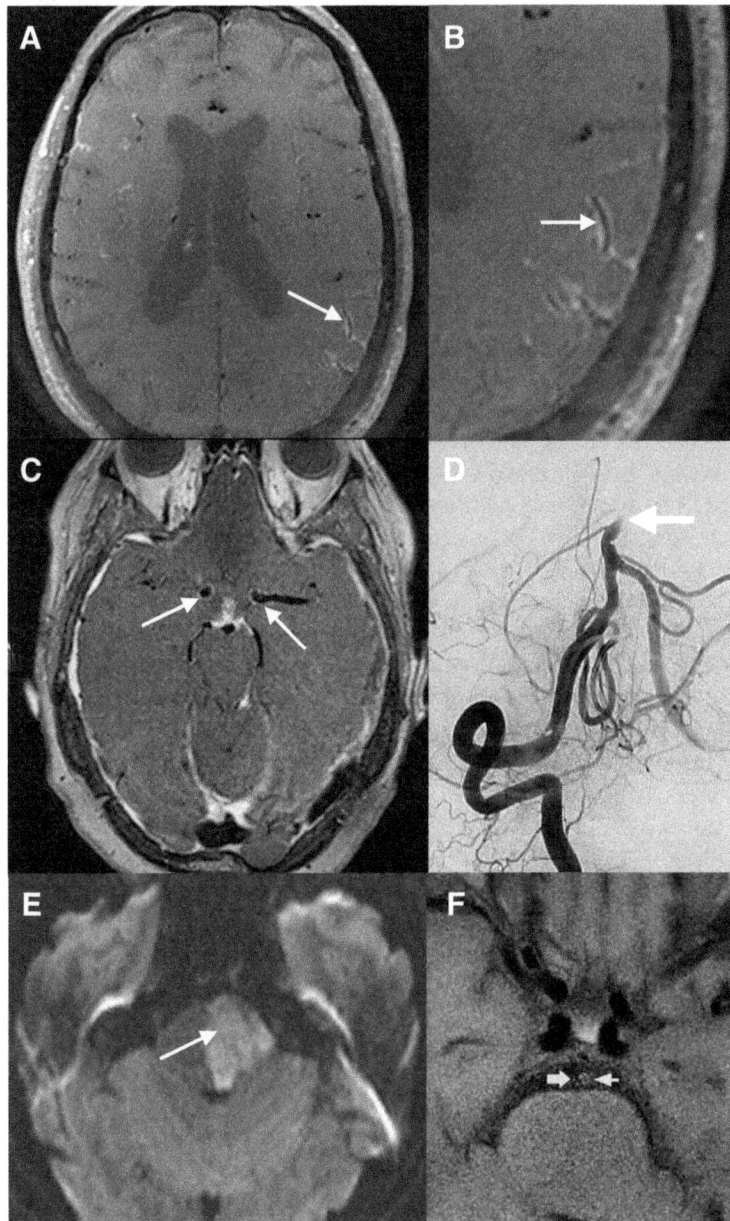

Fig. 3 a 3D axial T1-weighted post-contrast image showing the "tram track" appearance (*white arrow*) of a peripheral MCA branch with concentric enhancement from presumed cerebral vasculitis due to inflammatory amyloid angiopathy with adjacent leptomeningeal enhancement from recen superficial siderosis. **b** Higher magnification of the same patient showing the tram track appearance of concentric enhancement. **c** 3D axial T1-weighted post-contrast image in a second patient with bacterial meningitis and associated vasculitis, showing the concentric vessel wall enhancement in both terminal internal carotid artery segments (*white arrows*), which extends along the left middle cerebral artery vessel. **d** Lateral digital subtraction angiography showing a basilar artery dissection and near occlusion (minimal distal flow was seen on delayed imaging-not shown) (*white arrow*). **e** Axial diffusion-weighted image showing a pontine ischemic stroke (*white arrow*) which resulted from the dissection. **f** 3D axial T1-weighted image, proximal to occlusion, showing eccentric wall thickening with T1 hyperintense signal (*short white arrow*) representing arterial dissection, with the remaining patent lumen (*thick arrow*)

The vertebral arteries are prone to intracranial dissection, but their tortuous course, natural variation in caliber and small size make it difficult to reliably discern pathologic findings from normal variations or adjacent structures such as bone or venous plexuses [90]. Although studies have favorably compared IVWM of

intracranial vertebral artery dissection to other sequences [9, 91, 92] such as TOF MRA and other 3D techniques that do not suppress blood signal like spoiled gradient-recalled (SPGR), only one study attempted to show statistical superiority for the IVWM sequences [8]. In that study, which used a 1.5T MRI and included 18 patients with vertebral artery dissection and 12 controls, a 3D VRFA technique was statistically superior to SPGR in detecting the false lumen of the dissected artery [8].

Less has been published concerning IVWM and intracranial anterior circulation dissection. A case report described how IVWM led to stent placement in a patient with middle cerebral artery dissection and high-grade stenosis [93]. Other case reports have reported successful identification of middle and anterior cerebral artery dissection [94, 95]. None of these studies included a control group or reported rates of false negative IVWM findings, which does not provide support for the routine use of IVWM in patients suspected to have dissection. However, for patients who are strongly suspected of having intracranial dissection, such as trauma patients with cryptogenic ischemic stroke, but have negative CTA or MRA imaging, the definitive test is a digital subtraction angiogram, which carries a nontrivial risk of iatrogenic stroke or other complications [96]. Taking that into account, IVWM could be useful in this subset of patients who have had negative noninvasive screening for dissection, but a high clinical suspicion of dissection. IVWM may also be advantageous over other MRI techniques for the detection of subadventitial dissections, which may be occult on luminal imaging techniques if there is no associated luminal stenosis.

Comparisons to histopathology

Pathological studies comparing excised IAs to IVWM have generally shown excellent agreement between in-vivo and microscopic comparisons. Using rabbits with iatrogenic aneurysms, a study showed IA wall thickness was reliable at the dome of IA, but not the neck and at resolutions greater than one voxel, which modern scanning techniques are reducing to less than 0.5 mm [97]. Comparing 7T MRI on 2 patients with unruptured IAs prior to surgical clipping with histologic measurements on an ex vivo IVWM found excellent correlation for wall thickness measurements [98]. However, the study did not report other morphologic data such as wall enhancement or intramural pathology. If possible, future IVWM IA studies should include comparisons to surgical pathology, which would appear feasible given the number of patients who undergo clipping or other excision procedures, but is complicated by the difficulty of performing pathology on friable arterial vessel walls, often measuring <0.2 mm [99].

In comparison to the atherosclerosis pathology studies performed for IVWM of the carotid arteries, where carotid endarterectomy provides convenient tissue samples [100, 101], the large and medium diameter intracranial vessels, the major sites of atherosclerosis, are not typically available for pathology prior to autopsy.[14] As a result, the majority of studies comparing IVWM to intracranial atherosclerotic histopathology have used post-mortem MR acquisition. Two studies used cadaver intracranial vessel specimens to compare histopathologic findings to 7T IVWM [102, 103]. In those studies, IVWM was accurate at identifying increased wall thickness, areas of foamy macrophages, collagen deposition, luminal stenosis, or outer wall protrusion. However, the conclusions that can be drawn from post-mortem imaging, in the absence of blood or surrounding brain parenchyma and CSF, are not definitive. In one case report, the authors performed 3T IVWM of a patient with diffuse intracranial atherosclerosis and ischemic strokes shortly before they died of pneumonia and sepsis [104]. The plaque was not thought to be symptomatic, but had fibrofatty and calcific components on IVWM that corresponded to lipid and loose matrix, fibrous tissue and calcium on histopathology [104]. Intraplaque hemorrhage was not present in that patient's sample, so comparison was not possible.

Challenges with using IVWM for differentiating intracranial pathology (Fig. 4)

Although distinctive IVWM patterns have been described, the most important factor in using IVWM for reliable differentiation of intracranial pathology is interpreting it in conjunction with clinical information, as no single IVWM imaging finding has sufficiently accurate predictive ability. For example, concentric wall enhancement, usually categorized as continuous circumferential enhancement with the width of the thinnest enhancement being ≥50 % of the thickest segment, can be compared to eccentric enhancement, categorized as either clearly limited to one side of the vessel wall or the thinnest part of the wall enhancement being <50 % of the thickest point. Research shows that eccentric wall enhancement is present more often in intracranial atherosclerotic lesions than in autoimmune or infectious vasculitis [17]. However, concentric wall enhancement IVWM has also been reported in atherosclerotic stroke, RCVS, drug-induced vasculopathy, Graves disease and after both arterial thrombolysis and mechanical thrombectomy [20, 17, 72, 75, 105–107].

An example of how clinical information would help inform the utility of IVWM would be moyamoya disease, which would be expected to be more common in Asian patients with few vascular risk factors [108]. Angiographic imaging findings of moyamoya disease have been described as severely narrowed or occluded arteries of the proximal anterior circulation with extensive collateralization. Moyamoya disease can have similar IVWM findings to vasculitis such as mild concentric enhancement, but confined to the locations favored by the disease – distal ICA and the M1/A1 segments; or moyamoya can display stenosis alone without enhancement [7, 109]. Additional findings

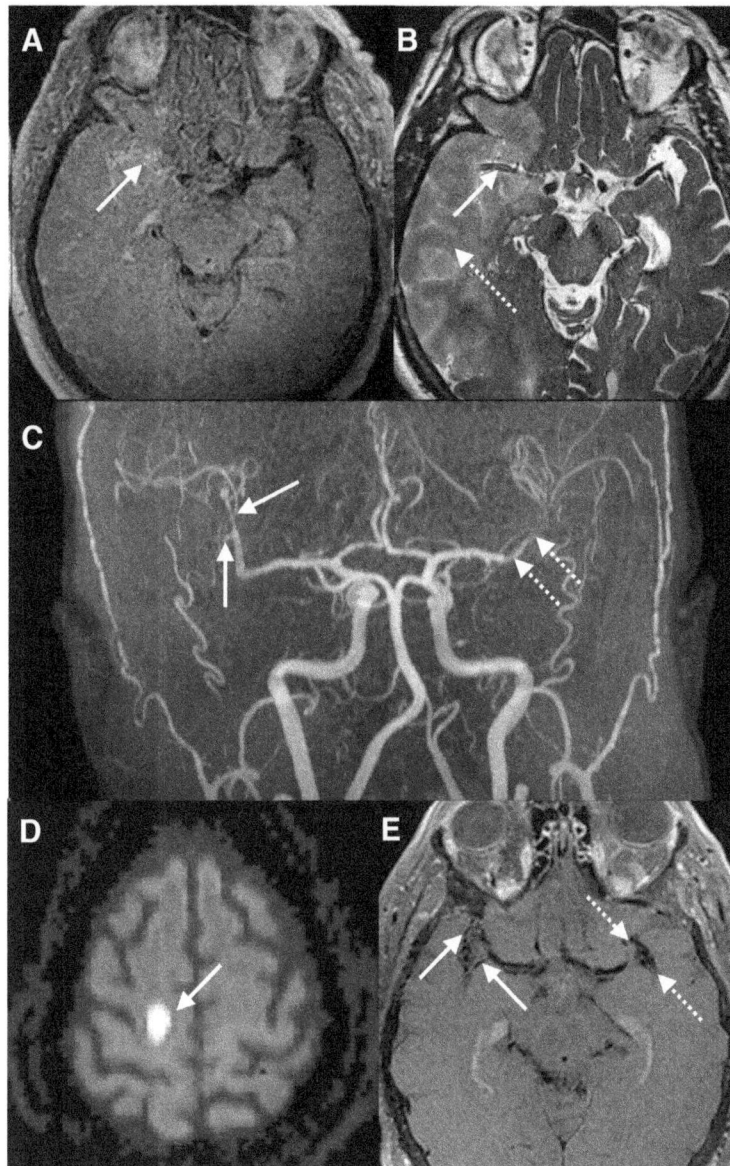

Fig. 4 a 3D axial T1-weighted post-contrast image showing diffuse vessel wall and luminal enhancement (*white arrow*) of the right M1 segment in a patient with left-sided weakness, sensory loss and neglect. **b** 3D axial T2-weighted image of the same section of the right M1 segment with hyperintense signal in the vessel lumen, consistent with occlusive thrombus from recently diagnosed atrial fibrillation, resulting in a large right MCA territory ischemic stroke (*dotted white arrow*). **c** Anterior-posterior digital subtraction angiogram in a second patient who presented with post-coital headache and was found to have multifocal luminal narrowing in the bilateral M2 branches (*dotted* and *solid white arrows*). **d** Axial diffusion-weighted image showing a right hemisphere ischemic stroke in the same patient. **e** 3D axial T1-weighted post-contrast image showing the absence of vessel wall enhancement at the M2 segments corresponding to the narrowing seen on the angiogram in image (**c**), consistent with reversible cerebral vasoconstriction syndrome, which should result in very subtle or no enhancement of the vessel wall at sites of vasospastic narrowing

include absence of wall thickening, collateralization and homogenous signal intensity of the arterial wall [110]. Other imaging features more common in moymoya disease include lack of eccentric lesions and focal enhancement, which help enable differentiation of moyamoya disease from intracranial atherosclerosis and other inflammatory etiologies [46, 109].

Imaging features of intracranial dissection, although exhibiting a pattern of eccentric wall thickening and intimal flap enhancement appearing similar to atherosclerosis, additionally often include crescentic mural T1 pre-contrast hyperintensity representing methemoglobin [46], which is less common and more superficial in intracranial atherosclerotic with intraplaque hemorrhage.

IVWM has also been used to differentiate vertebral and basilar artery hypoplasias from atherosclerosis based on the lack of wall thickening at a stenosis seen in hypoplasia [111, 112]. This may help predict the natural history of such lesions and inform the need for interventional angioplasty in patients with recurrent stroke despite maximal medical therapy.

Multicontrast IVWM, combining T1- with T2-weighted and other sequences, may also prove useful in differentiation of atherosclerosis, RCVS and vasculitis; diagnoses that can require costly or invasive workups [17, 74, 75]. The multicontrast approach will help to minimize the reliance on vessel wall enhancement for pathologic differentiation, which varies in duration in most published research and does not necessarily correlate with disease activity [75]. Indeed, a case report of radiation-induced vasculopathy described persistent IVWM concentric enhancement 2 years following the radiation exposure [113]. Using a multicontrast approach, future researchers can also unravel the natural history of the different intracranial pathologies seen on IVWM and ultimately develop protocols with sequences capable of reliably differentiating a diverse spectrum of intracranial pathology.

Conclusion

IVWM is not currently in wide clinical use, but the conditions for this transition are in place. 2D black blood IVWM techniques are readily available on all MRIs and can be performed at high resolution on 3T systems. All major MRI manufacturers have a 3D VRFA sequence that can be used at 3T, available as either a research or product sequence depending on the scanner make and model, allowing for black blood intracranial imaging with the requisite ability to construct multiplanar images with isotropic sub-millimeter resolution. At a minimum a TOF MRA and T1- or PD-weighted sequence with pre- and post-contrast imaging is required for IVWM, although additional information can be obtained by including a T2-weighted sequence and, in certain clinical scenarios, a 3D T1-weighted gradient echo sequence optimized for the detection of mural hemorrhage such as MP-RAGE. Overall scan time can be less than 30 min and incorporated into the billing format of a conventional MRA with contrast. While the current literature does not support conclusive delineation of intracranial pathology, IVWM allows radiologists to provide clinicians with important insights given the challenging clinical scenarios where IVWM is indicated, such as differentiating between vasculitis, RCVS and atherosclerosis.

Future research will clarify if the unique morphological findings seen on IVWM, such as unruptured IA enhancement or atherosclerotic plaque fibrous cap rupture, can predict future risk of morbidity and mortality from aneurysm rupture or ischemic stroke. There are ongoing prospective longitudinal studies that will begin to answer these questions and others, such as the ability of these morphological features to identify patients who would benefit from different management strategies. In this regard, IVWM has tremendous future potential to identify patients for clinical trials and as a surrogate biomarker outcome.

Abbreviations
BA, basilar artery; CSF, cerebrospinal fluid; CTA, computed tomography angiography; DANTE, delay alternating with nutation for tailored excitation; DWI, diffusion-weigthed imaging; IA, intracranial aneurysm; IPH, intraplaque hemorrhage; IVWM, intracranial vessel wall MRI; MCA, middle cerebral artery; MP-RAGE, magnetization-prepared rapid gradient-echo; MRA, magnetic resonance angiography; MSDE, motion sensitized driven equilibrium; PD, proton density; RCVS, reversible cerebral vasoconstriction syndrome; TOF, time-of-flight; VRFA, variable refocusing flip angle

Acknowledgements
None.

Funding sources
This publication was supported by the National Center for Advancing Translational Sciences of the National Institutes of Health under Award Number KL2TR001065. The content is solely the responsibility of the authors and does not necessarily represent the official views of the National Institutes of Health.

Authors' contributions
AD, LC, MP, and MMB helped conceive of the review, all drafted sections of the manuscript, helped edit it, and gave final approval.

Competing interests
The authors declare that they have no competing interests.

Disclosures
None.

Author details
[1]Department of Neurology, University of Utah, Salt Lake City, USA.
[2]Department of Neurosurgery, University of Utah, Salt Lake City, USA.
[3]Department of Radiology, University of Washington, Seattle, USA.

References
1. Jain K. Some observations on the anatomy of the middle cerebral artery. Can J Surg. 1964;7:134–9.
2. Qiao Y, Steinman DA, Qin Q, Etesami M, Schär M, Astor BC, et al. Intracranial arterial wall imaging using three-dimensional high isotropic resolution black blood MRI at 3.0 Tesla. J Magn Reson Imaging JMRI. 2011;34:22–30.
3. Crowe LA, Gatehouse P, Yang GZ, Mohiaddin RH, Varghese A, Charrier C, et al. Volume-selective 3D turbo spin echo imaging for vascular wall imaging and distensibility measurement. J Magn Reson Imaging JMRI. 2003;17:572–80.
4. Qiao Y, Zeiler SR, Mirbagheri S, Leigh R, Urrutia V, Wityk R, et al. Intracranial plaque enhancement in patients with cerebrovascular events on high-spatial-resolution MR images. Radiology. 2014;271:534–42.
5. Natori T, Sasaki M, Miyoshi M, Ohba H, Katsura N, Yamaguchi M, et al. Evaluating middle cerebral artery atherosclerotic lesions in acute ischemic stroke using magnetic resonance T1-weighted 3-dimensional vessel wall imaging. J Stroke Cerebrovasc Dis. 2014;23:706–11.

6. Portanova A, Hakakian N, Mikulis DJ, Virmani R, Abdalla WMA, Wasserman BA. Intracranial vasa vasorum: insights and implications for imaging. Radiology. 2013;267:667–79.

7. Ryoo S, Cha J, Kim SJ, Choi JW, Ki C-S, Kim KH, et al. High-resolution magnetic resonance wall imaging findings of Moyamoya disease. Stroke J Cereb Circ. 2014;45:2457–60.

8. Sakurai K, Miura T, Sagisaka T, Hattori M, Matsukawa N, Mase M, et al. Evaluation of luminal and vessel wall abnormalities in subacute and other stages of intracranial vertebrobasilar artery dissections using the volume isotropic turbo-spin-echo acquisition (VISTA) sequence: a preliminary study. J Neuroradiol J Neuroradiol. 2013;40:19–28.

9. Takano K, Yamashita S, Takemoto K, Inoue T, Kuwabara Y, Yoshimitsu K. MRI of intracranial vertebral artery dissection: evaluation of intramural haematoma using a black blood, variable-flip-angle 3D turbo spin-echo sequence. Neuroradiology. 2013;55:845–51.

10. Wang J, Helle M, Zhou Z, Börnert P, Hatsukami TS, Yuan C. Joint blood and cerebrospinal fluid suppression for intracranial vessel wall MRI. Magn Reson Med Off J Soc Magn Reson Med Soc Magn Reson Med. 2015;75:831–8.

11. Xie Y, Yang Q, Xie G, Pang J, Fan Z, Li D. Improved black-blood imaging using DANTE-SPACE for simultaneous carotid and intracranial vessel wall evaluation. Magn Reson Med. 2015.

12. Zhang L, Zhang N, Wu J, Zhang L, Huang Y, Liu X, et al. High resolution three dimensional intracranial arterial wall imaging at 3T using T1 weighted SPACE. Magn Reson Imaging. 2015;33:1026–34.

13. Wang J, Zhao X, Yamada K, et al. High-risk mid-cerebral artery atherosclerotic disease detection using Simultaneous Non-contrast Angiography and intraPlaque khemorrhage (SNAP) imaging. Proceedings of the International Society of Magnetic Resonance in Medicine. Salt Lake City, UT, USA; 2013.

14. Antiga L, Wasserman BA, Steinman DA. On the overestimation of early wall thickening at the carotid bulb by black blood MRI, with implications for coronary and vulnerable plaque imaging. Magn Reson Med. 2008;60:1020–8.

15. Busse RF, Brau ACS, Vu A, Michelich CR, Bayram E, Kijowski R, et al. Effects of refocusing flip angle modulation and view ordering in 3D fast spin echo. Magn Reson Med. 2008;60:640–9.

16. Fan Z, Zhang Z, Chung Y-C, Weale P, Zuehlsdorff S, Carr J, et al. Carotid arterial wall MRI at 3T using 3D variable-flip-angle turbo spin-echo (TSE) with flow-sensitive dephasing (FSD). J Magn Reson Imaging JMRI. 2010;31:645–54.

17. Mossa-Basha M, Hwang WD, De Havenon A, Hippe D, Balu N, Becker KJ, et al. Multicontrast high-resolution vessel wall magnetic resonance imaging and its value in differentiating intracranial vasculopathic processes. Stroke J Cereb Circ. 2015;46:1567–73.

18. Zhu C, Graves MJ, Yuan J, Sadat U, Gillard JH, Patterson AJ. Optimization of improved motion-sensitized driven-equilibrium (iMSDE) blood suppression for carotid artery wall imaging. J Cardiovasc Magn Reson Off J Soc Cardiovasc Magn Reson. 2014;16:61.

19. Yang Y, Liu F, Xu W, Crozier S. Compressed sensing MRI via two-stage reconstruction. IEEE Trans Biomed Eng. 2015;62:110–8.

20. Franke P, Markl M, Heinzelmann S, Vaith P, Bürk J, Langer M, et al. Evaluation of a 32-channel versus a 12-channel head coil for high-resolution post-contrast MRI in giant cell arteritis (GCA) at 3T. Eur J Radiol. 2014;83:1875–80.

21. Yang H, Zhu Y, Geng Z, Li C, Zhou L, Liu QI. Clinical value of black-blood high-resolution magnetic resonance imaging for intracranial atherosclerotic plaques. Exp Ther Med. 2015;10:231–6.

22. Kim SM, Ryu C-W, Jahng G-H, Kim EJ, Choi WS. Two different morphologies of chronic unilateral middle cerebral artery occlusion: evaluation using high-resolution MRI. J Neuroimaging Off J Am Soc Neuroimaging. 2014;24:460–6.

23. Hui FK, Zhu X, Jones SE, Uchino K, Bullen JA, Hussain MS, et al. Early experience in high-resolution MRI for large vessel occlusions. J Neurointerventional Surg. 2015;7:509–16.

24. Klein IF, Lavallée PC, Touboul PJ, Schouman-Claeys E, Amarenco P. In vivo middle cerebral artery plaque imaging by high-resolution MRI. Neurology. 2006;67:327–9.

25. Kim YS, Lim S-H, Oh K-W, Kim JY, Koh S-H, Kim J, et al. The advantage of high-resolution MRI in evaluating basilar plaques: a comparison study with MRA. Atherosclerosis. 2012;224:411–6.

26. de Havenon A, Yuan C, Tirschwell D, Hatsukami T, Anzai Y, Becker K, et al. Nonstenotic culprit plaque: the utility of high-resolution vessel wall mri of intracranial vessels after ischemic stroke. Case Rep Radiol. [Internet]. 2015 [cited 2015 Sep 18];2015. Available from: http://www.ncbi.nlm.nih.gov/pmc/articles/PMC4543789/.

27. Sui B, Gao P, Lin Y, Jing L, Qin H. Distribution and features of middle cerebral artery atherosclerotic plaques in symptomatic patients: a 3.0 T high-resolution MRI study. Neurol Res. 2015;37:391–6.

28. Zhao D-L, Deng G, Xie B, Ju S, Yang M, Chen X-H, et al. High-resolution MRI of the vessel wall in patients with symptomatic atherosclerotic stenosis of the middle cerebral artery. J Clin Neurosci Off J Neurosurg Soc Australas. 2015;22:700–4.

29. Chung GH, Kwak HS, Hwang SB, Jin GY. High resolution MR imaging in patients with symptomatic middle cerebral artery stenosis. Eur J Radiol. 2012;81:4069–74.

30. Xu W-H, Li M-L, Niu J-W, Feng F, Jin Z-Y, Gao S. Intracranial artery atherosclerosis and lumen dilation in cerebral small-vessel diseases: a high-resolution MRI Study. CNS Neurosci Ther. 2014;20:364–7.

31. Xu W-H, Li M-L, Gao S, Ni J, Zhou L-X, Yao M, et al. Plaque distribution of stenotic middle cerebral artery and its clinical relevance. Stroke. 2011;42:2957–9.

32. Kim BJ, Yoon Y, Lee D-H, Kang D-W, Kwon SU, Kim JS. The shape of middle cerebral artery and plaque location: high-resolution MRI finding. Int J Stroke Off J Int Stroke Soc. 2015;10:856–60.

33. Xu W-H, Li M-L, Gao S, Ni J, Zhou L-X, Yao M, et al. In vivo high-resolution MR imaging of symptomatic and asymptomatic middle cerebral artery atherosclerotic stenosis. Atherosclerosis. 2010;212:507–11.

34. Nishioka T, Luo H, Eigler NL, Berglund H, Kim C-J, Siegel RJ. Contribution of inadequate compensatory enlargement to development of human coronary artery stenosis: An in vivo intravascular ultrasound study. J Am Coll Cardiol. 1996;27:1571–6.

35. Schoenhagen P, Ziada KM, Kapadia SR, Crowe TD, Nissen SE, Tuzcu EM. Extent and direction of arterial remodeling in stable versus unstable coronary syndromes an intravascular ultrasound study. Circulation. 2000;101:598–603.

36. Klein IF, Lavallée PC, Mazighi M, Schouman-Claeys E, Labreuche J, Amarenco P. Basilar artery atherosclerotic plaques in paramedian and lacunar pontine infarctions: a high-resolution MRI study. Stroke J Cereb Circ. 2010;41:1405–9.

37. Lim S-H, Choi H, Kim H-T, Kim J, Heo SH, Chang D, et al. Basilar plaque on high-resolution MRI predicts progressive motor deficits after pontine infarction. Atherosclerosis. 2015;240:278–83.

38. Saam T, Hetterich H, Hoffmann V, Yuan C, Dichgans M, Poppert H, et al. Meta-analysis and systematic review of the predictive value of carotid plaque hemorrhage on cerebrovascular events by magnetic resonance imaging. J Am Coll Cardiol. 2013;62:1081–91.

39. McNally JS, Kim S-E, Yoon H-C, Findeiss LK, Roberts JA, Nightingale DR, et al. Carotid magnetization-prepared rapid acquisition with gradient-echo signal is associated with acute territorial cerebral ischemic events detected by diffusion-weighted MRI. Circ Cardiovasc Imaging. 2012;5:376–82.

40. McNally JS, McLaughlin MS, Hinckley PJ, Treiman SM, Stoddard GJ, Parker DL, et al. Intraluminal thrombus, intraplaque hemorrhage, plaque thickness, and current smoking optimally predict carotid stroke. Stroke J Cereb Circ. 2015;46:84–90.

41. Ota H, Yarnykh VL, Ferguson MS, Underhill HR, Demarco JK, Zhu DC, et al. Carotid intraplaque hemorrhage imaging at 3.0-T MR imaging: comparison of the diagnostic performance of three T1-weighted sequences. Radiology. 2010;254:551–63.

42. Ryu C-W, Jahng G-H, Kim E-J, Choi W-S, Yang D-M. High resolution wall and lumen MRI of the middle cerebral arteries at 3 tesla. Cerebrovasc Dis Basel Switz. 2009;27:433–42.

43. Vakil P, Ansari SA, Cantrell CG, Eddleman CS, Dehkordi FH, Vranic J, et al. Quantifying intracranial aneurysm wall permeability for risk assessment using dynamic contrast-enhanced MRI: a pilot study. AJNR Am J Neuroradiol. 2015;36:953–9.

44. Kim J, Jung K, Sohn C, Moon J, Han M, Roh J. Middle cerebral artery plaque and prediction of the infarction pattern. Arch Neurol. 2012;69:1470–5.

45. Yu JH, Kwak HS, Chung GH, Hwang SB, Park MS, Park SH. Association of intraplaque hemorrhage and acute infarction in patients with basilar artery plaque. Stroke J Cereb Circ. 2015;46:2768–72.

46. Swartz RH, Bhuta SS, Farb RI, Agid R, Willinsky RA, terBrugge KG, et al. Intracranial arterial wall imaging using high-resolution 3-tesla contrast-enhanced MRI. Neurology. 2009;72:627–34.

47. Skarpathiotakis M, Mandell DM, Swartz RH, Tomlinson G, Mikulis DJ. Intracranial atherosclerotic plaque enhancement in patients with ischemic stroke. Am J Neuroradiol. 2013;34:299–304.

48. Kim J-M, Jung K-H, Sohn C-H, Moon J, Shin J-H, Park J, et al. Intracranial plaque enhancement from high resolution vessel wall magnetic resonance imaging predicts stroke recurrence. Int J Stroke. 2016;11:171–9.

49. Yang W-Q, Huang B, Liu X-T, Liu H-J, Li P-J, Zhu W-Z. Reproducibility of high-resolution MRI for the middle cerebral artery plaque at 3T. Eur J Radiol. 2014;83:e49–55.

50. Kasner SE, Chimowitz MI, Lynn MJ, Howlett-Smith H, Stern BJ, Hertzberg VS, et al. Predictors of ischemic stroke in the territory of a symptomatic intracranial arterial stenosis. Circulation. 2006;113:555–63.

51. Hong K-S, Yegiaian S, Lee M, Lee J, Saver JL. Declining stroke and vascular event recurrence rates in secondary prevention trials over the past 50 years and consequences for current trial design. Circulation. 2011;123:2111–9.

52. Matouk CC, Mandell DM, Günel M, Bulsara KR, Malhotra A, Hebert R, et al. Vessel wall magnetic resonance imaging identifies the site of rupture in patients with multiple intracranial aneurysms: proof of principle. Neurosurgery. 2013;72:492–6. discussion 496.

53. Nagahata S, Nagahata M, Obara M, Kondo R, Minagawa N, Sato S, Sato S, Mouri W, Saito S, Kayama T. Wall enhancement of the intracranial aneurysms revealed by magnetic resonance vessel wall imaging using three-dimensional turbo spin-echo sequence with motion-sensitized driven-equilibrium: a sign of ruptured aneurysm? Clin Neuroradiol. 2014.

54. Kaminogo M, Yonekura M, Shibata S. Incidence and outcome of multiple intracranial aneurysms in a defined population. Stroke. 2003;34:16–21.

55. Navalitloha Y, Taechoran C, O'Chareon S. Multiple intracranial aneurysms: incidence and management outcome in King Chulalongkorn Memorial Hospital. J Med Assoc Thail Chotmaihet Thangphaet. 2000;83:1442–6.

56. Park S, Lee DH, Ryu C-W, Pyun HW, Choi CG, Kim SJ, et al. Incidental saccular aneurysms on head MR angiography: 5 Years' experience at a single large-volume center. J Stroke. 2014;16:189–94.

57. Chalouhi N, Ali MS, Jabbour PM, Tjoumakaris SI, Gonzalez LF, Rosenwasser RH, et al. Biology of intracranial aneurysms: role of inflammation. J Cereb Blood Flow Metab. 2012;32:1659–76.

58. Park JK, Lee CS, Sim KB, Huh JS, Park JC. Imaging of the walls of saccular cerebral aneurysms with double inversion recovery black-blood sequence. J Magn Reson Imaging. 2009;30:1179–83.

59. Tenjin H, Tanigawa S, Takadou M, Ogawa T, Mandai A, Nanto M, et al. Relationship between preoperative magnetic resonance imaging and surgical findings: aneurysm wall thickness on high-resolution T1-weighted imaging and contact with surrounding tissue on steady-state free precession imaging. Neurol Med Chir (Tokyo). 2013;53:336–42.

60. Edjlali M, Gentric J-C, Régent-Rodriguez C, Trystram D, Hassen WB, Lion S, et al. Does aneurysmal wall enhancement on vessel wall MRI help to distinguish stable from unstable intracranial aneurysms? Stroke J Cereb Circ. 2014;45:3704–6.

61. Su I-C, Willinsky RA, Fanning NF, Agid R. Aneurysmal wall enhancement and perianeurysmal edema after endovascular treatment of unruptured cerebral aneurysms. Neuroradiology. 2014;56:487–95.

62. McGuinness BJ, Memon S, Hope JK. Prospective study of early MRI appearances following flow-diverting stent placement for intracranial aneurysms. AJNR Am J Neuroradiol. 2015;36:943–8.

63. Fanning NF, Willinsky RA, terBrugge KG. Wall enhancement, edema, and hydrocephalus after endovascular coil occlusion of intradural cerebral aneurysms. J Neurosurg. 2008;108:1074–86.

64. Gory B, Sigovan M, Vallecilla C, Courbebaisse G, Turjman F. High-resolution MRI visualization of aneurysmal thrombosis after flow diverter stent placement. J Neuroimaging. 2015;25:310–1.

65. Coutinho JM, Sacho RH, Schaafsma JD, Agid R, Krings T, Radovanovic I, Matouk CC, Mikulis DJ, Mandell DM. High-Resolution Vessel Wall Magnetic Resonance Imaging in Angiogram-Negative Non-Perimesencephalic Subarachnoid Hemorrhage. Clin Neuroradiol. 2015.

66. Khan AA, Smith JDS, Kirkman MA, Robertson FJ, Wong K, Dott C, et al. Angiogram negative subarachnoid haemorrhage: outcomes and the role of repeat angiography. Clin Neurol Neurosurg. 2013;115:1470–5.

67. Lin N, Zenonos G, Kim AH, Nalbach SV, Du R, Frerichs KU, et al. Angiogram-negative subarachnoid hemorrhage: relationship between bleeding pattern and clinical outcome. Neurocrit Care. 2012;16:389–98.

68. Yu D-W, Jung Y-J, Choi B-Y, Chang C-H. Subarachnoid hemorrhage with negative baseline digital subtraction angiography: is repeat digital subtraction angiography necessary? J Cerebrovasc Endovasc Neurosurg. 2012;14:210–5.

69. Lh C. Vasculitis of the central nervous system. Rheum Dis Clin North Am. 1995;21:1059–76.

70. Hajj-Ali RA, Calabrese LH. Primary Central Nervous System Vasculitis. In: MS GSHM, MD CMW, MHS CALM, MD JJG, editors. Inflamm. Dis. Blood Vessels

[Internet]. Wiley-Blackwell; 2012 [cited 2015 Dec 30]. p. 322–31. Available from: http://onlinelibrary.wiley.com/doi/10.1002/9781118355244.ch29/summary.

71. Bley TA, Wieben O, Vaith P, Schmidt D, Ghanem NA, Langer M. Magnetic resonance imaging depicts mural inflammation of the temporal artery in giant cell arteritis. Arthritis Care Res. 2004;51:1062–3.

72. Küker W, Gaertner S, Nagele T, Dopfer C, Schoning M, Fiehler J, et al. Vessel wall contrast enhancement: a diagnostic sign of cerebral vasculitis. Cerebrovasc Dis Basel Switz. 2008;26:23–9.

73. Miller TR, Shivashankar R, Mossa-Basha M, Gandhi D. Reversible cerebral vasoconstriction syndrome, part 2: diagnostic work-up, imaging evaluation, and differential diagnosis. AJNR Am J Neuroradiol. 2015;36:1580–8.

74. Mandell DM, Matouk CC, Farb RI, Krings T, Agid R, TerBrugge K, et al. Vessel wall MRI to differentiate between reversible cerebral vasoconstriction syndrome and central nervous system vasculitis preliminary results. Stroke. 2012;43:860–2.

75. Obusez EC, Hui F, Hajj-Ali RA, Cerejo R, Calabrese LH, Hammad T, et al. High-resolution MRI vessel wall imaging: spatial and temporal patterns of reversible cerebral vasoconstriction syndrome and central nervous system vasculitis. AJNR Am J Neuroradiol. 2014;35:1527–32.

76. Pfefferkorn T, Linn J, Habs M, Opherk C, Cyran C, Ottomeyer C, et al. Black blood MRI in suspected large artery primary angiitis of the central nervous system. J Neuroimaging Off J Am Soc Neuroimaging. 2013;23:379–83.

77. Noh HJ, Choi JW, Kim JP, Moon GJ, Bang OY. Role of high-resolution magnetic resonance imaging in the diagnosis of primary angiitis of the central nervous system. J Clin Neurol Seoul Korea. 2014;10:267–71.

78. Saam T, Habs M, Pollatos O, Cyran C, Pfefferkorn T, Dichgans M, et al. High-resolution black-blood contrast-enhanced T1 weighted images for the diagnosis and follow-up of intracranial arteritis. Br J Radiol. 2010;83:e182–4.

79. Naggara O, Oppenheim C, Louillet F, Touzé E, Mas J-L, Leclerc X, et al. Traumatic intracranial dissection: mural hematoma on high-resolution MRI. J Neuroradiol J Neuroradiol. 2010;37:136–7.

80. Schievink WI. Spontaneous dissection of the carotid and vertebral arteries. N Engl J Med. 2001;344:898–906.

81. Flis CM, Jäger HR, Sidhu PS. Carotid and vertebral artery dissections: clinical aspects, imaging features and endovascular treatment. Eur Radiol. 2007;17:820–34.

82. Vertinsky AT, Schwartz NE, Fischbein NJ, Rosenberg J, Albers GW, Zaharchuk G. Comparison of multidetector CT angiography and MR imaging of cervical artery dissection. AJNR Am J Neuroradiol. 2008;29:1753–60.

83. Baliga RR, Nienaber CA, Bossone E, Oh JK, Isselbacher EM, Sechtem U, et al. The role of imaging in aortic dissection and related syndromes. JACC Cardiovasc Imaging. 2014;7:406–24.

84. Ben Hassen W, Machet A, Edjlali-Goujon M, Legrand L, Ladoux A, Mellerio C, et al. Imaging of cervical artery dissection. Diagn Interv Imaging. 2014;95:1151–61.

85. Ohkuma H, Suzuki S, Kikkawa T, Shimamura N. Neuroradiologic and clinical features of arterial dissection of the anterior cerebral artery. AJNR Am J Neuroradiol. 2003;24:691–9.

86. Hosoya T, Adachi M, Yamaguchi K, Haku T, Kayama T, Kato T. Clinical and neuroradiological features of intracranial vertebrobasilar artery dissection. Stroke. 1999;30:1083–90.

87. Ohkuma H, Suzuki S, Shimamura N, Nakano T. Dissecting aneurysms of the middle cerebral artery: neuroradiological and clinical features. Neuroradiology. 2003;45:143–8.

88. Kurino M, Yoshioka S, Ushio Y. Spontaneous dissecting aneurysms of anterior and middle cerebral artery associated with brain infarction: a case report and review of the literature. Surg Neurol. 2002;57:428–36.

89. Chun DH, Kim ST, Jeong YG, Jeong HW. High-resolution magnetic resonance imaging of intracranial vertebral artery dissecting aneurysm for planning of endovascular treatment. J Korean Neurosurg Soc. 2015;58:155–8.

90. Naggara O, Louillet F, Touzé E, Roy D, Leclerc X, Mas J-L, et al. Added value of high-resolution MR imaging in the diagnosis of vertebral artery dissection. Am J Neuroradiol. 2010;31:1707–12.

91. Han M, Rim N-J, Lee JS, Kim SY, Choi JW. Feasibility of high-resolution MR imaging for the diagnosis of intracranial vertebrobasilar artery dissection. Eur Radiol. 2014;24:3017–24.

92. Chung J-W, Kim BJ, Choi BS, Sohn CH, Bae H-J, Yoon B-W, et al. High-resolution magnetic resonance imaging reveals hidden etiologies of symptomatic vertebral arterial lesions. J Stroke Cerebrovasc Dis Off J Natl Stroke Assoc. 2014;23:293–302.

93. Lee H-O, Kwak H-S, Chung G-H, Hwang S-B. Diagnostic usefulness of high resolution cross sectional MRI in symptomatic middle cerebral arterial dissection. J Korean Neurosurg Soc. 2011;49:370.

94. Kwak HS, Hwang SB, Chung GH, Jeong S-K. High-resolution magnetic resonance imaging of symptomatic middle cerebral artery dissection. J Stroke Cerebrovasc Dis Off J Natl Stroke Assoc. 2014;23:550–3.

95. Chen H, Li Z, Luo B, Zeng J. Anterior cerebral artery dissection diagnosed using high-resolution MRI. Neurology. 2015;85:481.

96. Cloft HJ, Joseph GJ, Dion JE. Risk of cerebral angiography in patients with subarachnoid hemorrhage, cerebral aneurysm, and arteriovenous malformation a meta-analysis. Stroke. 1999;30:317–20.

97. Sherif C, Kleinpeter G, Loyoddin M, Mach G, Plasenzotti R, Haider T, et al. Aneurysm wall thickness measurements of experimental aneurysms: in vivo high-field MR imaging versus direct microscopy. Acta Neurochir Suppl. 2015;120:17–20.

98. Kleinloog R, Korkmaz E, Zwanenburg JJM, Kuijf HJ, Visser F, Blankena R, et al. Visualization of the aneurysm wall: a 7.0-tesla magnetic resonance imaging study. Neurosurgery. 2014;75:614–22. discussion 622.

99. Cahill J, Zhang JH. Subarachnoid hemorrhage is It time for a new direction? Stroke. 2009;40:S86–7.

100. Yuan C, Mitsumori LM, Ferguson MS, Polissar NL, Echelard D, Ortiz G, et al. In vivo accuracy of multispectral magnetic resonance imaging for identifying lipid-rich necrotic cores and intraplaque hemorrhage in advanced human carotid plaques. Circulation. 2001;104:2051–6.

101. Mitsumori LM, Hatsukami TS, Ferguson MS, Kerwin WS, Cai J, Yuan C. In vivo accuracy of multisequence MR imaging for identifying unstable fibrous caps in advanced human carotid plaques. J Magn Reson Imaging JMRI. 2003;17:410–20.

102. van der Kolk AG, Zwanenburg JJM, Denswil NP, Vink A, Spliet WGM, Daemen MJ AP, et al. Imaging the intracranial atherosclerotic vessel wall using 7T MRI: initial comparison with histopathology. AJNR Am J Neuroradiol. 2015;36:694–701.

103. Majidi S, Sein J, Watanabe M, Hassan AE, Van de Moortele P-F, Suri MFK, et al. Intracranial-derived atherosclerosis assessment: an in vitro comparison between virtual histology by intravascular ultrasonography, 7T MRI, and histopathologic findings. AJNR Am J Neuroradiol. 2013;34:2259–64.

104. Turan TN, Rumboldt Z, Granholm A-C, Columbo L, Welsh CT, Lopes-Virella MF, et al. Intracranial atherosclerosis: correlation between in-vivo 3T high resolution MRI and pathology. Atherosclerosis. 2014;237:460–3.

105. Yin J, Zhu J, Huang D, Shi C, Guan Y, Zhou L, et al. Unilateral symptomatic intracranial arterial stenosis and myopathy in an adolescent with Graves disease: a case report of an high-resolution magnetic resonance imaging study. J Stroke Cerebrovasc Dis Off J Natl Stroke Assoc. 2015;24:e49–52.

106. Guerrero WR, Dababneh H, Hedna S, Johnson JA, Peters K, Waters MF. Vessel wall enhancement in herpes simplex virus central nervous system vasculitis. J Clin Neurosci Off J Neurosurg Soc Australas. 2013;20:1318–9.

107. Power S, Matouk C, Casaubon LK, Silver FL, Krings T, Mikulis DJ, et al. Vessel wall magnetic resonance imaging in acute ischemic stroke: effects of embolism and mechanical thrombectomy on the arterial wall. Stroke J Cereb Circ. 2014;45:2330–4.

108. Ahn S-H, Lee J, Kim Y-J, Kwon SU, Lee D, Jung S-C, et al. Isolated MCA disease in patients without significant atherosclerotic risk factors: a high-resolution magnetic resonance imaging study. Stroke J Cereb Circ. 2015; 46:697–703.

109. Kim J-M, Jung K-H, Sohn C-H, Park J, Moon J, Han MH, et al. High-resolution MR technique can distinguish moyamoya disease from atherosclerotic occlusion. Neurology. 2013;80:775–6.

110. Yuan M, Liu Z, Wang Z, Li B, Xu L, Xiao X. High-resolution MR imaging of the arterial wall in moyamoya disease. Neurosci Lett. 2015;584:77–82.

111. Mariani LL, Klein I, Pico F. Hypoplasia or stenosis: usefulness of high-resolution MRI. Rev Neurol (Paris). 2011;167:619–21.

112. Zhu X-J, Wang W, Du B, Liu L, He X-X, Hu L-B, et al. Wall imaging for unilateral intracranial vertebral artery hypoplasia with three-dimensional high-isotropic resolution magnetic resonance images. Chin Med J (Engl). 2015;128:1601–6.

113. Li M, Wu S-W, Xu W-H. High-resolution MRI of radiation-induced intracranial vasculopathy. Neurology. 2015;84:631.

23

'Networks in the brain: from neurovascular coupling of the BOLD effect to brain functional architecture'

Luigi Barberini[1,2]* (iD), Francesco Marrosu[1], Iole Tommasini Barbarossa[3], Melania Melis[3], Harman S. Suri[4], Antonella Mandas[1], Jashit S. Suri[4], Antonella Balestrieri[1,5], Michele Anzidei[6] and Luca Saba[1,5]

Abstract

Background: Recently, many academic research groups focused their attention on changes in human brain networks related to several kinds of pathologies and diseases. Generally speaking, Network Medicine promises to identify the principles to understand, at the molecular level, the human life complex system. We applied the theoretical approach of the Network Medicine mainly to brain diseases, testing the potentiality of the method to produce an early and more in-depth diagnostic process. However, the range of our topics and application of the Network Medicine spans from common neurological and neuropsychological spectrum disorders to other physiological systems or district, only apparently out of the action range of the neurological one. In the areas of Neurology and Neuropsychology we are studying brain networks in Tourette Syndrome [TS] and Multiple Sclerosis [MS]. Moreover, we are studying brain networking related to genotype alteration responsible for different gustatory stimuli processing in the brain. Further, we recently started to study infective diseases and immunological system.

Main body of the abstract: The analysis of brain networks is made feasible by the development and application of imaging acquisition methods based on the Magnetic Resonance Imaging and functional MRI, as well as the availability of innovative calculation tools from graph theory and complex dynamical systems. This paper highlights the Network Medicine concepts and the application of the functional connectivity for the brain networks description. We will describe all these methods with a reduced use of formulas, along with some technical tools available in the WEB to perform the calculations of the related parameters. We will briefly describe the freely available software CONN used for calculating different connectivity parameters. In all these studies, the networks characterisation is performed using indexes from metric and topology of the brain networks. The possibility of early recognition of the diseases by the identification of the alteration in the network's parameters may significantly improve patient outcome, with also significant social community benefits. We intend to illustrate a possible pipeline for the Networks Brain application to neuroradiologists involved in the diagnosis of complex diseases.

Short conclusion: The multidisciplinary approach is one of the essential characteristics of journals in the imaging sciences field; the issues and the methodologies examined in this paper could be of great interest to the reader's community. Furthermore, until today very few studies focused on the network medicine and connectivity explored in functional MRI. Hence this might have an additional value for the journal.

* Correspondence: barberini@unica.it
[1]Department of Medical Sciences and Public Health, University of Cagliari, Cagliari, Italy
[2]Department of Nuclear Medicine, Universitary Hospital of Cagliari AOU, Cagliari, Italy
Full list of author information is available at the end of the article

Background

The brain is connected! The topology and the metric of these connections across Central Nervous System (CNS), and Peripheral Nervous System (PNS) reflect a holistic view of human functions and life. Modern Medicine needs to identify new paradigms for diagnostic, and therapeutic approaches, to consider human health differently. All the biological systems, regarded as fundamental constituents of living beings, are structured and connected. Indeed, the connection between the systems and the connection across the systems are present. Connections in humans can occur between different elementary units such as neurons, nephrons, cardiomyocyte, and so on, and among various tissues and organs, generally through a large variety of molecules. In this context, the problem is to identify the structures and the properties of these connections and to determine the mathematical laws describing their dynamic [1] . This approach may potentially answer to critical medical-related questions through the accurate description of the ways used by Biological Systems to perform the vital functions.

Characterization of the networks in and towards the brain may be useful to evaluate diseases alterations in other organs, hence to optimise early diagnostic tools and treatments. In this paper, we report some applications of brain networks analysis, based on the nuclear magnetic resonance imaging, for the assessment of several human pathological mechanisms. Magnetic resonance imaging may be considered as a relevant application tool for this innovative strategy for the brain functions evaluation.

fMRI and neurovascular coupling

Magnetic resonance technology may be used in brain imaging to realise structural images of the inner part of the brain and to quantify functional neuronal activity. The most diffused technique for neurons activity measurement is electroencephalography (EEG). However, EEG only allows for the investigation of the cortical neurons functions. Functional magnetic resonance imaging, or functional MRI (fMRI) [2], indirectly measures brain activity by detecting changes associated with local blood flow. It is a low sensitivity technique with signals dynamic spanning a broad temporal range. In fact, this technique relies on the fact that cerebral blood flow and neuronal activation are indirectly connected. When the need to perform a task activates a particular area of the brain, the blood flow toward that region increases to compensate the consumption of the oxygenated haemoglobin (oxyHb). Indeed, local blood flow in the brain is strictly related to oxygen ($O2$) and carbon dioxide ($CO2$) concentrations in tissues due to neurons energy consumption. This mechanism leads to regional differences in cerebral blood flow (CBF). Therefore, the Region of Interest (ROI), activated by the task, and the ones with low activity levels, because not involved, will show different blood flow dynamic.

We can describe the basic physiology of the "coupling" between neuronal activity and vascular brain system as follows: when a specific region of the brain increases its activity, responding to a task submitted to the subject, then the vascular system submits oxygen rich blood to this brain area. The higher local consumption of oxygen from the local capillaries leads to a decrease in oxyHb, and an increase in local deoxygenated haemoglobin (deoxy-Hb) concentration [3]. Following a time delay of a few seconds respect to the starting of the task elaboration, CBF increases as physiological reaction to deliver further oxyHb. This process causes an increased in the regional concentration of oxygenated haemoglobin due to the increase of CBF a few seconds after neuronal activation. In T2* contrast weighted EPI, commonly used in fMRI, the unbalanced growth of oxygenated haemoglobin local concentration, compared to the local oxygen consumption, causes an enhanced MRI signal intensity [4, 5].

This rapid unbalance in local tissue oxygenation induces a regional loss of coherence in the spin motion. Hence we can reveal a local variation in the Macroscopic Magnetization M [6], detachable in the Magnetic Resonance Imaging using the T2* contrast weighted Echo Planar Images (EPI) sequences. The variation of the local paramagnetic properties produces the loss of spin coherence. Since deoxyHb is paramagnetic and oxyHb is diamagnetic, the variation of the ratio between these two concentrations causes local dephasing of protons and modification of the signal detected from the tissues involved (blood-oxygen-level-dependent signal BOLD). Contrast for this kind of MR images is realised using T2*weighted sequences with the EPI pulses scheme used to observe this change [7]. Typical intensity of EPI sequences is in the range of 1–5% of the standard MRI signal, depending on the strength of the applied field.

Unfortunately, there are several limitations for BOLD effect-based fMRI and the scientific community is still debating on this topic [8]. Nevertheless, it is always considered as an essential tool for functional imaging, even when compared to other novel emerging functional techniques, such as Arterial Spin Labelling (ASL) [6–11].

Description of resting state experiments and default mode network

The bold signal can be detected not only during tasks performance but also in the so-called rest condition.

We can define the resting state as the mental state when a person may be awake and alert, but not focused on any activity requiring concentration or attention. In this condition, it is possible to consider spontaneous BOLD signal fluctuation. These fluctuations can be related to functional and physiological connections between different brain areas. These fluctuations were demonstrated in fMRI dataset in 1993 [12], but only recently these non-deterministic BOLD signal oscillations have been analysed with different mathematical techniques for the detection of functional connections of inter-hemispheric pathways. The analysis of non-deterministic BOLD signal oscillations aims to study physiological, pathologic, ageing- and drug-related changes in spontaneous blood oxygenation noise structure. Low-frequency resting state BOLD signals (typically <0.1 Hz) reveal coherent and spontaneous fluctuations that delineate the functional architecture of the human brain [13] . These fluctuations can bring pieces of information about brain activity also in the state of the brain defined as "resting state". Resting state fMRI (rsfMRI) is a method used to evaluate the global and local brain activity occurring when a subject is not performing specific tasks [14]. Along with BOLD signals oscillations, also the connectivity between different brain areas is active in the resting state.

The brain regions co-activated in rest condition define the default mode network (DMN) or default state network [14]: they are active in the default mode state of the brain, (intrinsic functional connectivity). Areas of the DMN are known to have activity highly correlated and distinct from other areas of the brain. It is considered necessary for several self-referential functions including imagination, conscious awareness, and conceptual processing. In particular, this pattern is most commonly observed to be active when a person is not focused on the outside world. The brain status in resting state is similar to the daydreaming, as a sort of wakeful rest, or, in other words, in the condition of mind-wandering. The Default Mode Network is also active when the individual is thinking about others or himself, triggering the action of recalling the past, and to plan for the future. Therefore, such network is activated "by default" when a person is not involved in a particular task. Therefore, DMN network is deactivated when the brain is required to perform some task, as in the Executive Attention Network (EAN) experiments [15]. Although DMN was initially noticed to be deactivated, also for specific goal-oriented tasks, sometimes referred to as task-negative network, it can be active in other goal-oriented tasks such as social working memory or autobiographical tasks. Moreover, in the network analysis is important the correlation "sign". DMN is negatively correlated with other networks in the brain such as attention networks. Interestingly, the researchers observed DMN abnormalities in several neuropsychological conditions, as in the attention deficit hyperactivity disorder (ADHD) [16]. For this reason, research on DMN in resting state is regarded as potentially valuable for the elucidation of brain disease mechanisms.

In summary, BOLD effect plays an important role also in the resting condition of brain activity, in the absence of an externally prompted task, because information of interest may usually be observed as oscillations, or spontaneous fluctuations in BOLD signals [17]. Resting state approach may be useful to explore the functional organisation in the brain and its alterations in neurological or psychiatric diseases. Over the last ten years, resting state functional connectivity research has revealed many networks, which are consistently found in healthy subjects, different stages of consciousness and across species, and represent specific patterns of synchronous activity. In particular, DMN highlighted essential aspects for the description of several neuro-psychological diseases; indeed, evidence supports disruptions of DMN in Alzheimer and ASD affected subjects.

Further, BOLD signal fluctuations can be used to highlight correlations in the activity of other brain areas. For these reasons, it is crucial to define areas or region of interest and the criteria for their spatial definition. Atlas with a much more spatially detailed between can be used in addition to the DMN in the resting state fMRI analysis.

All scans presented in this paper were obtained on a single 1.5-Tesla scanner using a gradient echo-planar imaging sequence for fMRI. The fMRI data were acquired using pre-settled sequences with TR/TE 3000/50, FA 90, a DFOV 22.8 cm × 22.8 cm on a matrix of 128 × 128, and thickness of 4 mm.

ROI and clusters-driven networking

The first step in fMRI statistical analysis is to create a statistical map, i.e. to identify which regions are "activated" above proper statistical thresholds. How to identify these regions of Interest (ROIs)? How to look for particular ROIs related to the nature of diseases? We need to introduce some aspects of the so-called "ROI analysis" [18]. ROIs can be identified and characterised with two different strategies: 1) by functional mapping of brain regions performed, validated and verified by means of several experiments and studies of the brain (Talairach Atlas); 2) by fMRI, focusing on the activated areas, corresponding to clusters of voxels, during the performance of a task. Although the presence of some disadvantages, this approach allows for the construction of brain networks from a different point of view, i.e. from functional spontaneous clustering of the brain. ROI and clustering-guided (or led) strategies may be used to investigate the alteration introduced by "external conditions" in the brain networks. Research in functional connectivity MRI (fcMRI) has recently focused on the exploration of method task-induced brain network, delivering significant results; further, this approach can also be applied in the rest conditions, and this is a promising pathway to get more in-depth knowledge about brain behaviours and performances. However, innovative mathematical methods and analysis are required to treat this information.

Data analysis, connectivity measures and fcMRI: Networking the brain functions: Towards a pipeline for brain networks analysis.

Connectivity measures may be used to test the alteration of brain connectivity in pathological occurrences. Resting state data in functional MRI (rsfMRI), as well as task-related designs, can be analysed with fcMRI. Different software for connectivity measures are freely available; however, the usual protocol to perform connectivity analyses comprises the following steps:

a) Functional data acquisition

Using the typical EPI MRI sequences, it is possible to collect data from experiments both with the resting-state conditions and with a task design.

b) Structural data acquisition.

To plot the functional results on the real brain anatomy of patient, anatomical MRI acquisition is performed for each subject. Also, this allows for the definition of the Grey Matter, White Matter and Cerebrospinal Fluid areas for the segmentation operation to perform noise corrections in the functional images.

c) ROI definition:

ROIs may be defined in different ways to achieve the best connections analysis model suitable for the aims of the study. It is possible to use text files with a list of the Montreal Neurological Institute (MNI) positions or a list of Talairach locations; also, on the web, there are several freely available tools for the conversion in these two References Systems (http://sprout022.sprout.yale.edu/mni2-tal/mni2tal.html).

Voxels position is related to functional areas using a complete list of Brodmann areas. This fact allows for voxel-to-voxel analysis as well as "seed areas" to voxel, and ROI-to-ROI analysis of connectivity properties at the single subject level and the group level.

In all our research projects, functional connectivity toolbox Conn (www.nitrc.org/projects/conn) [19] was employed; CONN has implemented the CompCor algorithm for physiological and other noise sources reduction strategies. CONN allows for removal of movement, temporal covariates accounting, and a temporal filtering of BOLD signal oscillations. Further, Conn noise reduction strategy allows for the physiological interpretation of anticorrelations, for it does not rely on global signal regression.

In CONN software the usual fMRI preprocessing is performed: spatial preprocessing procedures include slice-timing correction, realignment, coregistration, normalisation, and spatial smoothing. In addition to these steps, the CONN software employs segmentation of Grey Matter, White Matter, and CSF areas to use during removal of temporal confounding factors. Conn spatial preprocessing is implemented by SPM software (Wellcome Department of Imaging Neuroscience, London, UK; www.fil.ion.ucl.ac.uk/spm). Both SPM and Conn run in the Matlab calculation environment (The MathWorks, Natick, Massachusetts). Regarding statistical parametric mapping, this was performed in the framework of General Linear Model (GLM) (Friston et al. 1995) as implemented by FSL (FMRIB Software Library v5.0) by the Analysis Group (FMRIB, Oxford, UK). Usual random effects procedures, as developed by Holmes and Friston [20], to describe multi-subject functional neuroimaging data for valid population inference.

To avoid confounders and limit the noise for the evaluation of the neural activity and connectivity as possible, a robust statistical analysis must address the study of noise sources in fMRI. The first step of this procedure is the denoising of the BOLD signal, aimed to define, explore, and remove possible confounders such as patient movement induced alterations. Nevertheless, it is also possible to assess the spectral contribution of all the frequencies fluctuations of the BOLD signal in both resting state, and task-driven experiments: data filtering by separating bands components allows for the contributions exploration of low or fast components of the signals.

Usually, in fcMRI, two levels of the analysis may be identified: the first level for within-subject analysis, and the second level for between-subjects analysis. Notably, the former level defines and explores functional connectivity of different kinds of sources for each subject. Successively, a second-level analysis is performed to study between-subjects contrasts of interest, hence to define population phenotypes. These two processes highlight some variables that may be defined as covariates and included in the GLM model.

As previously reported, BOLD signals from voxels and ROIs of interest can be processed in CONN software using several indices of connectivity. Connectivity measure is performed at the voxel-to-voxel level and, to discuss connectivity properties in connection with spatially segregated brain functions, a seed to voxel, and ROI to ROI analysis can be performed. Usually, brain areas of interest were spatially labelled as in Broadmann areas atlas (BA) to characterise the source regions for the extraction of the time series of interest. These areas are subsequently used as labels for targets in ROI-to-ROI analysis, and seed to voxel analysis. All Ddata presented in this paper focuses on the zero-lagged bivariate-correlation and linear measure of functional connectivity between two sources, x and y, defined as [19]:

Equation 1 Bivariate correlation

$$r = (x^t \cdot x)^{\frac{1}{2}} \cdot b \cdot (y^t \cdot y)^{-\frac{1}{2}}$$

where.

Equation 2 Bivariate regression

$$b = \frac{x^t \cdot y}{x^t \cdot x}$$

This is the Voxel-Level Functional Connectivity MRI measurement derived from the Voxel-to-Voxel Connectivity Matrix r(x,y); in this project, the strength of the global connectivity pattern between each voxel and the rest of the brain with the Intrinsic connectivity contrast (ICC) [21] was characterised.

Equation 3 Intrinsic connectivity contrast index

$$C_n(G) = \frac{1}{|G|-1} \cdot |G_n|$$

Successively, it is possible to use the "cost function" as a measure, at ROI and network level, of the links properties. In particular, for ROI-level tests:

Equation 4 Cost function of the n node graph G

$$C(G) = \frac{1}{|G|} \cdot \sum_{n \in G} C_n(G)$$

while, for network-level measures, we can define:

Equation 5 Cost at network level

$$ICC = \frac{1}{|\Omega|} \sum_{y \in \Omega} |r(x,y)|^2$$

where $C_n(G)$ represents the cost in graph G, and |G| represents the number of nodes in graph G [19, 22].

The word "cost" is used to define the weight property of the link, a way to determine the intensity of the link between nodes and all over the network (or net path). The weight of a path in a graph can be defined as the sum of the weights of the traversed edges.

Indices like the Betweenness Centrality, an indicator of the number of "shortest paths" for a specific node, can be used to describe some "community" properties of the nodes. A node with high betweenness centrality has a great importance in the network.

All these parameters can give us the numeric evaluation of the topological properties of the network realised by the ROIs of the brain connected by the function execution task [23].

A display of fcMRI can be achieved through several representations employing CONN toolbox for Matlab. It is possible to show the performed graph-theory analysis of the ROIs networks, characterising the topological properties of the brain networks related to the disease; the characterisation is obtained through

graphics and pictures, as reported in the figures of the next paragraph.

This fact allows the researchers for several considerations about the areas involved and the functions performed by these regions. The definition of the network's organisation is related to the "self-organisation" property of the brain.

Self-organization is one of the emerging properties of the brain networks that can be related to the mechanism activated by the brain trying to solve the inefficiency associated with the action of the diseases in the brain.

This is a significant contribution arising from the application of the complex networks theory to the brain behaviour, and it refers to the so-called Networks Medicine.

Applications of networks analysis: Network medicine, and network-based approach to brain diseases. Ideas and hypothesis for the use of fcMRI

Network medicine represents the powerful tool to systematically investigate the molecular complexity of a particular disease, the molecular relationships between apparently distinct phenotypes, and the pathological alterations induced in functional brain networks [16]. The theoretical and methodological basis of this new discipline has been successfully tested in several clinical applications, and it may lead to the early identification of typical disease topology and pathways, increasing the specificity and the sensitivity of the current diagnostic methods. In this paper, some applications of this strategy/technique are proposed for the study of brain networks alterations induced in distinct phenotypes.

A first attempt to apply networks theory to fMRI signal was conducted to test the hypothesis of circuitry alterations in attention-control brain networks in TS. In particular, we can consider cortical-striatal-thalamic-cortical networking alterations and the potential involvement of the frontostriatal frontoparietal circuitries. A task driven experiment was designed for a modified finger tapping motor task. Randomized commands for patients in the MRI scanner trigger the switch from usual finger tapping to the ones with avoidance of middle finger/third digit tap. Therefore, this task should stimulate different control strength on the patient that can be quickly gained by Tourette patients due to their higher control ability. Task-induced activation or deactivation may be detected as circuitry alterations in the four major regions of interest constituting the default mode network (DMN), e.g. the posterior cingulate cortex (PCC), the cortex in the medial prefrontal region (MPFC), and left and right lateral parietal cortices (LLP and RLP). This scenario seems to be the proper environment for the application of Networks Theory to test the dynamic of the organisation and the properties of brain function. It is an ambitious task, especially considering that fMRI is a "noisy" low-intensity signals diagnostic method. After the characterisation of the Tourette Syndrome, a typical neurological diseases [24–26], we will present the study of the association between taste processing phenotypes and brain networks and the research about the immunological system disease and brain networks, to illustrate the connection potentiality in the diseases diagnosis process.

Tourette

One of the studies described in this article is based on the fMRI analysis of patients with TS during the performance of a complex motor task. Several studies about the TS emphasise the role of the cortical-striatal-thalamocortical brain circuits, particularly the subcortical components as the basal ganglia, and the cortical component as the prefrontal cortex [24, 25].

For this study, we acquired functional magnetic resonance imaging data from 11 individuals with Tourette's syndrome, and 11 healthy control subjects. Subjects were required to perform a complex motor task based on a switching on demand between two different conditions of finger tapping. These two different conditions required a high attention to motor strategy and a strength of maintenance this focus throughout the execution time of the task.

TS patients frequently present atypical brain connectivity [24]. However, the neural networks underlying their motor and vocal tic development are still poorly understood [25, 26]. In particular, this experiment focused on the front-striatal system networks, which are responsible for self-regulatory control [27]. The Fronto-striatal system includes lateral inferior prefrontal cortex, medial frontal gyrus, dorsolateral prefrontal cortex, lenticular nucleus (Pallido, and Putamen), and thalamus. Fronto-striatal systems are implicated in control, and inhibition of movements, and behaviours. Based on the literature, the hypothesis of an altered network functioning, responsible for setting specific actions in response to a particular stimulus, may be a satisfactory explanation for TS clinical manifestations.

The brain areas involved in attentional executive functions are the fronto-striatal and fronto-parietal systems. The former modulates the self-regulatory control, i.e. cognitive or affective self-monitoring, and motor area. The latter regulates the so-called "adaptive control", adjusting the transition from a movement to another [15, 28].

So we proposed the submission to pathological and healthy subjects of a motion task, with higher cost function related to the higher attention requested by motion

difficult; this should allow for revealing tic neural mechanisms in TS, mapping of connectivity within cortical-striatal-thalamic-cortical circuits [24, 28, 29]. Previous neuroimaging studies showed that attention task not only may stimulate/activate motion-selective cortical areas but also several others that seemed to be unrelated. Increasing or decreasing of activation in a cortical area is often attributed to attentional modulation of the cortical projections to that area. This fact leads to the idea that, in Tourette patients, attention is associated with changes in brain connectivity.

In our experiment, subjects completed a finger tapping motor task using both right and left hand and switching between the two conditions: usual finger tapping, and a finger tapping without opposition between thumb and medium fingers. Patients were not required to perform the task as quickly as possible. Participants completed a brief practice session before scanning to familiarise with stimuli and task requirements. The vocal command to switch between the two conditions was randomly submitted to increase the difficulty of the task.

All subjects were submitted to MRI analysis under the same stimulus conditions. The hypothesis is that the hemodynamic responses addressed by the attentional component of the task may reveal a cortical-striatal-thalamic-cortical network alteration.

We investigated the potential frequency-modulation of fcMRI measures related to a differential actions of brain circuitries using for each condition under study a specific band-pass filter [15] Additional information may be found in Buzsaki's paper, Science 2004 [17]. The following pictures show some preliminary results: differential networks between Tourette and control subjects, with associated parameters, which measure these differences.

Interestingly, although "cost function" is higher in TS than controls, the efficiency of the differential networks is higher in pathological subjects (Fig. 1). Furthermore, the degree of the network increases with the clustering coefficient, while network path lengths are similar in the two groups. To confirm such results, population size should be increased. Nevertheless, these data suggest that brain networks analysis may be a successful strategy for the characterisation of this condition.

Propylthiouracil

From the evolutionary point of view, the ability to perceive the bitter taste of bad food, leading to the rejection of the food, may be considered a sort of surviving ability, which propels natural selection. In this way, poisonous and dangerous food can be readily detected by their bitter taste, meaning that taste has a crucial role in evolution. Indeed, nutrition plays a vital role in evolution, and in the phenotype characterisation related to the diffusion of several pathologies. Nutrition and brain processes of taste perception are becoming prominent aspects in the diagnosis and prognosis of several neurological diseases. Nevertheless, there are few neuroimaging studies on taste perception and processing in the brain, and some of these studies are only related to the cortical brain areas [30]. To identify the areas involved in bitter taste perception and their connectivity, a population of 6 healthy volunteers were analysed through the functional magnetic resonance imaging techniques. The sensitivity to the bitter taste of thiourea compounds, such as 6-n-propylthiouracil (PROP), is a well-known example of genetic bitter taste variability. Individual differences in taste sensitivity to 6-n-propylthiouracil (PROP) may be associated with different activation patterns in the brain. Bitter taste sensitivity greatly varies among subjects and, in the case of PROP, a genetic modification related to the bitter sensitivity of the differently classified subjects was observed. For this study, the sensitive subjects group were organised and labelled as super testers, while insensitive ones, or "non-responsive", were labelled as non-tester. The term super-taster is used to distinguish individuals who perceive PROP as extremely bitter from those (medium tasters) who perceive it as moderately bitter. Several investigations attempted to elucidate molecular basis, genetic and psychophysical features of this human trait. Some studies consistently reported that PROP "supertasters" have a higher density of fungiform papillae on the anterior tongue surface, suggesting an anatomical difference in their peripheral taste system. Although human brain pathways involved in the complex gustatory circuitry are well known, it is still necessary to elucidate how the signals related to different food are processed in the brain. It is also important to establish whether such stimuli may influence different brain areas depending on the meaning that those food and taste have for each subject.

Preliminary data from functional magnetic resonance imaging (fMRI) acquired by our research group aimed at determining if individual genetic differences of taste perception of PROP can be represented in the brain by different activation patterns and connections. The four major regions of interest (ROIs) constituting the default mode network (DMN) are the medial prefrontal cortex (MPFC), the posterior cingulate cortex (PCC), the medial prefrontal, and left and right lateral parietal cortices (LLP and RLP). These regions were preliminary adopted in this study as brain activity sources for connectivity analysis. The complete set of Broadmann areas was considered as targets for connectivity analysis. Subjects underwent single fMRI run. During the scan, subjects were requested to stay still with relaxed muscles, and closed eyes. For each subject, fMRI study included 15 min recording of the brain activity at rest, followed by 15 min recording of the activity induced by PROP.

PROP administration occurred by placing on the tip of the tongue a filter paper disk impregnated with a 50 mM aqueous PROP solution.

The hypothesis for this experiment was that connectivity in appetitive and aversive neural circuits may correlate to the complexity of the complex neuronal circuits.

In this framework, it is possible to generate several schemes of experiments with coherent cognitive states to guide the autonomous behaviour of the subjects. Such processes may be strictly related to deeper structures of the brain, and, in turn, related to several areas of the prefrontal cortex. Analysis of neural signalling seems to highlight the role of the amygdala and orbitofrontal cortex, two brain areas involved in taste stimuli.

It seems that a dynamic relationship exists between circuits such as enhanced arousal or attention, potentially influencing behavioural choices, e.g. food intake or style [31].

These data underline the formidable challenges ahead in describing how the food taste neural circuits interact to produce a more complex and wide range of behaviours, also confirmed by others similar study [30].

In this preliminary fMRI project, six (1 males, and 5 females: age 28.6 ¬ ± 0.86 years) caucasian, non-smoker subjects were recruited according to standard procedures to perform a pilot study.

All subjects were genotyped for receptor TAS2R38 (the specific receptor of taste cells, which binds the thiocyanate group from PROP) using PCR techniques and then following the sequencing of the obtained fragments. Subjects were classified by their PROP taster status. The status was assigned through taste intensity rating in Labelled Magnitude Scale (LMS) using three suprathreshold PROP (0.032, 0.32, and 3.2 mM) and NaCl (0.01, 0.1, 1.0 M) solutions. Subsequently, three subjects classified as PROP super-tasters showed homozygous genotype for taster receptor variant (PAV/PAV), while the remaining three were classified as non-tasters and showed homozygous genotype for the non-taster receptor variant (AVI/AVI), .

In this pilot study, subjects underwent one fMRI run in the scanner. For the fMRI scan, subjects followed the procedure previously described. For each subject, the fMRI exam included a 15 min recording of the brain activity at rest followed by other 15 min of recording of the brain activity induced by PROP bitter taste stimulation. PROP stimulation was performed by placing a filter paper disk impregnated with 50 mmol/L of the compound on the tip of the tongue. Taste stimulation induced brain activity revealed by fMRI. Interestingly, interactions between PCC and other areas of the brain were observed and reported in Fig. 2.

Considering as Source the Posterior cingulate (PCC) cortex, some correlated target areas are: 1) Target

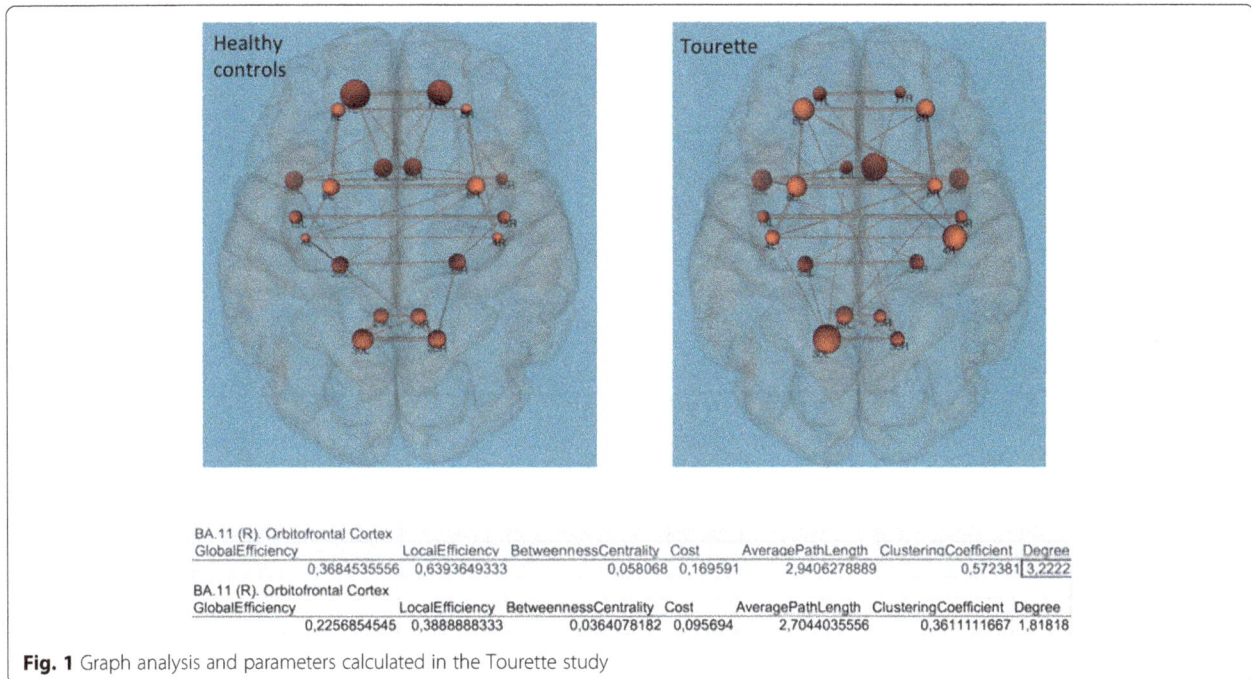

BA.11 (R). Orbitofrontal Cortex						
GlobalEfficiency	LocalEfficiency	BetweennessCentrality	Cost	AveragePathLength	ClusteringCoefficient	Degree
0,3684535556	0,6393649333		0,058068 0,169591	2,9406278889	0,572381	3,2222

BA.11 (R). Orbitofrontal Cortex						
GlobalEfficiency	LocalEfficiency	BetweennessCentrality	Cost	AveragePathLength	ClusteringCoefficient	Degree
0,2256854545	0,3888888333		0,0364078182 0,095694	2,7044035556	0,3611111667	1,81818

Fig. 1 Graph analysis and parameters calculated in the Tourette study

BA33(R,L): cingulate gyrus, in charge of functions as detection of errors, risk and conflict management, response inhibition, cognitive control, adaptation; an important part of the Limbic System. 2) Target BA43(R): subcentral areas with associated functions as "gustatory cortical area". 3) Target BA7(L): somatosensory associative cortex functions. 4) Target BA32(R): [15, 27, 32]. Functions: it appears to play an essential role in the regulation of the blood pressure and a wide variety of autonomic functions, such as the regulation of the heart rate. It is also involved in rational cognitive functions, such as reward anticipation, decision-making, empathy, impulse control, and emotion. All these functions have been related to the feeling reported by subjects after MRI examination, and to the actions activated and controlled by the brain in consideration of the requested response to the stimuli intensity experienced.

Using the Voxel to Voxel mapping for correlations representation it is possible to generate an SPM [20]style picture of direct and inverse correlation between activated Voxels, as reported in Fig. 3:

Using this representation it can be observed that the activation of LLP source was inversely correlated with Premotor Cortex (left), Dorsolateral Prefrontal Cortex (right) and Retrosplenial Cingulate Cortex (right), and directly with Primary Visual Cortex V1 (left). The MPFC source was inversely correlated with Somatosensory Associative Cortex (right) and Anterior Entorhinal Cortex (right). The PCC source was directly correlated to the Anterior Cingulate Cortex (right), Anterior Cingulate Cortex (left), Subcentral Area (right), Somatosensory Associative Cortex (left) and Dorsal Anterior Cingulate Cortex (right). The RLP source was directly correlated with Auditory Cortex (right) and Insula Cortex (left) [16, 17, 28].

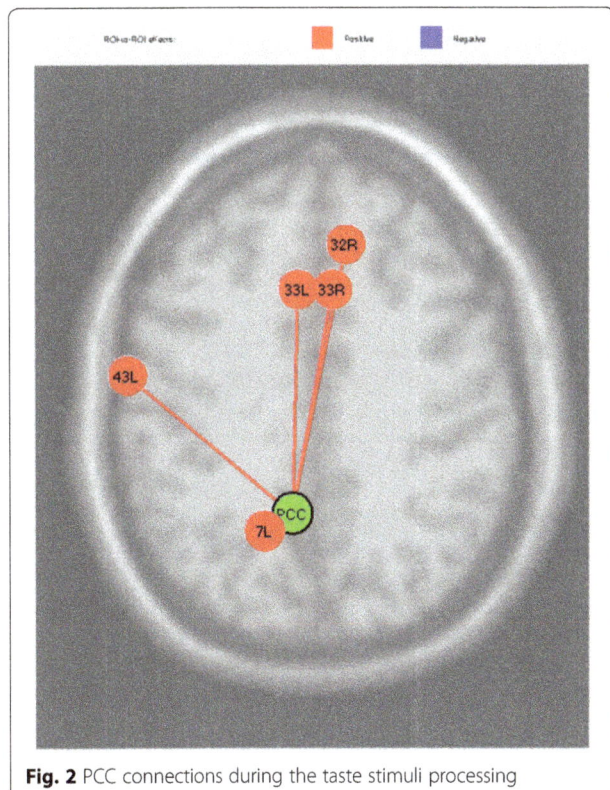

Fig. 2 PCC connections during the taste stimuli processing

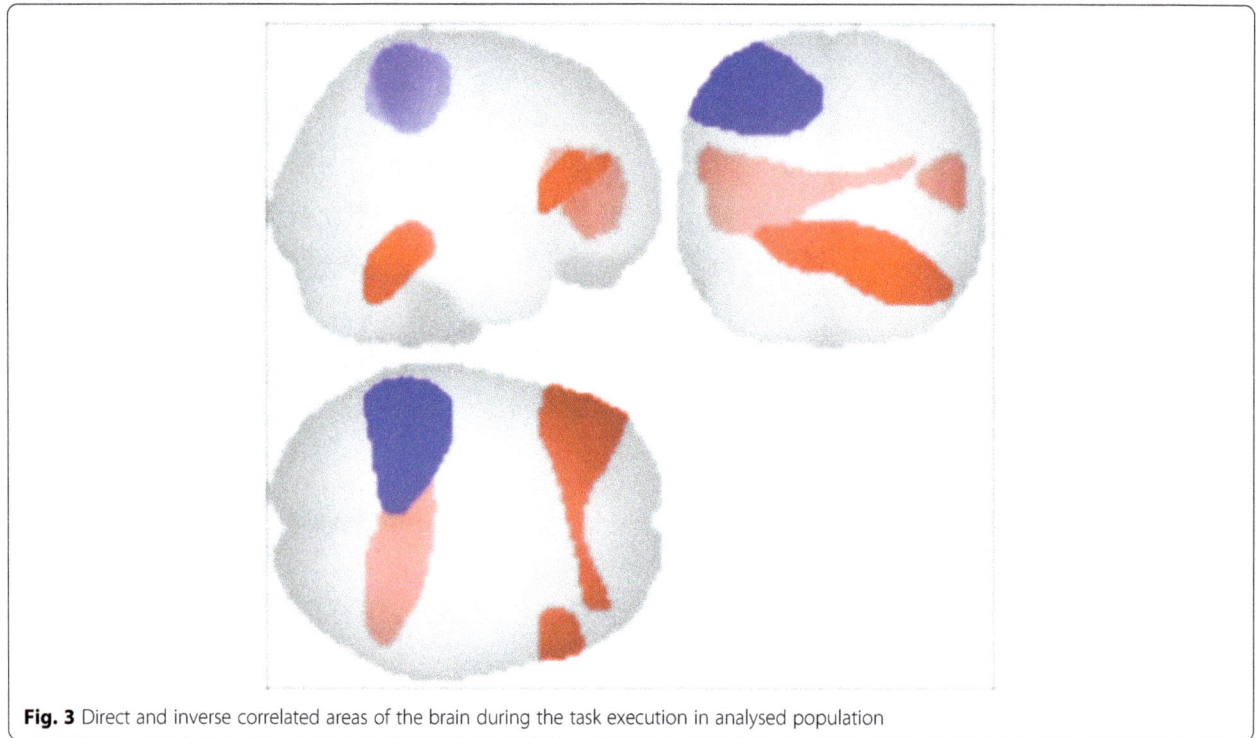

Fig. 3 Direct and inverse correlated areas of the brain during the task execution in analysed population

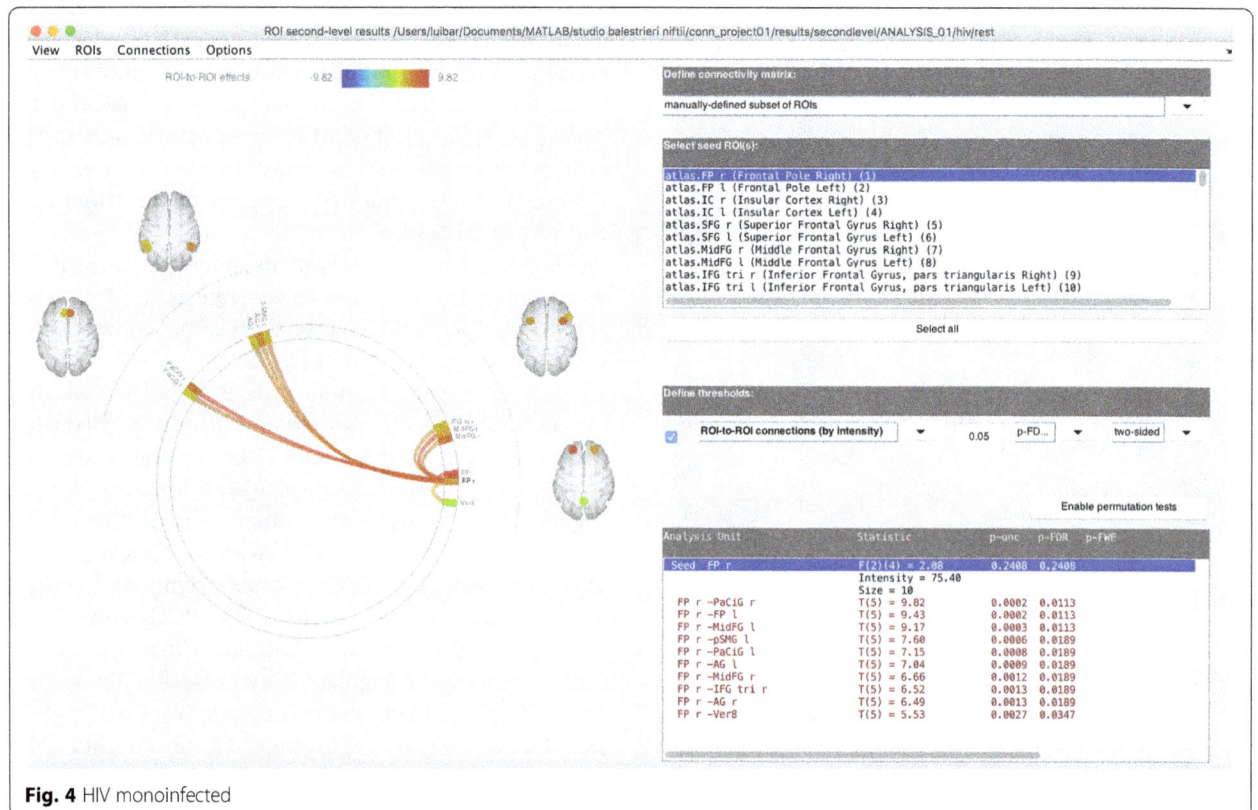

Fig. 4 HIV monoinfected

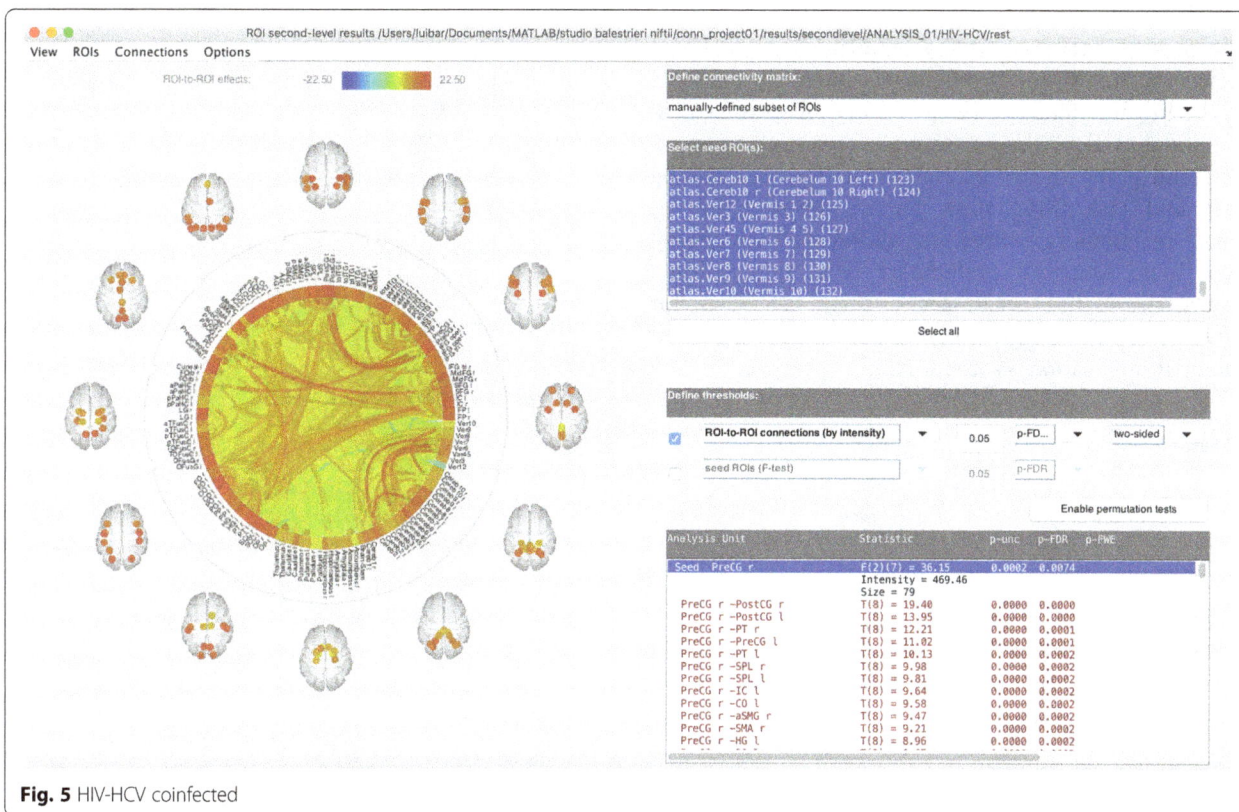

Fig. 5 HIV-HCV coinfected

In conclusion, preliminary results showed the different Cortical Areas in which PROP bitter taste signals are differently processed by the two genetic groups (PROP super-taster PAV/PAV subjects, and non-taster AVI/AVI subjects).

These preliminary results are consistent with individual differences in the ability to taste this compound, and highlight differences in neuronal connectivity indicating that super-tasters and non-tasters may also differ at the central level, and not only at the periphery. Further analysis with a larger population should be performed: nevertheless, this seems to be an exciting insight on eating behaviour and the food intake at brain level in humans [33, 34].

HIV-HCV study

The management of patients infected with hepatitis C virus (HCV) depends on comorbidity factors, and different phenotypes can have different disease progression. Data from studies on human immunodeficiency virus (HIV) comorbidity suggest that HIV/HCV-coinfected patients have different progress diseases compared to HCV-monoinfected patients. In fact, progression rate increases with older age, alcoholism, male sex, and HIV co-infection, with a higher risk of cirrhosis or decompensated liver than

HCV-monoinfected patients [35, 36]. Moreover, co-infected patients report cognitive alterations, and it is not evident the contributions of the single infections. Preliminary fcMRI data were collected from an undergoing study in our Research Unit to estimate the contribution of each kind of infection on drug activity against cognitive decay.

Although a limited number of patients was enrolled for this study, we observed different brain connectivity mapping between HIV monoinfected and HIV-HCV coinfected. These differences were found in areas not included in the DMN (MPFC, PCC, LLP and RLP), but in some other areas classified in the Atlas present in the CONN Toolbox.

Perturbations seem to be statistically stronger in other areas than DMN's ones. We report these activations to prove the sensibility of the method to study the alterations induced in the brain by immunological diseases.

The comparison of connectivity between HIV monoinfected and HIV-HCV coinfected can be compatible with a different brain networking of subjects in the groups (Figs. 4 and 5). It means that different brain areas can be involved in these two populations considering the differences in the cognitive, motor and somatosensory alterations. fcMRI can reveal these variations leading to a more focused and tailored therapy for the subjects.

Conclusions

The fc-MRI analysis offers a standard framework to perform a broad set of connectivity-based experiments on brain functions under a variety of pathological conditions. Calculation of several connectivity parameters and graph theory measurements for both resting state and task fMRI allow for the investigation of brain reactions/responses to different pathological alterations. Although preliminary data, the reported results show three examples of high reliability for different fcMRI measure conditions, suggesting their potential application as useful clinical practice.

Acknowledgements

Authors wish to thank Diana Caravana, Paolo Contu and Franco Conti, Technicians in MRI at the Department of Radiology – University of Cagliari AOU - Cagliari – Italy, for their contribution and expertise in the performing of the exams.

Funding

No source of funding to declare.

Author's contributions

LB performed the data analysis, was a major contributor in writing the manuscript. FM participated in the design of the study, analyzed and interpreted the data regarding the TOURETTE disease. ITB participated in the design of the study, analyzed and interpreted the data regarding the PROP test and was a contributor in the writing manuscript. MM participated in the design of the study, analyzed and interpreted the data regarding the PROP test. HSS participated in the design of the paper, and was a contributor in the writing manuscript. AM analyzed and interpreted the data regarding the HIV vs HIV-HCV study. JSS participated in the design of the paper, and was a contributor in the writing manuscript. AB performed the MRI examination of the HIV vs HIV-HCV study. MA suggested improvements in the MRI protocols applied. LS performed the MRI examination and was a contributor in the manuscript writing. All authors read and approved the final manuscript.

Authors' information

Not applicable.

Competing interests

The authors declare that they have no competing interests.

Author details

[1]Department of Medical Sciences and Public Health, University of Cagliari, Cagliari, Italy. [2]Department of Nuclear Medicine, Universitary Hospital of Cagliari AOU, Cagliari, Italy. [3]Department of Biomedical Sciences, University of Cagliari, Cagliari, Italy. [4]Diagnosis and Monitoring Division, AtheroPoint LLC, Roseville, CA, USA. [5]Department of Radiology, University of Cagliari AOU, Cagliari, Italy. [6]Department of Radiology, University of Rome "La Sapienza", Rome, Italy.

References

1. Albert-Laszlo Parabasi, "Network Science by Albert-László Barabási." [Online]. Available: http://barabasi.com/networksciencebook/.
2. J. C. Gore, "Principles and practice of functional MRI of the human brain.," J Clin Invest, Jul. 2003, vol. 112, no. 1, pp. 4–9.
3. X. Hu and E. Yacoub, "The story of the initial dip in fMRI.," NeuroImage, Aug. 2012, vol. 62, no. 2, pp. 1103–1108.
4. Logothetis NK, Auguth M, Oeltermann A, Pauls J, Trinath T. A neurophysiological investigation of the basis of the BOLD signal in fMRI. Nature. 2001;412(6843):150-7.
5. H. Yuan, C. Perdoni, L. Yang, and B. He, "Differential electrophysiological coupling for positive and negative BOLD responses during unilateral hand movements.," J Neurosci, Jun. 2011, vol. 31, no. 26, pp. 9585–9593.
6. Saba L. Magnetic Resonance Imaging Handbook. 2016. CRC Press; ISBN 9781482216288.
7. Bernstein MA, King KF, ZHOU XJ, Ehman RL, Bernstein MA, King KF, ZHOU XJ. Handbook of MRI pulse sequences. CRC Press Taylors and Francis Group; 2004. p. 1017. eBook ISBN: 9780080533124
8. S. Haller and A. J. Bartsch, "Pitfalls in fMRI," Eur Radiol, Nov. 2009, vol. 19, no. 11, pp. 2689–2706.
9. Friston KJ. Functional and effective connectivity in neuroimaging: a synthesis. Hum Brain Mapp. 1994;2:56–78.
10. K. J. Friston, "Functional and effective connectivity: a review," Brain Connect, vol. 1, no. 1, pp. 13–36, Jan. 2011.
11. J. A. Detre, H. Rao, D. J. J. Wang, Y. F. Chen, and Z. Wang, "Applications of arterial spin labeled MRI in the brain.," J Magn Reson Imaging, vol. 35, no. 5, pp. 1026–1037, May 2012.
12. Kiviniemi V, Kantola JH, Jauhiainen J, Tervonen O. Comparison of methods for detecting nondeterministic BOLD fluctuation in fMRI. Magn Reson Imaging. 2004;22(2):197–203.
13. Biswal B, Zerrin Yetkin F, Haughton VM, Hyde JS. Functional Connectivity in the Motor Cortex of Resting Human Brain Using Echo-Planar MRI. Magn Reson Med. 1995;34(4):537–41.
14. Greicius MD, Krasnow B, Reiss AL, Menon V. Functional connectivity in the resting brain: a network analysis of the default mode hypothesis. Proc Natl Acad Sci U S A. 2003;100(1):253–8.
15. N. U. F. Dosenbach, D. A. Fair, F. M. Miezin, A. L. Cohen, K. K. Wenger, R. A. T. Dosenbach, M. D. Fox, A. Z. Snyder, J. L. Vincent, M. E. Raichle, B. L. Schlaggar, and S. E. Petersen, "Distinct brain networks for adaptive and stable task control in humans.," Proc Natl Acad Sci U S A, vol. 104, no. 26, pp. 11073–11078, Jun. 2007.
16. De La Fuente A, Xia S, Branch C, Li X. A review of attention-deficit/ hyperactivity disorder from the perspective of brain networks. Front Hum Neurosci. 2013;7:192.
17. G. Buzsáki and A. Draguhn, "Neuronal oscillations in cortical networks.," Science, vol. 304, no. 5679, pp. 1926–1929, Jun. 2004.
18. R. A. Poldrack, "Region of interest analysis for fMRI.," Soc Cogn Affect Neurosci, vol. 2, no. 1, pp. 67–70, Mar. 2007.
19. Whitfield-Gabrieli S, Nieto-Castanon A. Conn: a functional connectivity toolbox for correlated and Anticorrelated brain networks. BRAIN Connect. 2012;3
20. Friston KJ, Holmes AP, Worsley KJ, Poline J-P, Frith CD, Frackowiak RSJ. Statistical parametric maps in functional imaging: a general linear approach. Hum Brain Mapp, vol. 1995:2.
21. R. Martuzzi, R. Ramani, M. Qiu, X. Shen, X. Papademetris, and R. T. Constable, "A whole-brain voxel based measure of intrinsic connectivity contrast reveals local changes in tissue connectivity with anesthetic without a priori assumptions on thresholds or regions of interest.," NeuroImage, vol. 58, no. 4, pp. 1044–1050, Oct. 2011.
22. Achard S, Bullmore E. "Efficiency and cost of economical brain functional networks," PLoS Comput. Biol. 2007;3(2):e17.
23. A.-L. Barabási, N. Gulbahce, and J. Loscalzo, "Network medicine: a network-based approach to human disease.," Nat Rev Genet, vol. 12, no. 1, pp. 56–68, Jan. 2011.
24. E. Stern, D. A. Silbersweig, K.-Y. Chee, A. Holmes, M. M. Robertson, M. Trimble, C. D. Frith, R. S. J. Frackowiak, "A functional Neuroanatomy of tics in Tourette syndrome," Arch Gen Psychiatry, vol. 57, no. 8, p. 741, Aug. 2000.

25.   Z. Wang, T. V Maia, R. Marsh, T. Colibazzi, A. Gerber, and B. S. Peterson, "The neural circuits that generate tics in Tourette's syndrome.," Am J Psychiatry, vol. 168, no. 12, pp. 1326–1337, Dec. 2011.

26.   A. Lerner, A. Bagic, E. A. Boudreau, T. Hanakawa, F. Pagan, Z. Mari, W. Bara-Jimenez, M. Aksu, G. Garraux, J. M. Simmons, S. Sato, D. L. Murphy, and M. Hallett, "Neuroimaging of neuronal circuits involved in tic generation in patients with Tourette syndrome," Neurology, vol. 68, no. 23, pp. 1979–1987, Jun. 2007.

27.   N. Mol Debes, M. Preel, and L. Skov, "Functional neuroimaging in Tourette syndrome: recent perspectives," Neurosci Neuroeconomics, vol Volume 6, pp. 1–13, Apr. 2017.

28.   J. A. Church, D. A. Fair, N. U. F. Dosenbach, A. L. Cohen, F. M. Miezin, S. E. Petersen, and B. L. Schlaggar, "Control networks in paediatric Tourette syndrome show immature and anomalous patterns of functional connectivity.," Brain, vol. 132, no. Pt 1, pp. 225–238, Jan. 2009.

29.   S. Bohlhalter, A. Goldfine, S. Matteson, G. Garraux, "Neural correlates of tic generation in Tourette syndrome: an event-related functional MRI study.," Brain, vol. 129, no. Pt 8, pp. 2029–2037, Aug. 2006.

30.   S. Bembich, C. Lanzara, A. Clarici, S. Demarini, B. J. Tepper, P. Gasparini, and D. L. Grasso, "Individual differences in prefrontal cortex activity during perception of bitter taste using fNIRS methodology.," Chem Senses, vol. 35, no. 9, pp. 801–812, Nov. 2010.

31.   E. R. Grimm and N. I. Steinle, "Genetics of eating behavior: established and emerging concepts.," Nutr Rev, vol. 69, no. 1, pp. 52–60, Jan. 2011.

32.   Roth RM, Saykin AJ, Flashman LA, Pixley HS, West JD, Mamourian AC. Event-related functional magnetic resonance imaging of response inhibition in obsessive-compulsive disorder. Biol Psychiatry. 2007;62(8):901–9.

33.   V. B. Duffy, A. C. Davidson, J. R. Kidd, K. K. Kidd, W. C. Speed, A. J. Pakstis, D. R. Reed, D. J. Snyder, and L. M. Bartoshuk, "Bitter receptor gene (TAS2R38), 6-n-Propylthiouracil (PROP) bitterness and alcohol intake," Alcohol Clin Exp Res, vol. 28, no. 11, pp. 1629–1637, Nov. 2004.

34.   T. Iole and L. Barberini, "Abstracts from the 24th annual meeting of the European chemoreception research organization (ECRO 2014), Dijon, France, September 10-13th, 2014," Chem Senses, vol. 40, no. 3, pp. 211–297, Mar. 2015.

35.   L. Aranzabal, J. L. Casado, J. Moya, C. Quereda, S. Diz, A. Moreno, L. Moreno, A. Antela, M. J. Perez-Elias, F. Dronda, A. Marin, F. Hernandez-Ranz, A. Moreno, and S. Moreno, "Influence of liver fibrosis on highly active antiretroviral therapy-associated hepatotoxicity in patients with HIV and hepatitis C virus Coinfection," Clin Infect Dis, vol. 40, no. 4, pp. 588–593, Feb. 2005.

36.   P. Labarga, V. Soriano, M. E. Vispo, J. Pinilla, L. Martín-Carbonero, C. Castellares, R. Casado, I. Maida, P. García-Gascó, and P. Barreiro, "Hepatotoxicity of antiretroviral drugs is reduced after successful treatment of chronic hepatitis C in HIV-infected patients," J Infect Dis, vol. 196, no. 5, pp. 670–676, Sep. 2007.

24

The relationship of cortical folding and brain arteriovenous malformations

Manish N. Shah[1*†], Sarah E. Smith[2†], Donna L. Dierker[2], Joseph P. Herbert[3], Timothy S. Coalson[2], Brent S. Bruck[4], Gregory J. Zipfel[4], David C. Van Essen[2] and Ralph G. Dacey Jr.[4]

Abstract

Background: The pathogenesis of human intracranial arteriovenous malformations (AVMs) is not well understood; this study aims to quantitatively assess cortical folding in patients with these lesions.

Methods: Seven adult participants, 4 male and 3 female, with unruptured, surgically unresectable intracranial AVMs were prospectively enrolled in the study, with a mean age of 42.1 years and Spetzler-Martin grade range of II-IV. High-resolution brain MRI T1 and T2 sequences were obtained. After standard preprocessing, segmentation and registration techniques, three measures of cortical folding, the depth difference index (DDI), coordinate distance index (CDI) and gyrification index (GI)), were calculated for the affected and unaffected hemispheres of each subject as well as a healthy control subject set.

Results: Of the three metrics, CDI, DDI and GI, used for cortical folding assessment, none demonstrated significant differences between the participants and previously studied healthy adults. There was a significant negative correlation between the DDI ratio between affected and unaffected hemispheres and AVM volume (correlation coefficient $r = -0.74$, $p = 0.04$).

Conclusion: This study is the first to quantitatively assess human brain cortical folding in the presence of intracranial AVMs and no significant differences between AVM-affected versus unaffected hemispheres were found in a small dataset. We suggest longitudinal, larger human MRI-based cortical folding studies to assess whether AVMs are congenital lesions of vascular development or *de novo*, dynamic lesions.

Keywords: AVM, MRI, Cortical folding, *de novo*, Congenital, Brain development

Background

Intracranial arteriovenous malformations (AVMs) are the direct communication of arteries to abnormally tortuous and dilated veins without an interposing capillary bed, often described as a tangle or "bag of worms" [1]. The mechanism of AVM formation is not well understood. Unlike their pulmonary or abdominal counterparts, brain AVMs have long been thought to be congenital malformations situated in often eloquent, functional brain parenchyma. Due to this direct, high-pressure, high-flow connection, patients are subject to hemorrhage, seizures and strokes [2]. If AVMs are truly congenital lesions of the

intracranial vascular system, there is a poorly understood interaction between the processes of AVM formation and cortical folding. Although the large vessels in the intracranial vascular system are mostly formed and have perforated the cortex by weeks 8–10 in utero, the brain begins its intricate folding process at weeks 24–34 (reviewed in [3–5]). To date, no hypothesis or human study explains what happens in the 16 week interval between intracranial vasculature maturation and cortical folding initiation [6]. There are no experimental animal AVM models within the brain parenchyma that expose either the mechanism of formation or the effect on cortical folding [7–10].

Cortical folding is a complex phenomenon that remains poorly understood. Our center has discovered cortical folding abnormalities in other diseases of the neurological system such as Williams' syndrome [11] and autism spectrum disorder [12]. Beginning at approximately 26 weeks

---

* Correspondence: manish.n.shah@uth.tmc.edu
†Equal contributors
[1]Departments of Pediatric Surgery and Neurosurgery, McGovern Medical School at UTHealth and UT MD Anderson Cancer Center, Pediatric Neurosurgery, 6431 Fannin St., MSB 5.144, Houston, TX 77030, USA
Full list of author information is available at the end of the article

gestation, cortical folding is thought to rely on a variety of factors including, but not limited to, gene expression, cortical growth, and tension from white matter fibers [13]. In addition, adequate oxygenation is necessary for proper neurodevelopment and cortical folding. Maintenance of tissue perfusion and adequate oxygenation relies heavily on changes at the microvascular level in response to various physiologic cues. The neuronal vasculature in particular is exquisitely sensitive to such signals, which include CO_2 and O_2 levels, mechanical distention and compression, and changes in local neuronal activity [14]. Dysregulation of the microvascular response to these factors results in an area of hypoperfusion. Brain tissue in an affected area is most at-risk for acute infarct or hypoperfusion when surrounding vasculature dilates in order to meet metabolic demand. Cortical steal syndrome occurs when increased resistance in the brain parenchyma relative to the surrounding normal vasculature causes a paradoxical drop in local perfusion pressure.

The extent to which AVMs induce this degree of local hypoxia is debated [2]. Cerebral hypoperfusion has been demonstrated in some patients [15], but not in others [16]. It appears that the main mechanism for maintenance of perfusion in brain surrounding AVMs in the latter group is neo-capillary formation [17]. This phenomenon is presumably the result of some initial hypoxic state that induces local vasculogenesis. Hypoxia and cerebral ischemia can cause cortical thinning due to selective neuronal loss [18–20]. Fierstra et al. demonstrated that cortical thinning is also seen in patients with cortical steal syndrome [21]. They proposed that repeated bouts of transient hypoperfusion associated with steal physiology, while insufficient to cause acute infarction, leads to selective neuronal loss over time.

It is likely that AVMs cause local tissue hypoxia at least initially and, as vasculogenesis precedes cortical folding by several months [6], AVMs could impact cortical development. The human brain has an overwhelming tendency to form complex cortical folds that are orderly in some respects but show a high degree of individual variability in most regions. If AVMs are true congenital lesions formed prior to cortical involution, their mechanical traction on adjacent brain parenchyma should substantially alter the process of cortical folding. This study aims to assess human cortical folding patterns with AVMs using advanced measurements of cortical shape and high-resolution MRI.

Methods
Participants
With institutional review board approval and informed consent, participants were prospectively enrolled in the study. A total of 7 otherwise healthy patients with surgically unresectable AVMs, incidentally found or presenting with seizures but without hemorrhage were enrolled. In addition, one healthy adult control subject was also enrolled, but was not used for the analysis. Some patients had recent stereotactic, focal irradiation to the AVM bed for treatment with Gamma Knife Radiosurgery, but there was no appreciable radiation effect on MRI.

The subject demographics and clinical characteristics are summarized in Table 1. The 7 subjects had a mean age of 42.1 years with 3 females and 4 males. The Spetzler-Martin grades ranges from II-IV. Five subjects initially presented incidentally or with headaches, one with seizures and one with facial numbness. Four of seven were treated with gamma knife stereotactic radiation, one had a hemorrhage and subsequent surgical resection and two had refused radiation treatment at last follow-up. Of the 5 treated patients, 3 had a positive response or elimination of the AVM, one subject had radiographic AVM growth and one subject expired after AVM rupture and hemorrhage. Overall, the seven subjects had an average clinical follow-up time of 17.8 months from last treatment.

The AVMs from the seven subjects varied greatly in terms of volume and location (see Table 1 and Fig. 1 for details). Three of seven subjects had a right cortical AVM, three had left cortical AVM, and one had a left cerebellar AVM. The location of the AVM (right or left) was defined as the affected hemisphere, while the opposite hemisphere was defined as the unaffected hemisphere.

Table 1 Characterization of the Seven AVM Subjects. This table indicates the cohort demographics, AVM characteristics, presentation, treatment and follow-up. Yrs = years, F/U = follow-up, mo = months

Subject	Age (yrs) /Gender	Grade	Location	Volume (cm3)	Presentation	Treatment	F/U (mo)	Outcome
RD02	46/M	4	Left Frontal	2.62	Incidental	Radiation	0	N/A
RD03	40/M	3	Left Motor	16.6	Seizures	Radiation	44	Response
RD04	43/M	3	Right Insular	11.5	Numbness	Radiation	39	Response
RD05	22/F	3	Right Motor	3.77	Incidental	None	0.1	N/A
RD06	47/M	4	Left Parietal	21.0	Headaches	Radiation	5.5	Expired
RD07	56/F	2	Vermian	7.63	Incidental	Surgery	18	Response
RD08	41/F	4	Right Temporal	37.4	Incidental	None	19	Growth

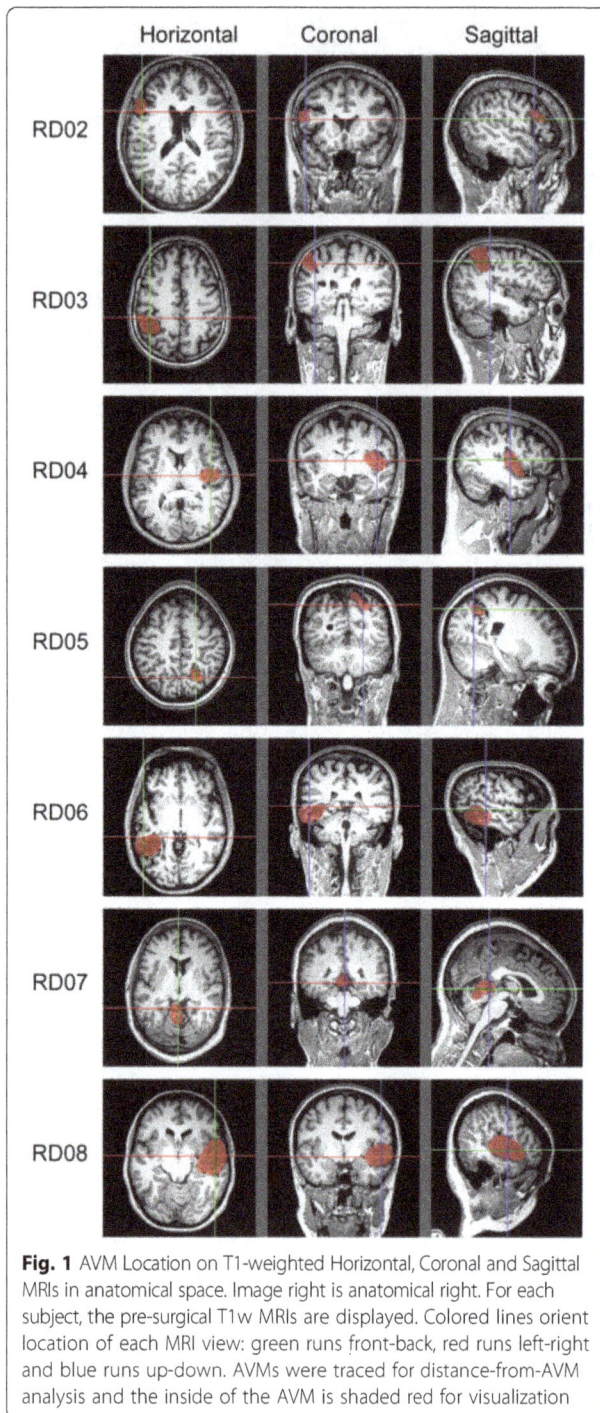

Fig. 1 AVM Location on T1-weighted Horizontal, Coronal and Sagittal MRIs in anatomical space. Image right is anatomical right. For each subject, the pre-surgical T1w MRIs are displayed. Colored lines orient location of each MRI view: green runs front-back, red runs left-right and blue runs up-down. AVMs were traced for distance-from-AVM analysis and the inside of the AVM is shaded red for visualization

phase oversampling for the MPRAGE and no oversampling for the SPACE sequences, as previously described by Glasser and Van Essen [22].

Segmentation and registration

The T1w images were segmented using Freesurfer version 5.1.0. The resulting surfaces were registered to the fs_LR atlas and sulcal depth maps generated using previously described methods [23]. Segmentations of the AVMs were manually traced using MRIcron [24].

Sulcal depth analysis

The PALS-B12.LR mean sulcal depth [25] was resampled to the fs_LR mesh using caret5 with an existing PALS-to-Conte69 deformation map [22]. This was the average of the sulcal depth maps for twelve human subjects, all healthy, right-handed adults aged 18–24 (six female, six

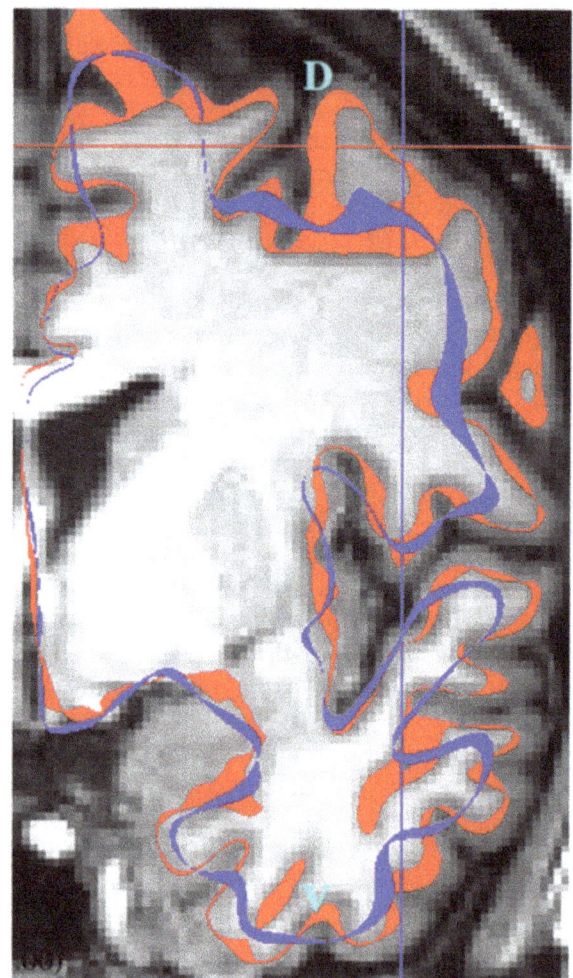

Fig. 2 A Representation of Cortical Folding Measures. This is a coronal MRI slice of patient RD05. The red line represents the subject's midthickness surface in Montreal Neurological Institute space. The blue line represents the HCP196 mean midthickness surface. D = dorsal; V = ventral

MRI acquisition

All 8 subjects had sagittally-acquired 3D T1-weighted magnetization-prepared rapid gradient echo (MPRAGE) sequences and 3D T2-weighted sampling perfection with application optimized contrast using different angle evolutions (SPACE) on a Siemens 3 T TIM Trio MRI scanner. A generalized autocalibrating partially parallel acquisition (GRAPPA) factor of 2 was used for both scans with 50 %

Table 2 Depth difference index (DDI), local (L) and remote (R) coordinate distance index (CDI and CDI), and gyrification index (GI) for Affected (A) and Unaffected (U) Hemispheres. Both DDI and CDI are vertex-wise differences (affected-unaffected) weighted by mean tile area and summed over vertices outside the medial wall (for DDI, vertices at least 20 mm from AVM)

Subject	DDI (A)	DDI (U)	L CDI (A)	L CDI (U)	R CDI (A)	R CDI (U)	GI (A)	GI (U)
RD02	3.081085	2.917788	5.818325	7.726299	6.756877	6.732552	2.1584	2.1512
RD03	2.696007	2.689072	7.650329	6.760775	6.052032	6.439287	2.1486	2.1609
RD04	2.905195	2.967963	8.866142	5.810119	9.404687	7.920285	1.9756	1.8767
RD05	3.352648	3.210038	7.815037	9.577932	7.498025	8.160805	2.2231	2.1589
RD06	3.219622	3.242632	12.84460	7.324401	11.34821	10.15757	1.5190	1.5667
RD07	2.640733	2.542771	5.383245	5.923716	5.747210	6.088752	1.8974	1.9363
RD08	3.171523	3.215196	11.91789	9.246596	13.68615	13.38209	1.5644	1.7112
Mean	3.009545	2.969351	8.613653	7.481405	8.641884	8.411620	1.9266	1.9374

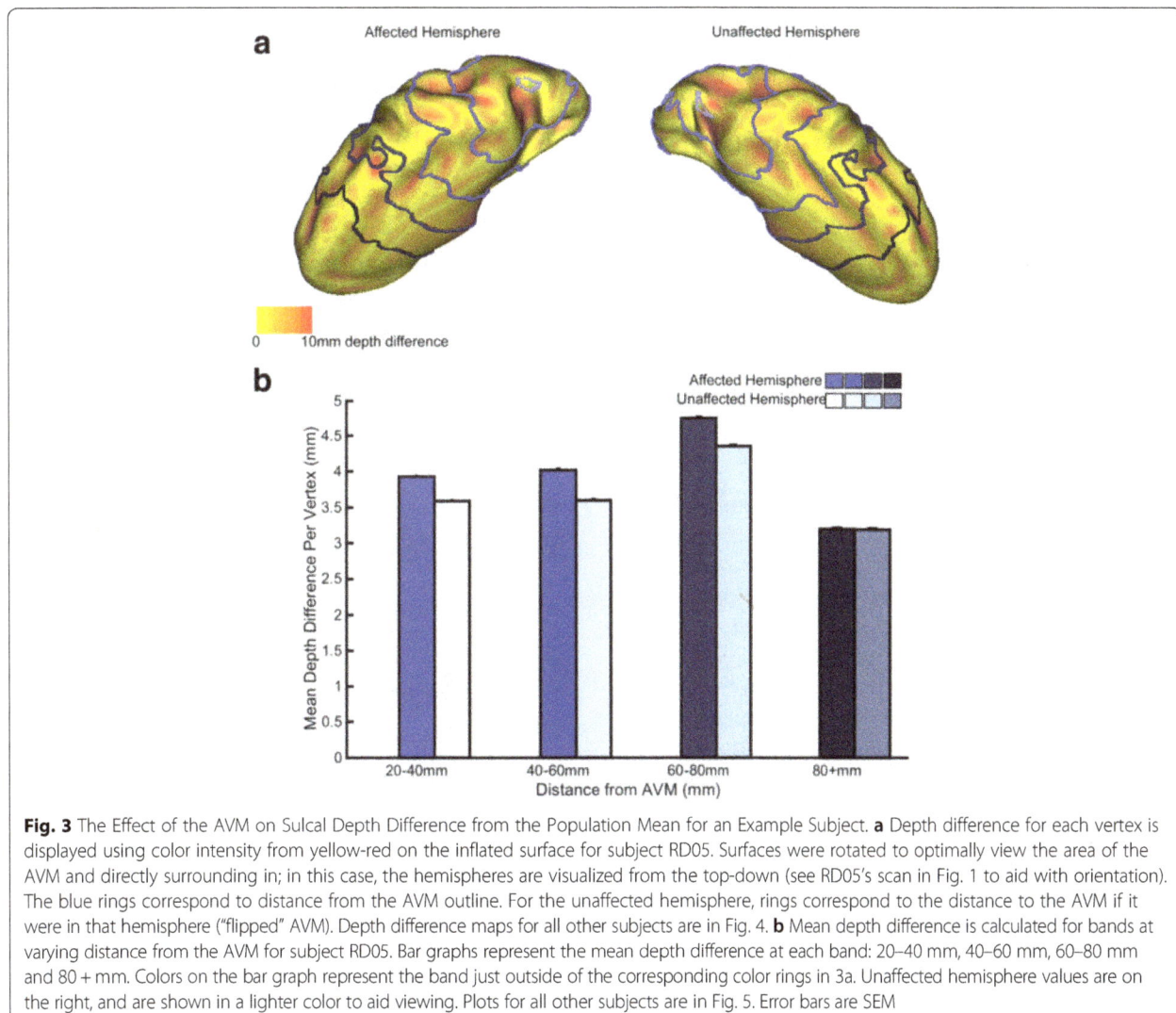

Fig. 3 The Effect of the AVM on Sulcal Depth Difference from the Population Mean for an Example Subject. **a** Depth difference for each vertex is displayed using color intensity from yellow-red on the inflated surface for subject RD05. Surfaces were rotated to optimally view the area of the AVM and directly surrounding in; in this case, the hemispheres are visualized from the top-down (see RD05's scan in Fig. 1 to aid with orientation). The blue rings correspond to distance from the AVM outline. For the unaffected hemisphere, rings correspond to the distance to the AVM if it were in that hemisphere ("flipped" AVM). Depth difference maps for all other subjects are in Fig. 4. **b** Mean depth difference is calculated for bands at varying distance from the AVM for subject RD05. Bar graphs represent the mean depth difference at each band: 20–40 mm, 40–60 mm, 60–80 mm and 80 + mm. Colors on the bar graph represent the band just outside of the corresponding color rings in 3a. Unaffected hemisphere values are on the right, and are shown in a lighter color to aid viewing. Plots for all other subjects are in Fig. 5. Error bars are SEM

male). For each vertex within each hemisphere, the difference between the subject's sulcal depth and the PALS-B12.LR mean sulcal depth was computed. The resulting depth difference reflects the degree to which cortical depth differs from the population mean at any given vertex. Figure 1 shows depth difference maps for each subject. For each hemisphere, a depth difference index (DDI) was computed by integrating across the surface (sum of the difference multiplied by a third of the area of the vertex's tiles), but excluding vertices in the fs_LR medial wall, and then dividing by the surface area outside of the medial wall. These DDIs were computed for both affected and unaffected hemispheres, and then input to a paired *t*-test.

In some subjects, cortex near the AVM was abnormal enough to perturb cerebral hull generation, which in turn confounded sulcal depth computation. Inspection of all hemispheres revealed that the confounds affected cortex within 15 mm of the AVM, so we restricted our DDI computation to vertices farther than 15 mm from the AVM boundary. For the unaffected hemisphere, the same ROI was used, to exclude equivalent cortex from the measure on the unaffected hemisphere (left and right hemispheres are in register with one another in fs_LR standard mesh surfaces).

Coordinate distance analysis

For this analysis, the per-vertex Euclidean distance between a normative reference average midthickness surface and the subject's own Montreal Neurological Institute (MNI)-space midthickness surface was used as a measure of folding abnormality. Figure 2 illustrates a patient's MNI-space surface, red, versus the normative reference midthickness, blue, in a coronal MRI slice.

The normative reference (RefSurf) was the mean midthickness surface from the Human Connectome Project (HCP) third release (Q1-2-3_Related196.L/R.midthickness. MSMSulc.164k_fs_LR.surf.gii), incorporating 196 healthy human young adults [26]. Each subject's midthickness surface (SubjectSurface) was normalized to MNI space by applying the talairach.xfm from the subject's freesurfer directory.

For each vertex i within each hemisphere, the distance between RefSurf[i] and SubjectSurface[i] was computed. For each hemisphere, a weighted sum of distance was computed across the hemisphere (sum of the distance multiplied by the mean of the area of the vertex's tiles), but excluding vertices in the fs_LR medial wall. Because this measure was not subject to the hull issues that limited DDI computation to vertices beyond 15 mm from the AVM, we computed it across two regions of interest: One local (within 15 mm of the AVM) and one remote ROI (further than 15 mm from the AVM). We hypothesized that differences in the affected hemisphere might

be more pronounced near the AVM. This measure, the coordinate distance index (CDI), was computed by dividing the weighted sum of distance by the surface area of the associated region. CDIs were computed for both affected and unaffected hemispheres and then input to a paired *t*-test.

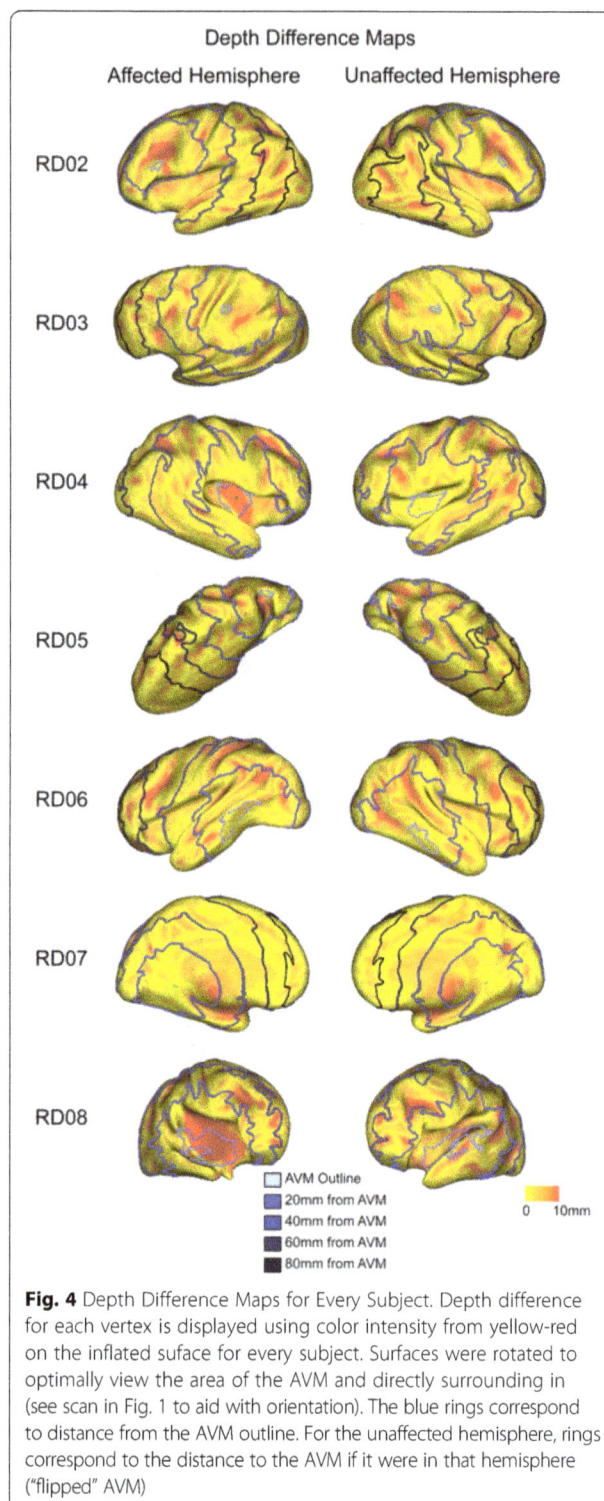

Fig. 4 Depth Difference Maps for Every Subject. Depth difference for each vertex is displayed using color intensity from yellow-red on the inflated suface for every subject. Surfaces were rotated to optimally view the area of the AVM and directly surrounding in (see scan in Fig. 1 to aid with orientation). The blue rings correspond to distance from the AVM outline. For the unaffected hemisphere, rings correspond to the distance to the AVM if it were in that hemisphere ("flipped" AVM)

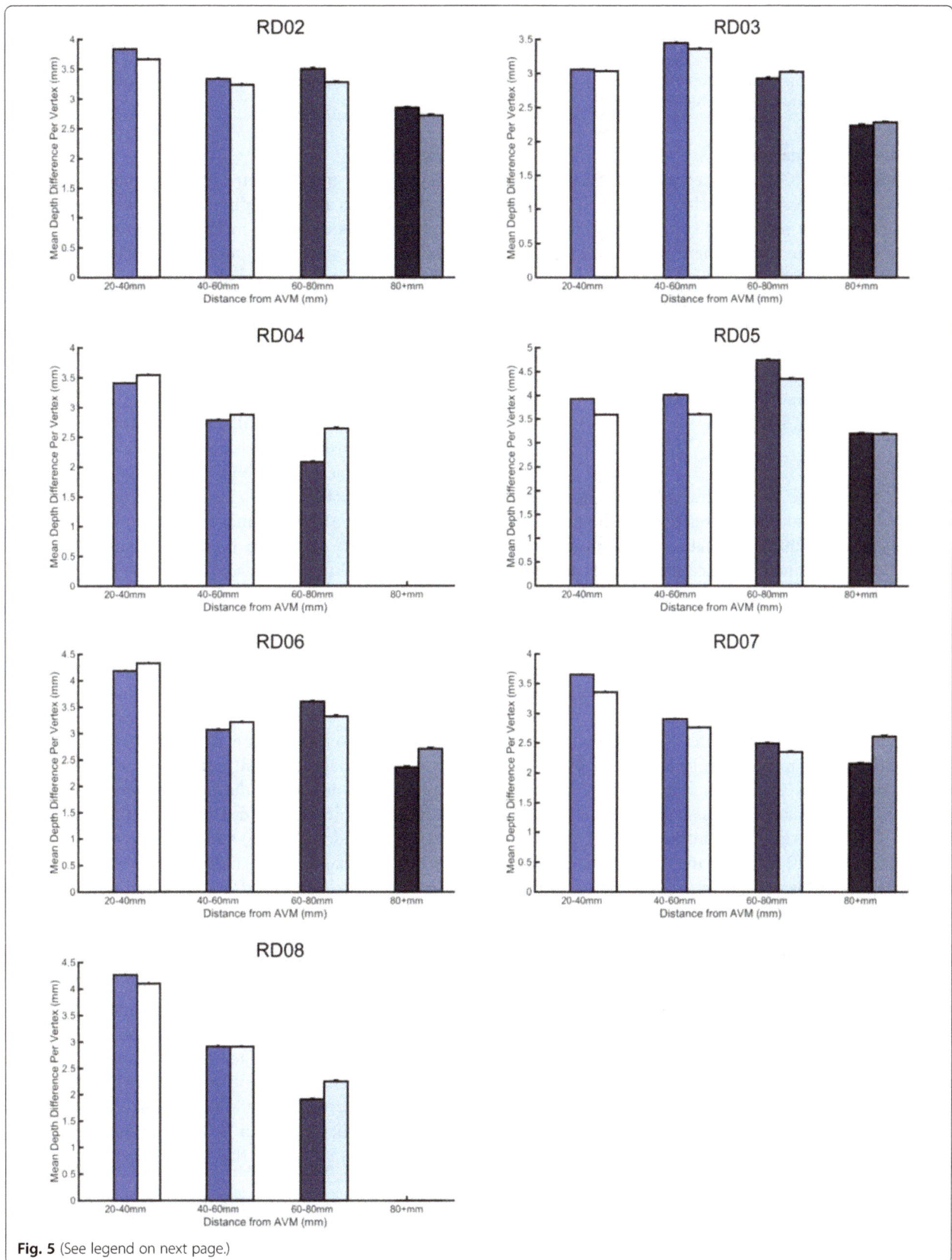

Fig. 5 (See legend on next page.)

(See figure on previous page.)
Fig. 5 Relationship between Distance from the AVM and Depth Difference for every subject. Mean depth difference is calculated for bands at varying distance from the AVM. Bar graphs represent the mean depth difference at each band: 20–40 mm, 40–60 mm, 60–80 mm and 80 + mm. Colors on the bar graph represent the band just outside of the corresponding color rings in Fig. 4. Unaffected hemisphere values are on the right, and are shown in a lighter color to aid viewing. Error bars are SEM

Gyrification index analysis

Gyrification index (GI) is defined as the ratio of cortical surface area to cerebral hull surface area [25, 27]. GI was computed for each subject, and then the GI for the affected and unaffected hemisphere was compared with a paired t test.

Power analysis

We assume and a one-tailed test with statistical significance, $\alpha = 0.05$ and a study power of $\beta = 0.80$. For a moderate effect size (50 %), we would need 21 participants (G*Power 3.1, [28]).

Results

In order to test whether the affected hemisphere had alterations in cortical folding relative to the unaffected hemisphere, we utilized 3 metrics - depth difference index (DDI), coordinate distance index (CDI) and gyrification index (GI). This data is presented in Table 2. With our small sample size of 7 subjects, none of these three metrics had a significant difference between the affected and unaffected hemisphere.

We next examined the relationship between depth difference (DDI prior to integration across all vertices) and distance from the AVM center. An example subject depth difference map is shown in Fig. 3a (maps for each subject are shown in Fig. 4). Qualitatively, variability makes it difficult to discern a spatial pattern for depth difference. We drew regions of interest (ROIs) in 20 mm bands starting 20–40 mm from the AVM (ROIs illustrated in Fig. 3a). We observed that most subjects had a difference between affected and unaffected sulcal depth which was more pronounced in ROIs closer to the AVM (see example in Fig. 3, RD05). Nonetheless, the existence of subjects for which this trend does not hold (ex. RD06, Fig. 5) indicates that other variables, such as AVM depth and location, may also affect cortical folding.

We also looked at whether there was a relationship between AVM volume and DDI. Fig. 6a is a scatter plot of AVM volume and DDI for the affected and unaffected hemispheres from each subject. There is a tight correlation in normalized sulcal depth between left and right hemispheres within a subject, which seemed to mask any effects of the AVM volume. To address this, we calculated the ratio of affected:unaffected DDI and compared this to AVM volume (Fig. 6b). Interestingly, with just 7 data points, this DDI ratio was inversely correlated with AVM volume (correlation coefficient $r = -0.74$, $p = 0.04$).

Discussion

This is the first morphometric study to quantitatively assess brain cortical folding differences in human subjects with brain arteriovenous malformations using Human Connectome Project (HCP) methodology [11, 22, 23]. We quantitatively assessed brain sulcal depth in 7 participants with AVMs compared to the mean depth of healthy young adults. We found no statistically significant differences between hemispheres containing the AVM and contralateral hemispheres in our sulcal depth analysis, coordinate distance analysis or gyrification index testing. However, the depth difference index (DDI) ratio (affected hemisphere/unaffected hemisphere) was larger in smaller AVMs and smaller in larger AVMs (both hemispheres had similar DDI). One hypothesis for why this may be occurring is that the larger AVMs are more likely to exert effects on the contralateral as well as ipsilateral hemisphere. However, as with distance from the AVM, the occurrence of significant outliers in this trend suggests that AVM volume is not the only factor influencing sulcal depth. The complexities of the interaction between AVM pathogenesis and cortical development are deserving of further study. Currently, the only mechanistic understanding of AVM pathogenesis comes from the observation of increased intracranial AVM prevalence in the main subtypes of an autosomal dominant syndrome with AVMs in various organs including the brain: Human Hereditary Telangiectasia (HHT1 and HHT2). HHT1 involves a mutation in endoglin (Eng) and HHT2 involves a mutation in actin-like kinase 1 (Alk1), both involved in the transforming growth factor beta (TGF-β) signaling cascade [29, 30]. As both Eng and Alk1 are expressed in endothelial cells, changes in their function and expression affect angiogenesis [31, 32]. A murine knockout of Alk1 needed angiogenic stimulation with VEGF for *de novo* formation of brain AVMs [33], potentially suggesting a "two-hit" model of AVM formation and explaining the relatively few congenital AVM cases. The vast majority of brain AVMs are present in the absence of HHT and there are no definitive human tissue studies implicating Alk1 in brain AVM formation [34, 35], leaving a major gap in the understanding of AVM pathogenesis.

Our results may support the *de novo* formation theory, as otherwise cortical folding differences would potentially be more evident. However, with only 7 patients at a single time instance, more longitudinal data is needed for such a conclusion. We originally hypothesized that sulcal depth

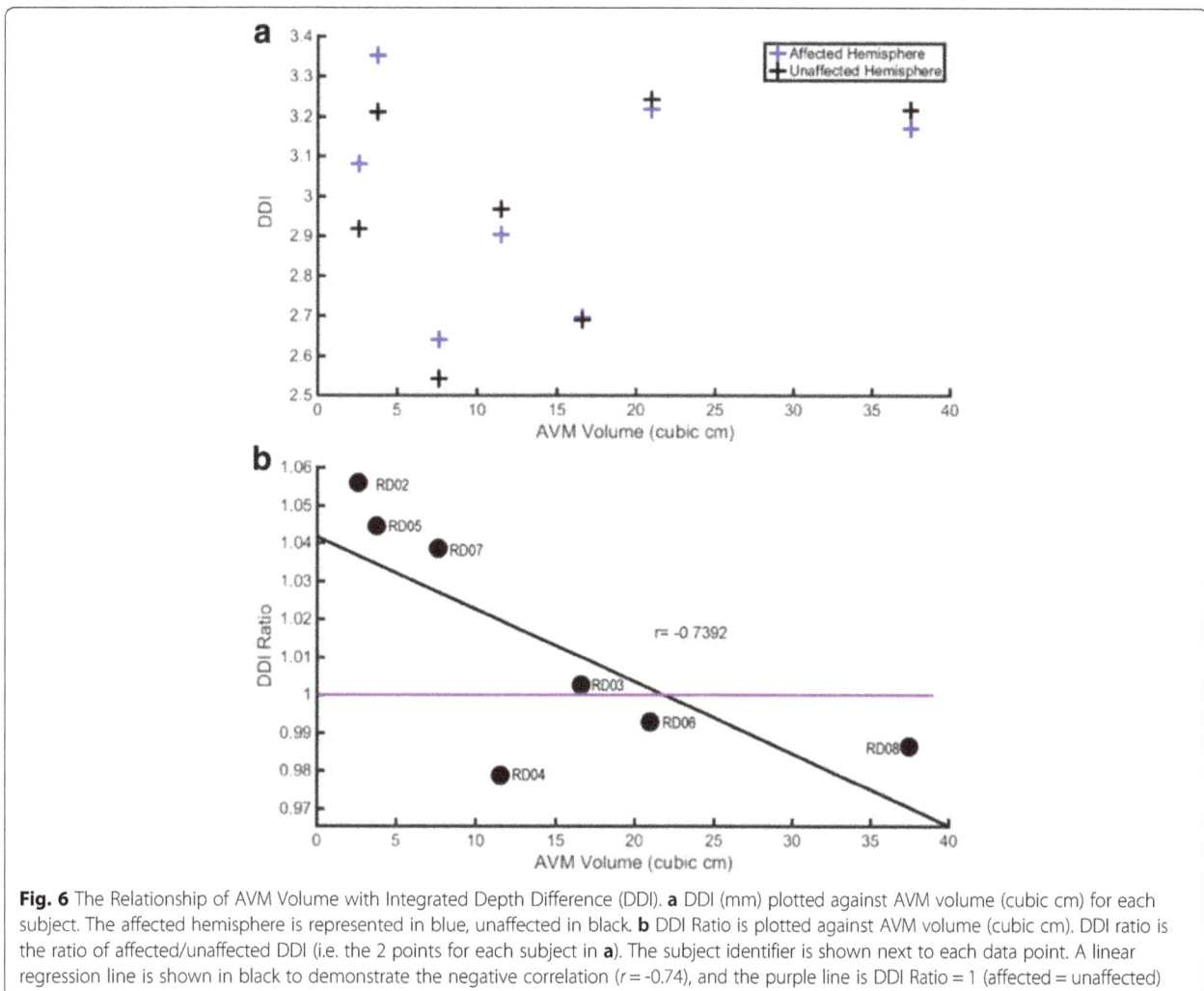

Fig. 6 The Relationship of AVM Volume with Integrated Depth Difference (DDI). **a** DDI (mm) plotted against AVM volume (cubic cm) for each subject. The affected hemisphere is represented in blue, unaffected in black. **b** DDI Ratio is plotted against AVM volume (cubic cm). DDI ratio is the ratio of affected/unaffected DDI (i.e. the 2 points for each subject in **a**). The subject identifier is shown next to each data point. A linear regression line is shown in black to demonstrate the negative correlation ($r = -0.74$), and the purple line is DDI Ratio = 1 (affected = unaffected)

differences would be confined to the cortex adjacent to the AVM. The AVM should provide local mechanical traction to folding and also a relative lack of perfusion caused by the absence of normal intervening capillaries. We were unable to define a spatial relationship of cortical folding differences caused by underlying AVMs, an important result that may suggest a decoupling of cortical folding and AVM pathogenesis. This lack of spatial relationship could be due to a much wider-spread pattern of cortical disruption, but it could also be that folding and AVM formation processes are independent.

Previous studies [36] have shown reorganization in eloquent areas overlying AVMs, which could have its basis in cortical folding but also in post-stroke cortical plasticity mechanisms that are also poorly understood [37]. Additionally, it is possible that extreme sulcal depth differences predispose AVM patients to ipsilateral seizure onset during the initial presentation in nearly 40 % of AVM patients [38], as many epilepsy etiologies are structural [39]. However, every healthy individual has a

distinct sulcal depth pattern and our comparisons employ the population mean. Further testing of sulcal depth and functional changes could further elucidate this relationship, especially if performed longitudinally in our AVM patient cohort.

Despite a large body of scientific literature, the pathogenesis of AVMs remains controversial [40, 41]. Our study raises several points essential to AVM pathogenesis. Although classically described as congenital malformations, there now exist many case reports of *de novo* AVM formation [42] on serial cerebral angiography. Our study represents a single point in time for each patient, and any structural differences seen in our population could be a result of a disordered cerebral circulation. However, there may be artifact in our calculation of sulcal depth related to gliosis developed alongside a *de novo* AVM and the subsequent changes in perfusion to the surrounding tissues. Such remodeling has previously been described in patients with cerebrovascular disease [43]. A longitudinal study looking at the evolution of sulcal depth differences in

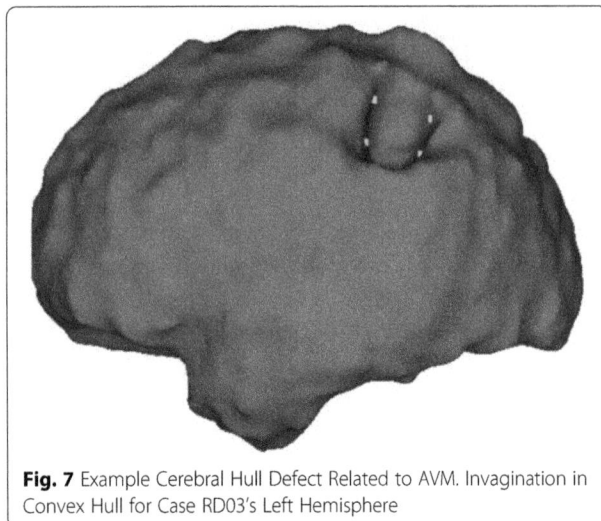

Fig. 7 Example Cerebral Hull Defect Related to AVM. Invagination in Convex Hull for Case RD03's Left Hemisphere

Acknowledgements
Not Applicable.

Funding
DCVE is supported by grant National Institutes of Health (NIH) R01-MH-60974.

Authors' contributions
MNS and SES are co-first authors and both equally designed the study, performed the analysis, analyzed the results and drafted the manuscript. DLD performed the analysis, analyzed results and helped draft the manuscript. JPH helped analyze results and draft the manuscript. TSC helped perform the analysis, analyze results and draft the manuscript. BSB helped collect data and draft the manuscript. GJZ helped analyzing results and drafting the manuscript. DCVE helped with study design, result analysis and manuscript drafting. RGD conceived and designed the study, analyzed results and helped draft the manuscript. All authors read and approved the final manuscript.

Authors' information
Not Applicable.

Competing interests
The authors declare that they have no competing interests.

Support
DCVE is supported by grant National Institutes of Health (NIH) R01-MH-60974.

Author details
[1]Departments of Pediatric Surgery and Neurosurgery, McGovern Medical School at UTHealth and UT MD Anderson Cancer Center, Pediatric Neurosurgery, 6431 Fannin St., MSB 5.144, Houston, TX 77030, USA. [2]Department of Neuroscience, Washington University, 660 S. Euclid Ave, St. Louis, MO 63110, USA. [3]Division of Neurosurgery, University of Missouri-Columbia, One Hospital Drive, 314 McHaney Hall, Columbia, MO 65212, USA. [4]Department of Neurological Surgery, Washington University, 660 S. Euclid Ave, St. Louis, MO 63110, USA.

patients with AVMs could be illuminating. The sulcal depth measure was confined to vertices outside a 15 mm radius of the AVM, due to problems generating the lesion's convex hull for analysis; Fig. 7 demonstrates a representative AVM-related hull defect. The presence of the AVM during cerebral hull generation in our study patients also likely confounds the gyrification index calculation. Morphometric measures that depend on nonlinear registration to an atlas target (e.g., deformation-based morphometry) may have similar confounds, to the extent that the AVM affects registration. Cortical thickness might be less affected overall and could be examined in future studies.

Our study might be simply underpowered to determine such a relationship with only six subjects with supratentorial AVMs. At our hypothesized moderate 50 % effect size, we would have needed 21 patients to have 80 % power to avoid a type II error. In addition to limiting the power of our study of sulcal depth differences, none of these patients presented with hemorrhage or focal neurological deficit. It is possible that these sequelae are in some way related to the minor folding differences we observed, but a larger study would be needed to determine what, if any, connection there is between the two.

Conclusions

This is the first study to quantitatively assess human developmental cortical folding in the presence of intracranial arteriovenous malformations. The study found no statistically significant cortical folding differences in the patient hemispheres with AVMs compared to their own contralateral hemispheres or compared to a previously obtained healthy, control dataset. However, longitudinal studies are recommended to definitively establish whether arteriovenous malformations are developmental, congenital lesions or dynamic, *de novo* entities.

References
1. McCormick WF. The pathology of vascular ("arteriovenous") malformations. J Neurosurg. 1966;24:807–16.
2. Moftakhar P, Hauptman JS, Malkasian D, Martin NA. Cerebral arteriovenous malformations. Part 2: physiology. Neurosurg Focus. 2009;26:E11.
3. Budday S, Steinmann P, Kuhl E. Physical biology of human brain development. Front Cell Neurosci. 2015;9:257.
4. Marin-Padilla M. The human brain intracerebral microvascular system: development and structure. Front Neuroanat. 2012;6:38.
5. Menshawi K, Mohr JP, Gutierrez J. A Functional Perspective on the Embryology and Anatomy of the Cerebral Blood Supply. J Stroke. 2015;17:144–58.
6. Nelson Jr MD, Gonzalez-Gomez I, Gilles FH. Dyke Award. The search for human telencephalic ventriculofugal arteries. AJNR Am J Neuroradiol. 1991;12:215–22.
7. Chaloupka JC, Vinuela F, Robert J, Duckwiler GR. An in vivo arteriovenous malformation model in swine: preliminary feasibility and natural history study. AJNR Am J Neuroradiol. 1994;15:945–50.
8. Kashba SR, Patel NJ, Grace M, Lee VS, Raoufi-Rad N, Amal Raj JV, Duong TT, Stoodley M. Angiographic, hemodynamic, and histological changes in an animal model of brain arteriovenous malformations treated with Gamma Knife radiosurgery. J Neurosurg. 2015;123:954-60.
9. Mut M, Oge K, Zorlu F, Undeger U, Erdem S, Ozcan OE. Effects of ionizing radiation on brain tissue surrounding arteriovenous malformations: an experimental study in a rat caroticojugular fistula model. Neurosurg Rev. 2004;27:121–7.
10. Qian Z, Climent S, Maynar M, Uson-Garallo J, Lima-Rodrigues MA, Calles C, Robertson H, Castaneda-Zuniga WR. A simplified arteriovenous malformation model in sheep: feasibility study. AJNR Am J Neuroradiol. 1999;20:765–70.

11. Van Essen DC, Dierker D, Snyder AZ, Raichle ME, Reiss AL, Korenberg J. Symmetry of cortical folding abnormalities in Williams syndrome revealed by surface-based analyses. J Neurosci. 2006;26:5470–83.

12. Nordahl CW, Dierker D, Mostafavi I, Schumann CM, Rivera SM, Amaral DG, Van Essen DC. Cortical folding abnormalities in autism revealed by surface-based morphometry. J Neurosci. 2007;27:11725–35.

13. Dubois J, Benders M, Borradori-Tolsa C, Cachia A, Lazeyras F, Ha-Vinh Leuchter R, Sizonenko SV, Warfield SK, Mangin JF, Huppi PS. Primary cortical folding in the human newborn: an early marker of later functional development. Brain. 2008;131:2028–41.

14. Hamel E. Perivascular nerves and the regulation of cerebrovascular tone. J Appl Physiol (1985). 2006;100:1059–64.

15. Homan RW, Devous Sr MD, Stokely EM, Bonte FJ. Quantification of intracerebral steal in patients with arteriovenous malformation. Arch Neurol. 1986;43:779–85.

16. Meyer B, Schaller C, Frenkel C, Schramm J. Physiological steal around AVMs of the brain is not equivalent to cortical ischemia. Neurol Res. 1998;20 Suppl 1:S13–7.

17. Meyer B, Schaller C, Frenkel C, Ebeling B, Schramm J. Distributions of local oxygen saturation and its response to changes of mean arterial blood pressure in the cerebral cortex adjacent to arteriovenous malformations. Stroke. 1999;30:2623–30.

18. Garcia JH, Lassen NA, Weiller C, Sperling B, Nakagawara J. Ischemic stroke and incomplete infarction. Stroke. 1996;27:761–5.

19. Saur D, Buchert R, Knab R, Weiller C, Rother J. Iomazenil-single-photon emission computed tomography reveals selective neuronal loss in magnetic resonance-defined mismatch areas. Stroke. 2006;37:2713–9.

20. Yamauchi H, Kudoh T, Kishibe Y, Iwasaki J, Kagawa S. Selective neuronal damage and borderzone infarction in carotid artery occlusive disease: a 11C-flumazenil PET study. J Nucl Med. 2005;46:1973–9.

21. Fierstra J, Poublanc J, Han JS, Silver F, Tymianski M, Crawley AP, Fisher JA, Mikulis DJ. Steal physiology is spatially associated with cortical thinning. J Neurol Neurosurg Psychiatry. 2010;81:290–3.

22. Glasser MF, Van Essen DC. Mapping human cortical areas in vivo based on myelin content as revealed by T1- and T2-weighted MRI. J Neurosci. 2011;31:11597–616.

23. Dierker DL, Feczko E, Pruett Jr JR, Petersen SE, Schlaggar BL, Constantino JN, Harwell JW, Coalson TS, Van Essen DC. Analysis of cortical shape in children with simplex autism. Cereb Cortex. 2015;25:1042–51.

24. Rorden C, Brett M. Stereotaxic display of brain lesions. Behav Neurol. 2000;12:191–200.

25. Van Essen DC. A Population-Average, Landmark- and Surface-based (PALS) atlas of human cerebral cortex. Neuroimage. 2005;28:635–62.

26. Van Essen DC, Smith SM, Barch DM, Behrens TE, Yacoub E, Ugurbil K, Consortium WU-MH. The WU-Minn Human Connectome Project: an overview. Neuroimage. 2013;80:62–79.

27. Hill J, Dierker D, Neil J, Inder T, Knutsen A, Harwell J, Coalson T, Van Essen D. A surface-based analysis of hemispheric asymmetries and folding of cerebral cortex in term-born human infants. J Neurosci. 2010;30:2268–76.

28. Faul F, Erdfelder E, Buchner A, Lang AG. Statistical power analyses using G*Power 3.1: tests for correlation and regression analyses. Behav Res Methods. 2009;41:1149–60.

29. Marchuk DA, Srinivasan S, Squire TL, Zawistowski JS. Vascular morphogenesis: tales of two syndromes. Hum Mol Genet. 2003;12 Spec No 1:R97–R112.

30. Kim H, Marchuk DA, Pawlikowska L, Chen Y, Su H, Yang GY, Young WL. Genetic considerations relevant to intracranial hemorrhage and brain arteriovenous malformations. Acta Neurochir Suppl. 2008;105:199–206.

31. Cheifetz S, Bellon T, Cales C, Vera S, Bernabeu C, Massague J, Letarte M. Endoglin is a component of the transforming growth factor-beta receptor system in human endothelial cells. J Biol Chem. 1992;267:19027–30.

32. Lamouille S, Mallet C, Feige JJ, Bailly S. Activin receptor-like kinase 1 is implicated in the maturation phase of angiogenesis. Blood. 2002;100:4495–501.

33. Chen W, Sun Z, Han Z, Jun K, Camus M, Wankhede M, Mao L, Arnold T, Young WL, Su H. De novo cerebrovascular malformation in the adult mouse after endothelial Alk1 deletion and angiogenic stimulation. Stroke. 2014;45:900–2.

34. Hashimoto T, Wu Y, Lawton MT, Yang GY, Barbaro NM, Young WL. Coexpression of angiogenic factors in brain arteriovenous malformations. Neurosurgery. 2005;56:1058–65. discussion 1058-1065.

35. Shenkar R, Elliott JP, Diener K, Gault J, Hu LJ, Cohrs RJ, Phang T, Hunter L, Breeze RE, Awad IA. Differential gene expression in human cerebrovascular malformations. Neurosurgery. 2003;52:465–77. discussion 477-468.

36. Alkadhi H, Kollias SS, Crelier GR, Golay X, Hepp-Reymond MC, Valavanis A. Plasticity of the human motor cortex in patients with arteriovenous malformations: a functional MR imaging study. AJNR Am J Neuroradiol. 2000;21:1423–33.

37. Liepert J, Miltner WH, Bauder H, Sommer M, Dettmers C, Taub E, Weiller C. Motor cortex plasticity during constraint-induced movement therapy in stroke patients. Neurosci Lett. 1998;250:5–8.

38. da Costa L, Wallace MC, Ter Brugge KG, O'Kelly C, Willinsky RA, Tymianski M. The natural history and predictive features of hemorrhage from brain arteriovenous malformations. Stroke. 2009;40:100–5.

39. Bhalla D, Godet B, Druet-Cabanac M, Preux PM. Etiologies of epilepsy: a comprehensive review. Expert Rev Neurother. 2011;11:861–76.

40. Kim H, Su H, Weinsheimer S, Pawlikowska L, Young WL. Brain arteriovenous malformation pathogenesis: a response-to-injury paradigm. Acta Neurochir Suppl. 2011;111:83–92.

41. Lasjaunias P. A revised concept of the congenital nature of cerebral arteriovenous malformations. Interv Neuroradiol. 1997;3:275–81.

42. Morales-Valero SF, Bortolotti C, Sturiale C, Lanzino G. Are parenchymal AVMs congenital lesions? Neurosurg Focus. 2014;37:E2.

43. Fierstra J, Maclean DB, Fisher JA, Han JS, Mandell DM, Conklin J, Poublanc J, Crawley AP, Regli L, Mikulis DJ, Tymianski M. Surgical revascularization reverses cerebral cortical thinning in patients with severe cerebrovascular steno-occlusive disease. Stroke. 2011;42:1631–7.

Permissions

All chapters in this book were first published in NI, by BioMed Central; hereby published with permission under the Creative Commons Attribution License or equivalent. Every chapter published in this book has been scrutinized by our experts. Their significance has been extensively debated. The topics covered herein carry significant findings which will fuel the growth of the discipline. They may even be implemented as practical applications or may be referred to as a beginning point for another development.

The contributors of this book come from diverse backgrounds, making this book a truly international effort. This book will bring forth new frontiers with its revolutionizing research information and detailed analysis of the nascent developments around the world.

We would like to thank all the contributing authors for lending their expertise to make the book truly unique. They have played a crucial role in the development of this book. Without their invaluable contributions this book wouldn't have been possible. They have made vital efforts to compile up to date information on the varied aspects of this subject to make this book a valuable addition to the collection of many professionals and students.

This book was conceptualized with the vision of imparting up-to-date information and advanced data in this field. To ensure the same, a matchless editorial board was set up. Every individual on the board went through rigorous rounds of assessment to prove their worth. After which they invested a large part of their time researching and compiling the most relevant data for our readers.

The editorial board has been involved in producing this book since its inception. They have spent rigorous hours researching and exploring the diverse topics which have resulted in the successful publishing of this book. They have passed on their knowledge of decades through this book. To expedite this challenging task, the publisher supported the team at every step. A small team of assistant editors was also appointed to further simplify the editing procedure and attain best results for the readers.

Apart from the editorial board, the designing team has also invested a significant amount of their time in understanding the subject and creating the most relevant covers. They scrutinized every image to scout for the most suitable representation of the subject and create an appropriate cover for the book.

The publishing team has been an ardent support to the editorial, designing and production team. Their endless efforts to recruit the best for this project, has resulted in the accomplishment of this book. They are a veteran in the field of academics and their pool of knowledge is as vast as their experience in printing. Their expertise and guidance has proved useful at every step. Their uncompromising quality standards have made this book an exceptional effort. Their encouragement from time to time has been an inspiration for everyone.

The publisher and the editorial board hope that this book will prove to be a valuable piece of knowledge for researchers, students, practitioners and scholars across the globe.

List of Contributors

Xinyi Leng, Hing Lung Ip, Yannie Soo, Thomas Leung and Ka Sing Wong
Department of Medicine and Therapeutics, the Chinese University of Hong Kong, Prince of Wales Hospital, Shatin, Hong Kong SAR, China

Fabien Scalzo, Albert K Fong and Mark Johnson
UCLA Stroke Center, University of California, CA 90095 Los Angeles, USA

David S Liebeskind
UCLA Stroke Center, University of California, CA 90095 Los Angeles, USA
UCLA Department of Neurology, Neuroscience Research Building, Suite 225, Los Angeles, CA 90095-7334, USA

Liping Liu
Department of Neurology, Beijing Tiantan Hospital, Capital Medical University, Beijing 100050 China

Edward Feldmann
Department of Neurology, Tufts University, Boston MA 02111, USA

Nam K. Yoon, Philipp Taussky and Min S.Park
Department of Neurosurgery, Clinical Neurosciences Center, University of Utah, Salt Lake City, Utah, USA

Scott McNally
Department of Radiology, University of Utah Health Care, Salt Lake City, Utah, USA

Fulvio Zaccagna, Beatrice Sacconi, Isabella Ceravolo, Andrea Fiorelli, Iacopo Carbone, Alessandro Napoli, Michele Anzidei and Carlo Catalano
Department of Radiological, Oncological and Anatomopathological Sciences, Sapienza – University of Rome, Viale Regina Elena 324, 00161 Rome, Italy

Luca Saba
Department of Radiology, Azienda Ospedaliero Universitaria (A.O.U.), di Cagliari-Polo di Monserrato, Italy

Pierleone Lucatelli, Michele Anzidei, Mario Bezzi and Carlo Catalano
Department of Radiological, Oncological and Anatomopathological Sciences – Radiology, 'Sapienza' University of Rome, Viale Regina Elena 324, 00161 Rome, Italy

Beatrice Sacconi
Department of Radiological, Oncological and Anatomopathological Sciences – Radiology, 'Sapienza' University of Rome, Viale Regina Elena 324, 00161 Rome, Italy
Center for Life Nano Science@Sapienza, Istituto Italiano di Tecnologia, Rome, Italy

Marinos Kontzialis
Department of Radiology, Rush University Medical Center, 1725 W. Harrison St., Chicago, IL 60612, USA

Bruce A. Wasserman
The Russell H. Morgan Department of Radiology and Radiological Sciences, Johns Hopkins University School of Medicine, 600 North Wolfe Street, Baltimore, MD 21287 USA

Nicholas A. Telischak and Max Wintermark
Department of Neuroradiology, S047 300 Pasteur Drive, Stanford, CA 94305, USA

Ying-Huan Hu, Shan Gao and Wei-Hai Xu
Department of Neurology, Peking Union Medical College Hospital, Chinese Academy of Medical Sciences and Peking Union Medical College, Shuaifuyuan 1, Dongcheng District, Beijing 100730, China

Jie Chen
Department of Neurology, Peking Union Medical College Hospital, Chinese Academy of Medical Sciences and Peking Union Medical College, Shuaifuyuan 1, Dongcheng District, Beijing 100730, China
Department of Neurology, Beijing Tiantan Hospital, Capital Medical University, Beijing 10050, China

Michal Sharon, Robert Yeung, Liying zhang, Sean P. Symons and Richard I. Aviv
Department of Diagnostic Imaging, Division of Neuroradiology, Room AG 31, Sunnybrook Health Sciences Centre, 2075 Bayview Ave, Toronto, ON M4N 3M5, Canada

Karl Boyle and Mark I. Boulos
Department of Medicine, Division of Neurology, Sunnybrook Health Sciences Centre, 2075 Bayview Ave, Toronto, ON M4N 3M5, Canada

Dan C. Huynh, Rita Vitorino, Daniel Efkehari, Jesse Knight, Thien J. Huynh, Sean Symons and Richard I. Aviv
Division of Neuroradiology, Department of Medical Imaging, University of Toronto and Sunnybrook Health Sciences Centre, 2075 Bayview Avenue, Room AG 31, Toronto, ON M4N 3M5, Canada

Mark W. Parsons
Department of Neurology, John Hunter Hospital, The University of Newcastle, Newcastle, NSW, Australia

Max Wintermark
Department of Radiology, Neuroradiology Division, Stanford University, California, USA

Achala Vagal
Department of Radiology, Section of Neuroradiology, University of Cincinnati College of Medicine, Cincinnati, OH, USA

Christopher D. d'Esterre
Calgary Stroke Program, Department of Radiology, University of Calgary, Alberta, Canada

Andrew Bivard
Melbourne Brain Centre, University of Melbourne, Melbourne, VIC, Australia

Rick Swartz
Department of Medicine (Neurology), Sunnybrook Health Sciences Centre, University of Toronto, Toronto, ON, Canada

Dale Connor, Thien J. Huynh, Sivaniya Subramaniapillai, Sean P. Symons and Richard I. Aviv
Division of Neuroradiology and Department of Medical Imaging, Sunnybrook Health Sciences Centre, University of Toronto, 2075 Bayview Avenue, Room AG 31, Toronto, ON M4N 3M5, Canada

Andrew M. Demchuk
Calgary Stroke Program, Department of Clinical Neurosciences, Department of Radiology, Hotchkiss Brain Institute, University of Calgary, Calgary, Canada

Dar Dowlatshahi
Department of Medicine (Neurology), University of Ottawa, Ottawa Hospital Research Institute, Ottawa, Canada

David J. Gladstone
Division of Neurology, Department of Medicine, and Brain Sciences Program, Sunnybrook Health Sciences Centre, University of Toronto, Toronto, Canada

Hemant Sarin
Charleston, West Virginia (WV), USA

Patrick Turski, Andrew Scarano, Eric Hartman and Zachary Clark
Department of Radiology, University of Wisconsin School of Medicine and Public Health, Madison, Wisconsin, USA

Leonardo Rivera, Yijing Wu, Oliver Wieben and Kevin Johnson
Department of Medical Physics, University of Wisconsin School of Medicine and Public Health, Madison, Wisconsin, USA

Tilman Schubert
Department of Clinic of Radiology and Nuclear Medicine, Basel, Switzerland

Eytan Raz
Department of Radiology, New York University School of Medicine, 660 First Avenue, New York, NY 10016, USA

Michele Anzidei and Michele di Martino
Departments of Radiological Sciences, University of Rome La Sapienza, Viale Regina Elena 324, Rome 00161, Italy

Michele Porcu
Department of Imaging, Azienda Ospedaliero Universitaria (A.O.U.), di Cagliari – Polo di Monserrato, s.s. 554 Monserrato, Cagliari 09045, Italy

Pier Paolo Bassareo and Giuseppe Mercuro
Department of Cardiology, Azienda Ospedaliero Universitaria (A.O.U.), di Cagliari – Polo di Monserrato, s.s. 554 Monserrato, Cagliari 09045, Italy

Jasjit S.Suri
Monitoring and Diagnostic Division, AtheroPoint(TM) LLC, Roseville, CA, USA
Point of Care Devices, Global Biomedical Technologies, Inc, Roseville, CA, USA
Electrical Engineering Department (Affl.), U of Idaho, Moscow

Jie Sun, Daniel S. Hippe, Baocheng Chu and Chun Yuan
Department of Radiology, University of Washington, 850 Republican St, WA, Seattle 98109, USA

Hunter R. Underhill
Department of Pediatrics, Univeristy of Utah, Salt Lake City, UT, USA

Tobias Saam
Institute for Clinical Radiology, Ludwig-Maximilians-Univeristy Hospital Munich, Munich, Germany

Norihide Takaya
Department of Cardiology, Juntendo Univeristy, Tokyo, Japan

Jianming Cai
Department of Radiology, PLA General Hospital, Beijing, China

Minako Oikawa-Wakayama
Department of Radiology, Japanese Red Cross Sendai Hospital, Sendai, Japan

Wei Yu and Li Dong
Department of Radiology, Beijing Anzhen Hospital, Beijing, China

Thomas S. Hatsukami
Department of Surgery, Univeristy of Washington, 850 Republican St, WA, Seattle 98109, USA

Hui Chen, Nan Liu, Ying Li, Fei Chen and Guangming Zhu
Department of Neurology, Military General Hospital of Beijing PLA, Beijing 100700, China

Nicoletta Anzalone, C. De Filippis, F. Scomazzoni, G. Calori, A. Iadanza, F. Simionato and C. Righi
Neuroradiology Department, Biostatistic Department, S Raffaele Hospital, Milan, Italy

Max Wintermark
Department of Radiology, Division of Neuroradiology, Stanford University, 300 Pasteur Drive, Stanford 94305-5105, CA, USA

Christian Federau
Department of Radiology, Division of Neuroradiology, Stanford University, 300 Pasteur Drive, Stanford 94305-5105, CA, USA
University Hospital Center and University of Lausanne (CHUV-UNIL), Lausanne, Switzerland

Luca Saba
Department of Radiology, Azienda Ospedaliero Universitaria di Cagliari, Cagliari, Italy

Audrey Nguyen
University of Lausanne, Faculty of Biology and Medicine, Rue du Bugnon 21, Lausanne 1011, Switzerland

Soren Christensen
Stanford Stroke Center, Stanford University School of Medicine, Stanford, CA, USA

E. Prasanna Venkatesan and Lexi Wilson
Calgary Stroke Program, Department of Clinical Neurosciences, University of Calgary, Calgary, Canada

Emmad Qazi
Calgary Stroke Program, Department of Clinical Neurosciences, University of Calgary, Calgary, Canada
Department of Radiology, University of Calgary, Calgary, Canada

Fahad S. Al-Ajlan
Calgary Stroke Program, Department of Clinical Neurosciences, University of Calgary, Calgary, Canada
Department of Radiology, University of Calgary, Calgary, Canada
Department of Neurosciences, King Faisal Specialist Hospital and Research Centre, PO Box 3354 Riyadh11211, MBC 76, Riyadh, Saudi Arabia

Bijoy K. Menon
Calgary Stroke Program, Department of Clinical Neurosciences, University of Calgary, Calgary, Canada
Department of Radiology, University of Calgary, Calgary, Canada
Department of Community Health Sciences, University of Calgary, Calgary, Canada
Hotchkiss Brain Institute, Calgary, Canada

Chi Kyung Kim
Calgary Stroke Program, Department of Clinical Neurosciences, University of Calgary, Calgary, Canada
Department of Neurology, Korea University Guro Hospital, Seoul, South Korea

Robert J.van Oostenbrugge
Department of Neurology, Cardiovascular Research Institute Maastricht (CARIM), Maastricht University Medical Center, Maastricht, The Netherlands

Debbie Beumer
Department of Neurology, Cardiovascular Research Institute Maastricht (CARIM), Maastricht University Medical Center, Maastricht, The Netherlands
Department of Neurology, Erasmus MC University Medical Center, Rotterdam, The Netherlands

Susanne Fonville and Diederik W. J. Dippel
Department of Neurology, Erasmus MC University Medical Center, Rotterdam, The Netherlands

Maxim J. H. L. Mulder and Ghesrouw Saiedie
Department of Neurology, Erasmus MC University Medical Center, Rotterdam, The Netherlands
Department of Radiology, Erasmus MC University Medical Center, Rotterdam, The Netherlands

Wim H. van Zwam
Department of Radiology, Cardiovascular Research Institute Maastricht (CARIM), Maastricht University Medical Center, Maastricht, The Netherlands

Aad van der Lugt
Department of Radiology, Erasmus MC University Medical Center, Rotterdam, The Netherlands

Philip J. Homburg
Department of Rehabilitation, Erasmus MC University Medical Center, Rotterdam, The Netherlands

Luca Saba, Michele Porcu, Antonella Balestrieri and Alessio Mereu
Department of Radiology, Azienda Ospedaliero Universitaria (A.O.U.), di Cagliari – Polo di Monserrato, s.s. 554 Monserrato, Cagliari 09045, Italy

Michele Anzidei, Marco Francone and Pierleone Lucatelli
Department of Radiological, Oncological and Pathological Sciences, Sapienza University of Rome, Rome, Italy

Carlo Nicola de Cecco
Department of Radiological Sciences, Oncology and Pathology, University of Rome Sapienza-Polo Pontino, Latina, Italy

Roberto Sanfilippo and Roberto Montisci
Department of Vascular Surgery, Azienda Ospedaliero Universitaria (A.O.U.), di Cagliari – Polo di Monserrato, s.s. 554 Monserrato, Cagliari 09045, Italy

Jasjit S. Suri
Stroke and Monitoring Division, AtheroPoint, Roseville, CA, USA

Max Wintermark
Department of Radiology, Neuroradiology Section, Stanford University, Stanford, California, USA

Karl Boyle and Raed A. Joundi
Department of Medicine, Division of Neurology, Sunnybrook Health Science Centre and University of Toronto, 2075 Bayview Avenue, Toronto M4N 3M5, Canada

Richard I. Aviv
Department of Medical Imaging, Division of Neuroradiology, Sunnybrook Health Science Centre and University of Toronto, 2075 Bayview Avenue, Toronto M4N 3M5, Canada

Adam de Havenon and Lee Chung
Department of Neurology, University of Utah, Salt Lake City, USA

Min Park
Department of Neurosurgery, University of Utah, Salt Lake City, USA

Mahmud Mossa-Basha
Department of Radiology, University of Washington, Seattle, USA

Francesco Marrosu and Antonella Mandas
Department of Medical Sciences and Public Health, University of Cagliari, Cagliari, Italy

Luigi Barberini
Department of Medical Sciences and Public Health, University of Cagliari, Cagliari, Italy
Department of Nuclear Medicine, Universitary Hospital of Cagliari AOU, Cagliari, Italy

Antonella Balestrieri and Luca Saba
Department of Medical Sciences and Public Health, University of Cagliari, Cagliari, Italy
Department of Radiology, University of Cagliari AOU, Cagliari, Italy

Iole Tommasini Barbarossa and Melania Melis
Department of Biomedical Sciences, University of Cagliari, Cagliari, Italy

Harman S. Suri and Jashit S. Suri
Diagnosis and Monitoring Division, AtheroPoint LLC, Roseville, CA, USA.

Michele Anzidei
Department of Radiology, University of Rome "La Sapienza", Rome, Italy

Manish N. Shah
Departments of Pediatric Surgery and Neurosurgery, McGovern Medical School at UTHealth and UT MD Anderson Cancer Center, Pediatric Neurosurgery, 6431 Fannin St., MSB 5.144, Houston, TX 77030, USA

Sarah E. Smith, Donna L. Dierker, Timothy S. Coalson and David C. Van Essen
Department of Neuroscience, Washington University, 660 S. Euclid Ave, St. Louis, MO 63110, USA

Joseph P. Herbert
Division of Neurosurgery, University of Missouri-Columbia, One Hospital Drive, 314 McHaney Hall, Columbia, MO 65212, USA

Brent S. Bruck, Gregory J. Zipfel and Ralph G. Dacey Jr.
Department of Neurological Surgery, Washington University, 660 S. Euclid Ave, St. Louis, MO 63110, USA

Index

www.ingramcontent.com/pod-product-compliance
Lightning Source LLC
Chambersburg PA
CBHW080655200326
41458CB00013B/4868